NEUROPHYSIOLOGY

NEUROPHYSIOLOGY

Third edition

R H S Carpenter

Lecturer in Neurophysiology, University of Cambridge;
Fellow and Director of Medical Studies, Gonville and Caius College, Cambridge

A member of the Hodder Headline Group
LONDON • SYDNEY • AUCKLAND
Co-published in the USA by Oxford University Press, Inc., New York

© 1996 R H S Carpenter

First published in Great Britain in 1984
Second Edition 1990

Third Edition published 1996 by Arnold,
a member of the Hodder Headline Group,
338 Euston Road, London NW1 3BH

Reprinted 1996

Co-published in the United States of America by
Oxford University Press, Inc.,
198 Madison Avenue, New York, NY 10016
Oxford is a registered trademark of Oxford University Press

Whilst the advice and information in this book is believed to be true and
accurate at the date of going to press, neither the authors nor the publisher
can accept any legal responsibility or liability for any errors or omissions
that may be made.

British Library Cataloguing in Publication Data
A catalogue record for this book is available from the British Library

Library of Congress Cataloging-in-Publication Data
A catalog record for this book is available from the Library of Congress

ISBN 0 340 60880 3

Typeset in 9/11 pt Palatino by GreenGate Publishing Services, Tonbridge, Kent
Printed and bound in Great Britain by The Bath Press, Avon

CONTENTS

Preface to the first edition   **vii**
Preface to the second and third editions   **viii**
Acknowledgements and Using NeuroLab   **ix**

PART 1 NEURAL MECHANISMS

1 THE STUDY OF THE BRAIN
The history of the brain   **3**
Central neurones   **7**
Anatomical methods   **10**
Physiological methods   **14**

2 COMMUNICATION WITHIN NEURONES
The flow of electrical current along nerves   **19**
The dependence of potential
on ionic permeabilities   **21**
The dependence of ionic permeability
on potential   **25**
Conduction velocity   **29**
Threshold properties   **33**
Neural codes   **36**

3 COMMUNICATION BETWEEN NEURONES
Common features of all neurones   **43**
Sensory receptors   **47**
Synaptic transmission   **54**

PART 2 SENSORY FUNCTIONS

4 SKIN SENSE
Sensory modalities   **73**
Types of receptor   **74**
Central projections   **77**
Neural responses   **79**
Central responses   **84**
Pain   **84**

5 PROPRIOCEPTION
Muscle proprioceptors   **90**
Joint receptors   **94**
Conscious proprioception   **94**
The vestibular apparatus   **95**

6 HEARING
The nature of sound   **101**
Sound spectra   **103**
The structure of the ear   **106**
Fourier analysis by the cochlea   **108**
Responses from auditory fibres   **110**
Spatial localization of sound   **114**
Central pathways and responses   **116**

7 VISION
Light and dark   **122**
Image-forming by the eye   **124**
The retina   **129**
Retinal interneurones   **135**
Mechanisms of adaptation   **137**
Visual acuity   **141**
Visual form recognition   **149**
Colour vision   **155**
Visual localization   **160**
Visual proprioception   **164**

8 SMELL AND TASTE
Smell   **170**
Taste   **179**

PART 3 MOTOR FUNCTIONS

9 TYPES OF MOTOR CONTROL
Difficulties in studying motor systems   **187**

Motor control and feedback   **189**
The hierarchy of control   **195**

10 LOCAL MOTOR CONTROL
Motor neurones   **200**
Descending pathways   **201**
Sensory feedback from muscles   **205**

11 THE CONTROL OF POSTURE
The importance of support   **214**
Vestibular contribution to posture   **216**
Visual contributions to posture   **219**
Neck reflexes   **222**
Posture as a whole   **223**

12 GLOBAL MOTOR CONTROL
Motor cortex   **226**
Cerebellum   **231**
Basal ganglia   **238**

PART 4 HIGHER FUNCTIONS

13 RECOGNITION AND MEMORY
CEREBRAL CORTEX
Prefrontal cortex   **248**
Parietal cortex   **251**
Temporal lobe   **258**

14 MOTIVATION AND BEHAVIOUR
Motivation   **273**
Emotion   **275**
The hypothalamus   **278**
Sleep and cortical arousal   **283**
A last look at the brain   **286**

Index   **291**

PREFACE TO THE FIRST EDITION

The supervision system practised at Cambridge and elsewhere brings many benefits both to teacher and taught: not least, that lecturers are brought face to face with the results of deficiencies in their own teaching in a peculiarly immediate and painful way. What has seemed to many supervisors a most worrying trend over the last 10 years or so is the extent to which a student may come away from a series of lectures on (let us say) the circulation with an impressive amount of detailed information, including perhaps the minutiae of experiments published only a month or two previously, yet with little sense of what might be called *function*: of what the circulation really does, of how it responds to actual examples of changed external conditions, and how it relates to other major systems. And in the case of the central nervous system things seem even worse: a student may acquire an immensely detailed knowledge of the anatomical intricacies of the motor system, yet not be able to tell you even in the broadest terms what the cerebellum actually does or have the slightest feel for what kinds of processes must be involved in such an act as throwing a cricket ball. The result is much knowledge, but little understanding, and very little sense of ignorance.

I believe this to be the result of two factors. The first is, paradoxically, that over the last decade or so, universities and teaching hospitals have quite rightly begun to take teaching much more seriously than once was the case, and consequently a perfectly laudable sense of competition has developed amongst lecturers to gain the approval of their audiences. But students – at least in the short term – tend to form judgements rather on the basis of the number of 'facts' that they have succeeded in copying down in the course of a lecture: the more recent these facts are, the better they are pleased. Lecturers naturally respond to this by filling their lectures with increasing amounts of detail, at the expense of fundamental principles. The students' notebooks swell with quantities of undigested information, but they are bewildered – even resentful – when asked simple but basic questions like 'How does a man stand upright?'. This change in emphasis has made physiology less enjoyable either to study or teach than it used to be, as well as less educational: there is no time and little motivation to ask questions of oneself and all is reduced, in the end, to rote-learning.

The second factor that has debased the intellectual quality of much of our teaching is the increasing emphasis that is put on mechanism instead of function. More time is often spent in talking about the detailed physics of nerve conduction than in discussing exactly what information is being carried by nerves, how it is coded, and how the nervous system is actually used. Again, lecturers' fear of instant student opinion is perhaps partly the cause: most students get immediate and easy satisfaction (of a limited kind) by seeing the detailed steps that cause a particular phenomenon, and if all can be reduced to a series of biochemical reactions, then so much the better. To understand whole systems and their interactions requires rather more effort of thought, and one can never be sure one is right. But in the long run, and most particularly for medical students, it is precisely the large-scale functioning of physiological systems that is important. A doctor needs to have a feel for what is likely to be the consequence of chronic heart failure in terms of problems of fluid balance or what may happen if his asthmatic patient decides on a holiday in the Andes. Whether the cardiac action potential is due mainly to calcium or to sodium, and whether or not the substantia nigra projects to the red nucleus are for him matters of singularly little interest or significance.

This book is an attempt to go counter to this trend by starting from the premise that a more satisfactory way to teach physiology is to build a scaffold of general principles on which factual details may later be hung as the need arises, and to prefer to consider *what* systems do rather than *how* they do it. However, this is largely a matter of emphasis and organization rather than of content, and the reader will find details of mechanism if they are required. Above all, the aim has been to recreate something of the intellectual excitement of the study of physiology that has been lost sight of in recent years, and to encourage the student to think and to question. If it is at all successful in this, the thanks should go not to me but rather to those past and present students of mine for whose intellectual stimulation I am – as all teachers must surely be – deeply grateful.

R H S Carpenter
Cambridge, 1984

PREFACE TO THE SECOND EDITION

A second edition has provided an opportunity to remedy some defects in the first. One of which I was particularly conscious was that in trying to achieve a connected and coherent narrative, I had sometimes neglected to be sufficiently exhaustive in enumerating the factual detail that is so greatly enjoyed by both students and examiners. This has now been rectified by the use of boxes containing tables and other systematic information outside the text itself. In addition, a number of topics receive a wider coverage; these include pain, subcortical visual mechanisms, eye movements, central auditory mechanisms and the hypothalamus. Finally, an attempt has been made in the last chapters to distil from the preceding ones some kind of answer to that troublesome question that students so frequently ask: what *principles* govern the processes that convert patterns of sensory information into patterns of behaviour? What, in short, does the brain *do*?

As always, I owe a special debt to my long-suffering students for acting as guinea pigs for certain lines of approach, and for their encouragement and criticism

R H S Carpenter
Talloires, August 1989

PREFACE TO THE THIRD EDITION

Most of neurophysiology is concerned with dynamics, with sensory coding, with feedback, with plasticity and stability. These are easy concepts to teach to a few students round a table, with a plentiful supply of paper to scribble on, less easy to convey in a book. But the coming of age of the personal computer has changed all that, and with NeuroLab you have the opportunity – the first of its kind – to experiment with model systems and see for yourself how they respond, as well as having the chance to try out experiments and demonstrations on yourself. It has been fun to develop, and I am certain that you will find it fun to use. Meanwhile, the text has been thoroughly revised and updated, with some changes of emphasis, and a more extensive use of supplementary notes indicated with the symbol shown to the right. The increasingly molecular approach to much of neurophysiology is an unwelcome trend in many ways, not least for medical students who face the 'anatomization' of yet another area of study – how soon will it be before they are required to memorize stretches of DNA? But it has also brought with it some unifying simplifications which have helped to bring a little more tidiness to certain areas.

Once again, to my students huge thanks for their stimulation and support, particularly in fine-tuning NeuroLab to meet their needs.

R H S Carpenter
Studland, 1995

ACKNOWLEDGEMENTS

It is a pleasure to acknowledge my indebtedness to Dr Susan Aufgaerdem, Professor George L. Engel, Mr Austin Hockaday, Dr J. Keast-Butler, Dr Richard Kessel, Dr Peter Lewis, Dr J. Purdon Martin, Dr N. R. C. Roberton, Dr T. D. M. Roberts and Mr Peter Starling for their help in providing illustrations; to the editors and to the staff of Arnold and GreenGate Publishing Services for their valuable help; to various authors and publishers where mentioned for permission to reproduce material; and above all to the late Dr R. N. Hardy, who died so tragically while the original book was in its final stages: his friendly encouragement, and his qualities of wisdom and humanity are sadly missed by all who knew him.

USING NEUROLAB

Installation

NeuroLab runs on a PC, the faster the better: on a 386 or on SX machines some of the demonstrations may run a little slowly. NeuroLab requires Windows 3.1 or better, and it must have at least a VGA display (SVGA is better); for the colour demonstrations to work properly you need 256 colours rather than 16. A SoundBlaster card or equivalent is not essential, but is highly desirable for the hearing experiments. A mouse is essential. Note that NeuroLab makes considerable demands on the computer's capabilities, and some machines may not be able to carry out all its commands, particularly where this involves animation or changes to the palette.

Installation is simple. Insert the diskette into your floppy drive, and in Windows go to the Program Manager window. From the File menu, select Run. In the Command Line field, type "a:setup" (or a different letter if your floppy drive is not drive a:), then click on OK. The process of installation will then proceed automatically, prompting you for instructions from time to time. When it has finished, the NeuroLab and NeuroLab Help icons will be added to the group that you have chosen.

Running NeuroLab

These instructions assume that you are familiar with ordinary Windows terminology. If you would like to see a visual demonstration of some of the NeuroLab controls (buttons, thermometers, panels, sliders, radio buttons and so on), double click on the NeuroLab Help icon.

To run NeuroLab, just double-click on the NeuroLab icon. The main menu window will then appear, consisting of a large number of icon pushbuttons, with titles. Each of these corresponds to one of the NeuroLab exhibits (an exhibit is a set of demonstrations or experiments on a particular topic). Click once on a button, and the corresponding exhibit will appear in its own window. Each exhibit is described at the appropriate place in the book, and references to exhibits are marked in the text with the symbol shown to the right. When you have finished with an exhibit, click on Quit. The NeuroLab menu window will still be there, and you can select another exhibit, or alternatively click on the Quit button to leave NeuroLab completely.

You can have several exhibits running at once if you wish; you can also shrink an exhibit to an icon if you want to put it into temporary abeyance.

Because we have no control over the conditions of use or the configuration of the computer you are using, we cannot accept liability if any part of NeuroLab fails to run properly; but if you experience difficulty with installation you may request help by e-mail: rhsc1 @ cus.cam.ac.uk.

Dark mysteries are here – old pathways, secret places
Under the tangled cortex, grown snugly thick now –
Intricately synapsed: electrode-proof

PART

1

NEURAL MECHANISMS

1 THE STUDY OF THE BRAIN

The history of the brain 3
Central neurones 7

Anatomical methods 10
Physiological methods 14

This book is about trying to understand the human brain. Is this ludicrously overambitious?

Your brain is a machine whose complexity far exceeds anything made by humans. It is made up of units – cells called *neurones* – that provide both the pathways by which information is transmitted within it and also the computing machinery that makes it work. There are quite a lot these neurones: about 30 times as many as the entire population of this planet. A typical neurone is wired up to a couple of thousand of its neighbours, and it is the pattern of these connections that determines what the brain does. So the study of the brain is like the study of human society: for a society can only be fully understood if we comprehend not just the behaviour of isolated individuals but also the interactions that each of them makes with those with whom they are in contact. Consequently understanding the brain is a task as daunting as trying to comprehend the behaviour of the entire human race, its politics, its economics, and all other aspects of what it does; in fact, about 30 times more difficult. As a result, the study of the brain has in some respects a closer affinity with 'arts' subjects like history than it does with much conventional science. For many people this is part of its attraction.

Our brains *need* to be complex: part of what they do is to embody a kind of working model of the outside world that enables us to imagine in advance what would be the result of different courses of action. It follows that the brain must be at least as complicated as the world we experience. How has such complexity come about? The evolutionary history of the brain is not well understood, but was probably something like the account that follows.

THE HISTORY OF THE BRAIN

The co-ordination of a single-celled organism such as an amoeba is essentially chemical: its brain is its nucleus, acting in conjunction with its other organelles. But a multicellular organism clearly needs some system of communication between its cells, particularly when, as in Hydra, they are specialized into different functions: secretion, movement, nutrition, defence and so on. In small and slow creatures, such communication may still be chemical: cells in one part may release chemical messengers – hormones or *transmitters* – that determine what another part does (Fig. 1.1). But as an organism gets bigger, *time* becomes a problem. Because the time taken for diffusion is proportional to the square of the distance travelled, it takes a disproportionately longer time for a chemical signal released at one end of it to reach the other. If speed of response is not particularly important, and if in addition there is some kind of fluid circulation that will increase the rate of dispersion of chemical transmitters, this kind of communication may still be satisfactory even in very large organisms. Our own hormonal control systems are, of course, precisely of this kind.

But such systems are not only slow, they are also imprecise. When a sudden fright leads to release of adrenaline into our blood, it acts indiscriminately on the whole body. For fast and localized action, we need an arrangement that will release the transmitter as rapidly as possible at the site where it is required, and nowhere else. This function of *localized* secretion is carried out by the nerve cells or neurones, cells that have reached out to touch their targets so they can instil their transmitters directly and confidentially: a whisper in the ear instead of a shout (Fig. 1.1).

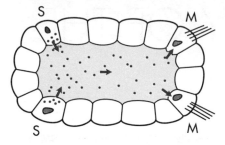

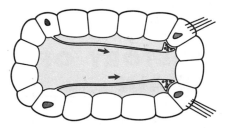

Fig. 1.1 **(a)** A hypothetical multicellular organism with sensory cells (S) that control motor cells (M) by releasing a chemical transmitter or hormone (red) into the common fluid space. **(b)** Direct connections between sensory and motor cells by means of nerve axons, providing communication that is both quicker and more specific. Their ultimate action on the motor cells is still chemical.

Without spatial selectivity of this kind, we would need as many different transmitter substances as target organs, whereas in fact, as we shall see, all the thousands of millions of skeletal muscle cells in our bodies are controlled by just one chemical transmitter: acetylcholine.

Neurones are of ectodermal origin, and some remain in epithelia as *sensory receptors* that are sensitive to mechanical or chemical stimuli, to temperature or to electromagnetic radiation. Others migrate inward, and become specialized as *interneurones* that respond only to the chemicals released locally by sensory neurones or other interneurones. They in their turn release transmitter at their terminals, which form junctions called *synapses* either with interneurones or with effectors such as muscles or secretory cells. So interneurones provide the communication channels by which information is passed rapidly from one part of the central nervous system to another, through mechanisms that form the subject of Chapters 2 and 3. In Hydra, for example, we find a network of such intercommunicating neurones, making contact on the one hand with sensory cells on its surface that respond to touch and chemical stimuli, and on the other with muscle cells and secretory glands. Hydra's brain is thus spread more or less

uniformly throughout its body, with only a slight increase in density in the region of its mouth: yet even such a relatively undifferentiated structure can generate co-ordinated, even 'purposeful' behaviour.

The next step in the evolution of the nervous system came with the increasing specialization of sensory organs, particularly of *teloreceptors* such as eyes and olfactory receptors. For an animal that normally moves in one particular direction, such organs tend to develop at the front end, and the result of the consequent extra influx of sensory information to a localized region is an increased proliferation of interneurones in the head. In Planaria we have the

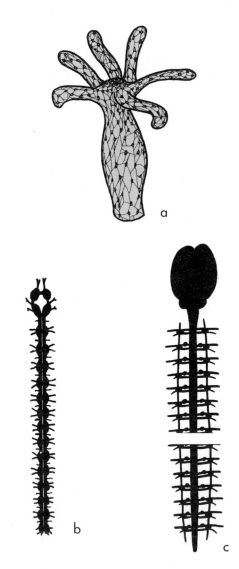

FIG. 1.2 Schematic representation of Hydra nerve-net **(a)**, and central nervous systems of earthworm **(b)** and Man **(c)**. (Partly after Buchsbaum, 1971)

first true brain of this kind, a dense concentration of neurones close to the eyes and sensory lobes of the head, giving rise to a pair of nerve cords that run down the body and send off side branches connecting with other neurones and effector cells. In segmented animals like the earthworm, the nerve cords show a series of swellings or ganglia, one to each segment. Each is a kind of brain in its own right, and a decapitated earthworm is still capable of many kinds of segmental and intersegmental co-ordination. Though our bodies are not of course segmented, our nerve cord, the *spinal cord*, still shows some segmental properties, particularly in the organization of the incoming and outgoing fibres, and in the existence of corresponding chains of ganglia along each side (Fig. 1.2). We shall see later, in Chapter 10, that our spinal cord is also capable of a limited degree of brainlike activity. The primitive nerve net has not been altogether superseded, but survives as an adjunct to the central nervous system in the diffuse networks near the viscera that control movements of the gut and some other visceral functions.

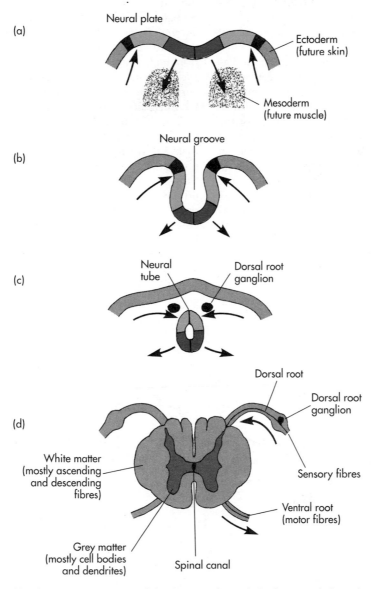

FIG. 1.3 (a)–(c) Highly schematic representation of development of neural tube from neural plate, showing relative positions of sensory (pink) and motor (red) regions. (d) Cross-section of adult human spinal cord, at the level of the second thoracic vertebra.

The subsequent development of the brain is rather more complex, and not well understood. By looking at its evolutionary history in conjunction with the sequence of its growth in foetal development, one can postulate a framework that may help to relate the primitive nervous system to the more intricate structure of the adult human brain.

The central nervous system is derived from a narrow strip of ectoderm, the *neural plate,* which runs down the middle of the vertebrate embryo's back. The centre of this strip becomes depressed into a trough or groove, and eventually its edges come to meet in the middle to form a closed structure, the *neural tube* (Fig. 1.3). It is natural for sensory fibres from the skin to enter at the margins of the neural plate, and for motor fibres to the more medial musculature to leave the plate nearer the midline, and as a consequence one finds that it is in the dorsal half of the neural tube that the sensory fibres terminate (their cell bodies lying in the *dorsal root ganglia* on each side of the tube), while the cell bodies of the efferent motor fibres lie in the ventrolateral part of the neural tube, and this arrangement is evident in the adult spinal cord (Fig. 1.3d). Here one can see in cross-section the *ventral and dorsal horns,* consisting of masses of *grey matter* (mostly cell bodies), a less prominent central region concerned with the neural control of visceral function, and a surrounding sheath consisting of *white matter,* mainly bundles of nerve fibres running longitudinally up and down the cord.

At the head or cephalic end of the neural tube, a modification of this basic plan occurs. The central fluid-filled canal, which is very small in the spinal cord, widens out at two separate points to form hollow chambers or *ventricles:* at the same time it migrates back to the dorsal surface of the neural tube, so that the ventricles are open on their dorsal side. This surface is covered by the *choroid* membrane, the site of production of the cerebrospinal fluid that fills the canals and ventricles of the brain. The more caudal of the ventricles is called the fourth ventricle, and the region around it is the *hindbrain* or rhombencephalon; it is connected to the more rostral third ventricle by the *cerebral aqueduct.* The region round the aqueduct is called the *midbrain* or mesencephalon, and that round the third ventricle is the *forebrain or* prosencephalon (Fig. 1.4). Subsequently, the third ventricle produces a pair of swellings at the front end, which become inflated into the *lateral ventricles:* the neural tissue surrounding them forms the *cerebral hemispheres* (telencephalon) while the rest of the forebrain is called the diencephalon.

The hindbrain is likewise divided into two regions: the caudal part is called the *medulla,* and the rostral part (metencephalon) is marked by the outgrowth of the *cerebellum* over the dorsal surface, and a massive bundle of fibres associated with it, the *pons,* on the ventral surface (Figs1.4 and 1.5). In less developed species such as fish all these structures are easily recognizable without dissection, but in humans the extraordinary ballooning growth of the cerebral hemispheres has not only engulfed the other surface features (leaving only the cerebellum and medulla peeping out at the back), but the massive

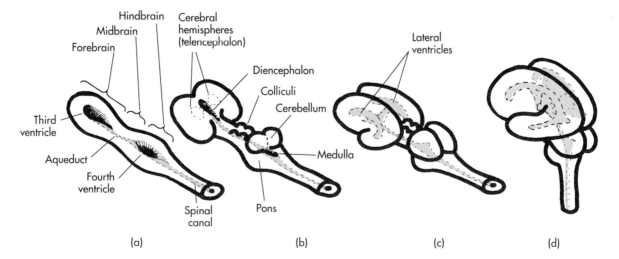

FIG. 1.4 The notional steps leading from neural tube to human brain. **(a)** The opening of the canal to form the third and fourth ventricles. **(b, c)** The growth of the cerebellum, and of the cerebral hemispheres with their associated lateral ventricles. **(d)** Human brain, showing greatly enlarged cerebral hemispheres, and flexion of the neural tube.

fibre tracts needed to connect the cerebral hemi-spheres to each other and to the rest of the brain have tended to elbow older structures out of the way and have often considerably distorted their shape. Another factor that makes the anatomy of the human brain somewhat confusing is that the neural tube has become bent forward: while the axis of the hindbrain is near vertical, that of the forebrain is horizontal (Fig. 1.4).

The most important areas of the human brain are shown in the sagittal and transverse sections of Figure 1.5. The *cerebellum* is an important co-ordinating system for posture and for motor movements in general (Chapter 12) that arose originally as an adjunct to the vestibular apparatus, a sensory organ concerned with balance and the detection of movement (Chapter 5). Important landmarks on the dorsal surface of the midbrain are the four humps (corpora quadrigemina) formed by the *superior and inferior colliculi,* primitive sensory integrating areas for vision and hearing respectively; in higher vertebrates their function is mainly that of organizing orienting reactions and other semireflex responses to visual and auditory stimuli. In the diencephalon, on each side of the third ventricle, lie the two halves of the *thalamus,* a dense group of nuclei whose neurones partly act as relays for fibres that project upward to the cerebral hemispheres. Close to them but more lateral is the *corpus striatum*, an old area that is concerned with the control of movements (Chapter 12). Also in the diencephalon, but lying on the floor of the third ventricle, is the *hypothalamus,* the brain's interface with the hormonal and autonomic systems that control the body's internal homeostasis (Chapter 14). More laterally, various nuclei, fibre tracts and other areas form a loosely defined system called the *limbic system* which connects with the hypothalamus, with the olfactory areas, and with many other regions of the brain; they are concerned with such functions as emotion, motivation and certain kinds of memory (Chapter 14). Finally, there is the *cerebral cortex*, which covers the lateral ventricles and is deeply convoluted and furrowed in higher vertebrates, enabling a large superficial area of tissue to be crammed into a relatively small volume. Its role in carrying out some of the most complex things we do is discussed in Chapter 13.

The divisions of the brain described so far are very gross ones, and for the most part quite obvious to the naked eye. Finer anatomical distinctions can only be made by looking at the neurones themselves, and the way their populations vary from one region to another.

Box 1.1 Some important structures within the three divisions of the primitive brain

Hindbrain	*Myelencephalon:*
	Medulla
	Vestibular nuclei
	Medullary reticular formation
	Metencephalon:
	Pontine nuclei and reticular formation
	Cerebellum
Midbrain	*Mesencephalon:*
	Tectum (colliculi)
	Red nucleus
	Substantia nigra
	Mesencephalic reticular formation
Forebrain	*Diencephalon:*
	Thalamus
	Hypothalamus
	Septum
	Telencephalon:
	Corpus striatum
	Hippocampus
	Amygdala
	Cerebral cortex

CENTRAL NEURONES

Neurones from different parts of the nervous system show a wide range of shapes and sizes (Fig. 1.6). What they have in common is a compact cell body containing the nucleus, and a number of projecting filaments that generally show extensive branching: these projections form the pathways by which information from different sources is gathered together by the neurone, and then transmitted in turn to some other region. In a 'classic' neurone, one projection (the *axon*) forms the output of the cell, and the others *(dendrites)* form the input. However, there are many exceptions to this rule: the dorsal root ganglion cells, for instance, have no dendrites at all and the cell body simply lies to one side of a single continuous axon (Fig. 1. 6b); and in many sites within the brain the dendrites are known to act as outputs as well as inputs.

The axon is specialised for carrying information rapidly over long distances, and may often be very

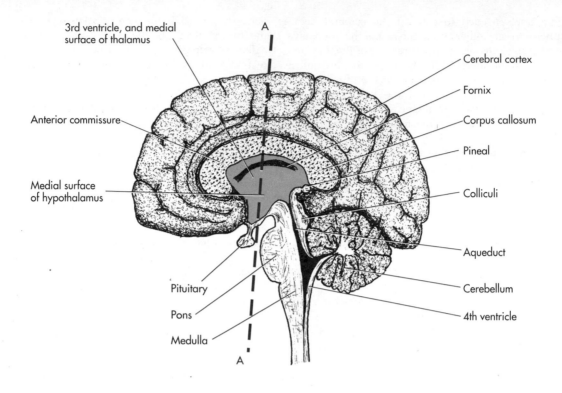

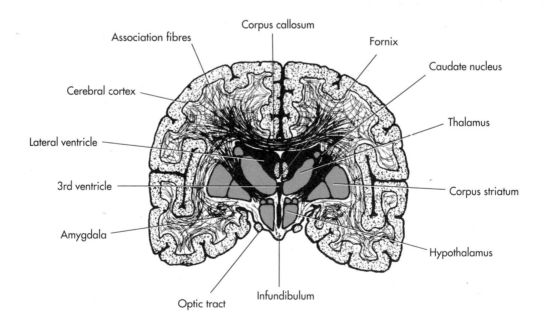

FIG. 1.5 Semi-schematic sections of the human brain. **(a)** Sagittal, showing medial aspect; **(b)**, transverse, in the plane A–A.

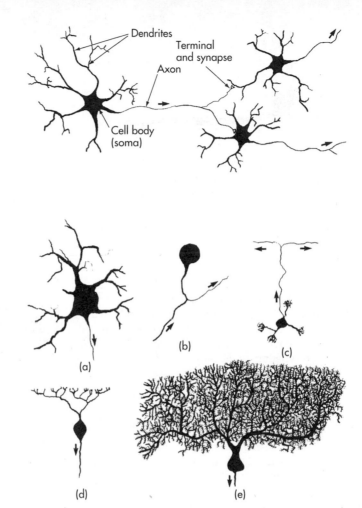

FIG. 1.6 Top, schematic representation of a 'classic' central neurone synapsing with two others, in one case on a dendrite and in the other on the cell body or soma. Right, some typical and somewhat idealized central neurones: **(a)** motor neurone; **(b)** dorsal root (unipolar) neurone ; **(c)** granule cell (cerebellum); **(d)** bipolar cell, retina; (e) Purkinje cell, cerebellum. The arrows indicate the axon.

long indeed – as, for example, those that carry muscle commands all the way from the cerebral cortex to the bottom of the spinal cord. Apart from very short ones, their information is in the form of propagated *action potentials*, discussed in Chapter 2. The larger axons are frequently swathed in layers of *myelin,* a lipid substance that speeds up the conduction of action potentials by acting as an electrical insulator: these layers are the result of accessory *Schwann cells* sending out myelin-rich processes that wrap themselves round and round the axons to form a kind of Swiss roll (Fig. 1.8); the myelin is interrupted at regular intervals, at the *nodes of Ranvier*. Schwann cells are a specialized form of the *glial cells* that make up the bulk of nervous tissue, whose functions include regulation of the brain's ionic environment and possibly more complex functions as well.

Within neurones are found the usual intracellular organelles and other components, including 10 nm *neurofilaments* extending linearly along axons and dendrites as well as within the cell body, and the larger microtubules *(neurotubules)* that seem to be associated with the transport of substances to and from nerve terminals, at a rate of some 3 mm/h. The far end of the axon is usually branched, and its terminals make synaptic contact either with the dendrites or the bodies of other neurones, with secretory cells or (in the case of *motor neurones*) with muscle cells. At this point the signal – previously electrical – makes the terminal release a tiny quantity of chemical transmitter, which then acts on the postsynaptic cell.

We shall see later that it is the *pattern* of excitation – in time or space – arriving at the dendrites and body of a neurone that determines whether or not it in turn sends action potentials down its axon. In that respect, a neurone is a kind of miniature brain in its own right that makes decisions on the basis of the

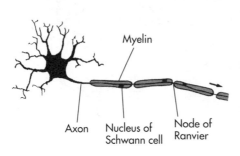

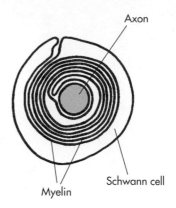

FIG. 1.7 Diagram of a neurone with myelinated axon (not to scale: the distance between the nodes of Ranvier is typically of the order of 1 mm, while the cell body might be 20–80 μm in diameter).

FIG 1.8 Schematic cross-section of myelinated axon, showing the layers of myelin formed by the Schwann cell wrapping itself round and round.

pattern of activity at its inputs. Thanks to the work of biophysicists who have studied the way in which different synaptic inputs to a neurone interact with one another, we have a fair idea of the general rules that determine whether or not a cell will respond to a given pattern of excitation. In particular, we know that these rules depend very critically on the shape of the dendritic tree and the distribution of synapses upon it. For instance, two synapses interact in a very different way if they lie near one another on a single branch, rather than far apart on separate branches (discussed in Chapter 3). It follows from this that a full understanding of the function of a single neurone requires detailed knowledge of the size and shape of its dendrites, and of the origin of all the thousands of afferent fibres synapsing with it. Even for one neurone, this would be an impossibly daunting task, let alone for the hundred thousand million or so that constitute the brain. In practice, one cannot hope to do much more than try to identify neurones that are typical of a particular area, and form some idea of their 'average' properties. We are helped in this by the fact that neurones are to a large extent grouped in homogeneous communities called *nuclei,* groups of similar cells projecting to the same area of the nervous system and whose afferent fibres likewise have common origins. The existence of nuclei implies that of the *tracts* that join them, and much of the work of neuroanatomists is to identify the inputs and outputs associated with particular nuclei.

ANATOMICAL METHODS

Just looking with the naked eye at sections of the brain, one can make out the grosser nuclei and tracts but a microscope is needed to make out the details of neuronal connections. Since neuronal tissue is virtually transparent, some kind of stain is needed; the problem then is that if we stain all the nerve cells, the brain is such a densely knotted structure that the whole thing will simply come out black and we shall be no better off: what is needed is a *selective* stain. One such is the *Golgi silver stain*, which has the odd property that it is only taken up by a very small percentage of the neurones in the tissue to which it is applied, apparently at random; those cells that do take it up do so completely, resulting in a complete and often very beautiful delineation of their dendritic structure (see, for example, Fig. 12.8). Another technique is to inject a dye such as procion yellow into a neurone through a micropipette inserted into it; this dye then diffuses into most parts of the cell but not outside it, and provides a good way of marking a cell whose electrical responses have previously been recorded with the same micropipette. Some marker substances are transported along axons, either from the cell body to the terminals (orthograde) or in the opposite direction (retrograde). One example is *horseradish peroxidase* (HRP); after extracellular injection at a particular site, it is taken up by axon terminals and carried back to the cell body. In this way one may identify the origin of efferents to a particular region of the brain (HRP also acts like the Golgi silver stain in that it can be used to delineate a cell's dendritic and axonal ramifications). Similarly, labelled amino acids (tritiated leucine, for example) are taken up by cell bodies and transported towards the terminals, enabling one to identify the areas to which a particular nucleus projects.

A related technique for tracing axonal pathways is to study the *degeneration* that results from injury to a nerve fibre. Two kinds of degeneration follow damage to an axon: *orthograde* or Wallerian degeneration, distal to the cut, and *retrograde* degeneration, in the direction of the cell body. In the first case, one may use the Nauta stain that identifies certain of the degeneration products; in retrograde degeneration one may see various characteristic changes in the cell body (Fig. 1.9). Sometimes these degenerative changes may actually extend beyond the synapse to affect the next neurone along, and are then described as transneuronal orthograde or retrograde degeneration. In monkeys, for instance, removal of the eye results in shrinkage of the neurones in the thalamus with which the fibres from the eye make contact. Thus by making a lesion in a particular nucleus one may in principle trace both the afferent and efferent pathways associated with it, and in some cases one may identify the second-order cells with which these fibres synapse as well. A problem with degeneration studies, but not with HRP or labelled amino acids, is that they do not distinguish between fibres that genuinely begin or end in a particular region and those *fibres of passage* that merely happen to pass through it. Finally, one may select cells that are associated with a particular protein – typically a peptide transmitter (see Chapter 3) – by means of immunohistochemical stains, labelled antibodies that enable one to identify groups of cells within a nucleus that share a common function.

A wiring diagram is not enough

If these anatomical techniques were perfect, and if we had the patience to identify each of the 10^{11} or so individual pathways in the central nervous system, we would end up with something like a wiring diagram of the brain. Would we really be much the wiser as a result? It is true that we could in principle then apply our knowledge of the biophysical properties of individual neurones to calculate how the whole thing would react to any given pattern of stimulation at the sensory receptors: the problem is, of course, the almost inconceivable difficulty of ever actually carrying out such a calculation. With modern computers, the accurate simulation of the behaviour of even a few dozen neurones connected together in a realistic network is about the limit of what can be achieved within a reasonable period of time. Thus it is not so much that we know too little of the behaviour of individual neurones but rather that we lack the conceptual techniques for analysing their behaviour as a whole.

The brain is in fact composed of elements that are essentially rather simple, but joined together in ways that are extremely complex. In that respect it has certain similarities with a digital computer. Figure 1.10 shows the circuit diagram of a tiny part of a very small computer, of the circuits that perform the relatively trivial task of getting data from the keyboard. Without knowing very much about logic circuits, one can see at once that there is a relatively limited number of types of element in the circuit (the logic gates), and it is clear that the function of the whole circuit must reside in the way that these standard units are connected to one another. Now a full understanding

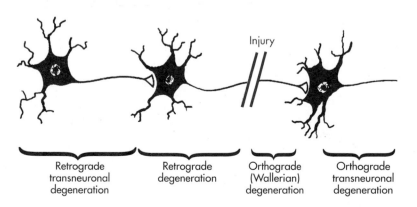

FIG. 1.9 Schematic representation of the types of degeneration that may follow injury to a neurone.

of the details of this circuit's operation requires a certain degree of intellectual effort, and to master the computer of which it forms a part might take years of study, yet the brain is thousands of millions of times larger in scale.

Another example of a highly complex system made out of vast numbers of quite simple elements is provided by substances like foam rubber (Fig. 1.11). Here too, the shape and behaviour of each individual element – each bubble – is unique, yet determined by relatively simple physical laws. But it would clearly be a hopeless task to attempt to work out the overall properties of a slab of such foam – its elasticity, for example – by painstakingly considering one bubble at a time and calculating its effects on each of its neighbours. An alternative to a *reductionist* approach of this sort is to step back a little from the system, until the differences between each of its elements become blurred, and then try to derive some description of their average behaviour *en masse* without the necessity of considering each one in detail. A well-known example of this kind of *holistic* approach is the

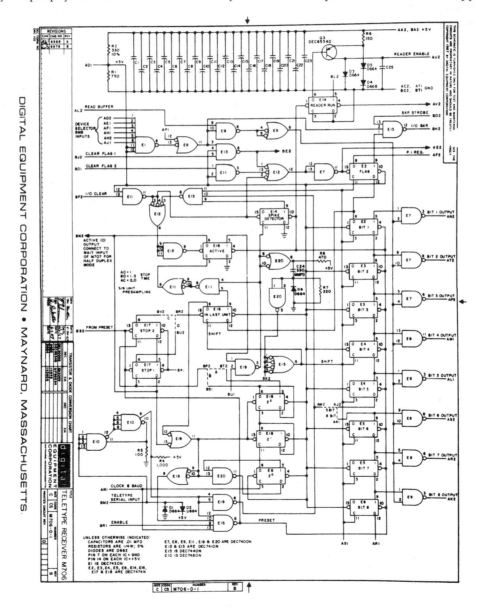

FIG. 1.10 Logic diagram of a very minor part (the keyboard receiver) of a very small computer. (Courtesy of Digital Equipment Corporation)

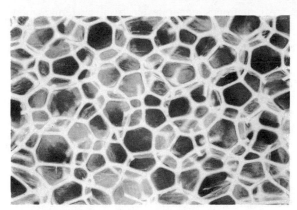

FIG. 1.11 Microphotograph of foam rubber.

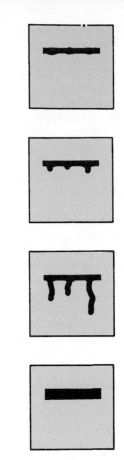

FIG. 1.12 A system which amplifies patterns. We make a horizontal dribble of ink on a vertical card (a). Drops begin to form at points where there happens to be more ink (b), and in doing so they draw ink away from neighbouring regions, thus exaggerating the original non-uniformity (c). A prediction of the behaviour of the ink based only on averages (d) is the one result that is *never* observed!

study of the physical properties of gases. Gases exert a pressure because their molecules are constantly rushing about and bumping against the walls of their containers, generating an average force that depends on their velocity or temperature, and on how many of them there are. If one knew the exact position and velocity of every single molecule of such a gas, then in principle one could compute each of their individual trajectories and hence predict their collisions with the walls and with each other: one would then have a perfect understanding of the gas. But this is clearly out of the question. A more sensible approach is to turn the large numbers involved into an actual advantage, by considering only the 'lumped' properties of the molecules, their average behaviour as a whole, and then derive statistical descriptions of the way in which pressure depends on volume and temperature through the methods of statistical mechanics.

Might we hope – by analogy – to be able to develop a sort of statistical mechanics for neurones? Unfortunately, the one thing we cannot do with neurones is to take averages: it is precisely the *differences* between them – the patterns of their activity – that are significant. It is as unhelpful to talk about the average behaviour of a sheet of cells in the retina or cerebral cortex as it would be to talk about an average page of this book or an average Beethoven piano sonata. In fact we shall see again and again that at every level of the brain there are special mechanisms of *lateral inhibition* whose specific function is to exaggerate differences of activity between neighbouring neurones and thus to enhance or amplify any patterns that may exist, and such mechanisms make the whole system more uncomputable than ever.

A simple example may illustrate why this is. Suppose we take a piece of card, dribble a line of ink across it, and then up-end it (Fig. 1.12). The ink starts to run down in an irregular way that is partly a function of the amount of ink at different points along the line. But as soon as a drop starts to form at the lower edge, it begins to draw ink off from neighbouring regions, thus reinforcing itself at their expense. We end up with a series of discrete trickles, in which the pattern of 'activity' (quantity of ink at different distances) has been automatically amplified. A description in terms of average behaviour would be meaningless: on average, the ink descends uniformly along all its length, the one thing that is never actually observed. Here, and in the brain, we are dealing with one of those fashionably chaotic systems in which the tiniest initial perturbations may generate incalculably large effects.

Another reason why we cannot take averages is that one person's neuronal connections are different from another's, both at the level of individual nerve cells but also to a certain extent at grosser levels. One example concerns a part of the cerebral cortex called the motor area where – as we shall see in Chapter 12 – the movements of various parts of the body are represented in a systematic pattern. These 'motor maps' differ quite markedly not only from one individual to another, but even in the same individual when measured on different occasions, partly as a function of use and disuse. This is very far from being an isolated example: we shall see later that connections in many parts of the brain are to a large extent determined by experience, and that it is precisely this *plasticity* of function that enables us to learn to adapt our behaviour to circumstances. So the functioning of the brain is probably as much a matter of how it has been *programmed* as of its hardware – of the general outline of its wiring specified by genetic instructions – and these programs are necessarily as varied as the experiences of the brain's owner. The same computer processor chip may be used for writing a book or for playing *Sonic the Hedgehog*: no amount of peering at it down a microscope will tell us *which,* for it is a matter of how it is programmed. So even supposing we did manage to make some sense of the wiring diagram of A's brain, it is not at all obvious that it would throw much light on the functioning of B's.

So there are many levels at which one may try to investigate the brain, and corresponding to them, a number of distinct branches of the neurosciences have emerged. To pursue the computer analogy a little further, biophysicists investigate the properties of the individual logic gates; neuroanatomists trace the connections that link one unit to another; psychologists describe the programs in the machine and how they got there; and pharmacologists study the colours of the wires. The task of neurophysiologists has generally been to try to bridge the levels at which the other disciplines perform their investigations, by trying to correlate anatomical structure with patterns of neuronal activity, and neural events with overt behaviour and sensation. Such, at least, is the intention of this book.

PHYSIOLOGICAL METHODS

There are essentially three techniques that are used to try to correlate the activity of particular neurones with particular functions: they are *recording, stimulation,* and *lesions.*

All neurones generate electrical currents when they are active, and these electrical effects may be picked up by means of *electrodes.* We may have *gross* electrodes that look at the average responses of many hundreds of neurones at once or *microelectrodes* that are small enough to impale single nerve cells and record their activity in isolation from whatever else may be going on around them. Though 'micro', intracellular electrodes are not much smaller than the neurones themselves, and there is a danger of bias in making such recordings since populations of smaller cells may be missed entirely. Some workers have experimented with arrays of electrodes, which have the advantage that one may then be able to observe something of the spatial pattern of activity. For trying to deduce the function of a whole nucleus by recording from a single cell is rather like reading a book by looking at just one letter on each page. Electrical recording has proved most successful at the sensory or input side of the brain, since one may then find out what a particular cell responds to by presenting it with a variety of different sensory stimuli: the difficulties of recording from the motor side are considered in Chapter 9.

Local metabolic effects may also be used to pinpoint neural activity. One example is to treat an animal with labelled *deoxyglucose* (DOG), and then present it with a particular task, such as looking at a specific kind of visual stimulus. Those cells that are most active during that period take up the DOG preferentially, and their localization becomes apparent when the brain is subsequently sectioned. Another highly fashionable technique is the brain scan, using either PET (positron emission tomography) or MRI (magnetic resonance imaging), which both provide dynamic graphical pictures of local changes in cerebral blood flow. Though it cannot provide accurate localization or follow very fast events, it has the advantage that changes in the pattern of activity can be observed in conscious human subjects: some examples are described on p.256.

Experimental *stimulation* of the brain may be electrical, using gross- or micro-electrodes, or sometimes by local microinjection of pharmacological agents or other substances. Stimulation is a natural way to try to investigate the motor system, though for reasons discussed more fully in Chapter 9 it has not often proved a very helpful technique. Stimulation of single cells is usually inadequate to achieve any overt response at all, while simultaneous stimulation of large numbers of them with large electrodes and heavy currents has proved in general to be too 'unphysiological' to give meaningful results. However, stimulation at one site while recording

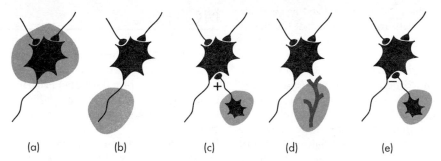

(a)   (b)   (c)   (d)   (e)

FIG. 1.13 If a lesion causes the loss of a particular function, it may indeed be because it has directly interfered with the area responsible for that function (a); but equally, it may be that it has merely interrupted fibres of passage (b), or has abolished a tonic 'permissive' input (c), or has interfered with blood supply (d). A lesion that abolishes a source of tonic inhibition may give rise to 'release', the appearance of new and abnormal reactions (e).

from another is often a good way to establish the existence of functional connecting pathways.

Finally *lesions:* apart from their use in demonstrating anatomical pathways through degeneration, they may also be used to try to associate particular functions with particular regions of the brain. If destruction of a specific area X of the brain results in the loss of some function Y, then it might seem reasonable to conclude that Y is localized in X. The trouble is, however, that there are many other ways in which such a result might be explained. The function Y might in fact be localized somewhere else altogether but with connecting fibres that merely happen to run through the region X, or perhaps requiring some kind of tonic permissive influence from X; or a lesion at X may simply interfere with the blood supply to the true area of localization of Y (Fig. 1. 13). Paradoxically, one is on safer ground if one finds that a lesion in area X has absolutely *no* effect whatever on function Y, for then one can be fairly sure (unless the function is localized at two independent sites that somehow work in parallel) that Y is not localized in X.

Chemical lesions – the blocking of particular pathways by the local application of appropriate pharmacological agents – have the advantage of being both more specific and more reversible, as well as being free of some of the objections outlined above. Sometimes the result of a lesion is not the abolition of a function but the sudden appearance of new behaviour not previously seen, a phenomenon called *release* (Fig. 1.12). Again, it is easy to jump to erroneous conclusions. If you remove one of the circuit boards from your hi-fi and it starts to make a whistling noise, is it fair to conclude that the function of the board you removed was to inhibit whistling? Yet it is still commonly said that because the effect of lesions in certain parts of the corpus striatum is a

jerkiness in moving and tremor at rest, the function of those areas is to smooth out movements and inhibit tremor!

Part of the problem is undoubtedly that the whole notion of localization of function in centres is too crude and simple-minded, a hangover from the days of phrenology, with its picture of the brain divided up into a number of discrete little compartments with highly specialized functions (Fig. 1.14); the relative ease with which beautifully coloured pictures of localized cortical activity can be obtained with modern brain scanning techniques has led to a revival of this simple-minded approach. Some classic experiments once performed on rats by the psychologist Karl Lashley cast doubt on such a view of localization. He made lesions of different sizes in the cerebral

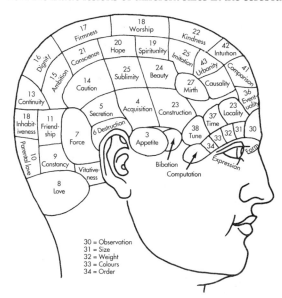

FIG. 1.14 Phrenological head: an early attempt at cerebral localisation (Fowler).

cortex, avoiding the regions specialized as primary areas of input and output, and found that the defect of performance in a task like learning to run a maze depended more or less on the quantity of cortex removed, and surprisingly little on the region where it was taken from. Although when we record at one particular time from a neurone in a particular region of the cortex it may seem to be doing something very specific, it is likely that large areas of the cortex are not in fact rigidly committed to specialized tasks but may change their function as the result of experience or of damage to neighbouring areas. For instance, the map of the human body found in sensory cortex readjusts itself in a matter of days after amputation of a limb. The situation is reminiscent of that in the old electromechanical telephone exchanges, where automatic switches called selectors had the job of connecting one subscriber to another in response to signals from the telephone dial. But there was not one set of selectors for each subscriber: if so, the total number of selectors required would have become astronomical. Instead, they were lumped together in a common pool: on lifting your receiver, a device called a line-finder hunted through the available bank of equipment until it found one free, and then gave you the dialling tone. This meant that in the course of a day, any one selector could be used by a large number of subscribers. If we were to drop hand grenades into the exchange and blow up a certain proportion of the selectors, the service would get worse for *all* subscribers, in that they would be more likely to find all the lines engaged. This kind of *plasticity* – the ability of one area to take over the function of another that is out of action – is often found at higher levels of the brain (as, for example, in recovery from stroke), and makes deductions from lesions more difficult still.

Thus there are profound intellectual and technical difficulties with all the methods of investigation currently in use, and the history of brain science has not been a simple linear progression. It is as if we try to find out how our pocket calculator works by sticking nails in it and then measuring their voltages or passing large currents through them, or by noting its reaction to having bits knocked off it with a hammer. Astonishing, in fact, that we know anything at all about the brain.

References

Buchsbaum, R. (1951) *Animals without Backbones*. Penguin, Harmondsworth.
Fowler, O. S. (undated) *The Human Science of Phrenology*.
Lashley, K. S. (1929) *Brain Mechanisms and Intelligence*. University of Chicago Press, Chicago.

NOTES

Page 3 Brain mirroring the world Santiago Ramón y Cajal (1852–1934), whose contributions to neuroanatomy won him the Nobel Prize in 1906, wrote in *Charlas de Café*: 'As long as our brain is a mystery, the universe, the reflection of the structure of the brain, will also be a mystery'.

Page 7 Neuroanatomy There is a huge range of excellent textbooks of neuroanatomy to choose from. A very full text with much reference to medical material is Brodal, A. (1981) *Neurological Anatomy in Relation to Clinical Medicine* (Oxford University Press, Oxford). Nauta, W. J. H. and Freitag, M. (1986) *Fundamental Neuroanatomy* (W. H. Freeman, New York) is slimmer but has fine illustrations and a synoptic approach that helps conceptual understanding. Another thoughtful account is Jones, E. G. (1983) *The Structural Basis of Neurobiology* (Elsevier, New York). For absolutely stunning pictures in full colour, England, M. A. and Wakely, J. (1991) *A Colour Atlas of the Brain and Spinal Cord* (Wolfe, London) is highly recommended. If you are lucky enough to find a copy of Chandler Elliott, H. (1963) *Textbook of Neuroanatomy* (Pitman, London), turn to and admire the extraordinary clear diagrams of the development of the ground-plan of the brain, which have not been bettered in more recent books.

Page 7 The neurone A very clear account of the cell biology of the neurone, with good illustrations, is Levitan, I. B. and Kaczmarek, L. K. (1991) *The Neuron: Cell and Membrane Biology* (Oxford University Press, Oxford).

Page 13 Reductionism and holism A recurring theme in Hofstadter (1979) *Gödel, Escher, Bach: an Eternal Golden Braid* (Harvester, New York), a brilliant tour-de-force and one of the great popular scientific works of the last few decades.

Page 13 Pattern generation and amplification A readable and clear account of the formation of natural patterns – the generation of complexity through simple interactions – is Stevens, P. S. (1976) *Patterns in Nature* (Peregrine, Harmondsworth).

Page 14 Neural programming The field of neural networks is now a hugely popular one, with many books aimed at different levels of technical expertise. A recent book for the mathematically inclined is Hassoun, M. H. (1993) *Associative Neural Memories: Theory and Implementation* (Oxford University Press, Oxford). Another recent book designed specifically to link the computational approach to the way the brain actually works is Churchland, P. S. and Sejnowski, T. J. (1994) *The Computational Brain* (MIT

Press, Cambridge, Mass). Edelman, G. M. (1989) *Neural Darwinism: the Theory of Neuronal Group Selection* (Oxford University Press, Oxford) is an account of a rather specific proposal for how the general rules of neuronal programming might be implemented. Finally, an example plucked almost at random of how 'neural' networks in manmade computers may be set to work to carry out tasks of extreme complexity: Svärdström, A. (1993) Neural network feature vectors for sonar targets classification. *Journal of the Acoustic Society of America 93*, 2656–2665.

Page 14 Neurophysiology No book better encapsulates the purely physiological approach to brain function than Walsh, E. G. (1964) *Physiology of the Nervous System* (Longmans, London) – sadly, long out of print. If you find a copy, snap it up.

Page 15 Interpretation of lesions There is an apocryphal story of the man who demonstrated his findings about the auditory system of the grasshopper at a meeting of the Royal Society. 'Gentlemen,' he said, 'I have here a grasshopper that I have trained to jump whenever I clap my hands.' He claps, and the grasshopper jumps. 'Now, gentlemen, I shall cut off its legs – so – and you will now observe that when I clap my hands it no longer jumps. It is therefore clear that grasshoppers hear with their legs.' Perhaps the logical flaw is obvious here – the fact that grasshoppers do hear with their legs is beside the point! Yet hardly less glaringly flawed deductions have quite often found their way into the literature.

Page 15 PET scans – dynamic phrenology? See, for instance, Raichle, M. E. (1994) Visualizing the mind. *Scientific American* April, 36-42.

Page 16 The telephone exchange as a metaphor of the brain There has been a tendency throughout history for the brain to be likened to the latest piece of technology. Telephone exchanges, with their thousands of incoming and outgoing wires and their awesomely intricate and ever-changing patterns of connections, were as popular in the early years of this century as images of 'how the brain works' as were computers in the 1970s. Now the boot is on the other

foot, for neural network computers were based on neurophysiology rather than the other way round.

Page 16 The vicissitudes of neuroscience Recently documented in an admirably complete, thoughtful and readable account with a wealth of illustrations: Finger, S. (1994) *Origins of Neuroscience: a History of Explorations into Brain Function* (Oxford University Press, Oxford).

NEUROLAB

Brain anatomy

Pages 7, 10

This is designed for quick self-testing on the essentials. Click on one of the circles round the edge and the name of the corresponding structure will appear in the window at top right. Alternatively, you can do it the other way round. Click on the button at the right of the name-bar; a list of structures will appear that you can scroll through with the scroll-bar. Click on one of them, and the corresponding indicator will appear on the left. To see a transverse rather than a sagittal section, click on the long button at bottom right. As with all the NeuroLab exhibits, click on the Quit button when you have finished.

Neural network

Page 14

Click in the boxes on the left; the input pattern is transformed as it passes from layer to layer, ending up on the right as a count of how many boxes have been checked. This is not a true neural net, in the sense that it learns for itself; it has been programmed to do it. But it shows how a network of simple neural elements (each has a threshold and fires when the number of active inputs exceeds that threshold) can perform quite a complex function. If you press Learning, you can experiment with a neural network that really does learn: it is described on p. 272.

2 COMMUNICATION WITHIN NEURONES

The flow of electrical current along
   nerves 19
The dependence of potential on ionic
   permeabilities 21
The dependence of ionic permeability
   on potential 25

Conduction velocity 29
Threshold properties 33
Neural codes 36

Although it had been known for nearly 2000 years that nerves served to communicate between the body and the brain, the question of *how* they did it was settled only some 40 years ago. Nervous conduction is now one of the best understood processes in the whole field of physiology, and its elucidation has been a major triumph for that branch of the subject known as biophysics – the application of purely physical methods to biology.

The problem posed by nerves is simply the means by which they convey information from one end to the other. That there was some link between *electricity* and nervous and muscular action had been sensed as far back as the end of the eighteenth century, with Galvani's celebrated observation of the twitching of frogs' legs when in contact with certain combinations of metals. Further understanding had to wait for the development of galvanometers sensitive enough to register the passage of very small electrical currents; by the end of the nineteenth century it was clear not only that nerves and muscle could be activated by electrical stimulation but conversely, that their normal activity was always accompanied by changes in electrical potential. It did not follow, of course, that these electrical changes were the *cause* of neural communication, since activity of many other kinds of tissue also gave rise to electrical effects. It was not until 1939 that it was finally established that electrical

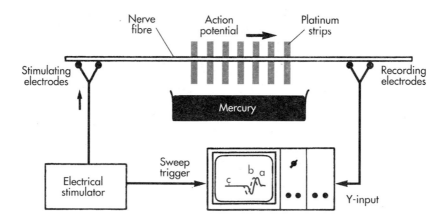

FIG 2.1 Knock-down proof that action potentials depend on electrical currents. A nerve is stimulated electrically (left) and the electrical response recorded (right) on an oscilloscope: **(c)** is the stimulus artefact that results from direct electrical conduction down the nerve. After a latent period, there is a diphasic action potential **(a)**. On raising the trough of mercury, so that the platinum strips are in electrical continuity, the latent period is reduced **(b)**. (After Hodgkin, 1939)

currents were not only generated as a side effect of nervous conduction but were also *necessary* for conduction to take place at all.

If we lay one end of a nerve across a pair of electrodes, and stimulate the other end electrically (Fig. 2.1), after a short latency or delay due to the time taken for excitation to travel from the stimulating to the recording electrodes we see a characteristic transient change in the voltage across the recording electrodes, the biphasic *action potential*. If now we lay a series of platinum strips across the nerve, the latency remains unchanged. But on making electrical contact between the strips, for example by immersing their ends in a bath of mercury, it is found that the latency is immediately reduced, but returns to its previous value as soon as the mercury is removed. Clearly the presence of the mercury increases the apparent conduction velocity of the nerve; this can only be because it allows currents to pass more easily from one part of the nerve's surface to another. In other words, the currents generated by an active nerve are not just an accidental byproduct of transmission, like the noise from a car: they are an essential determinant of the entire process.

THE FLOW OF ELECTRICAL CURRENT ALONG NERVES

Now nerve fibres, with their conductive central core of axoplasm surrounded by an insulated membrane often reinforced with extra non-conductive layers of myelin, are clearly very like ordinary insulated wires. Could action potentials simply be transmitted by passive conduction, in the same way that signals pass along a telephone wire? For most nerves, the answer is a clear no: action potentials show a number of properties that do not fit such a simple model, and in fact it turns out that they are actually conducted very much better than they would be if the nerve fibres were merely acting like simple electric wires.

To get an idea of how bad a passive conductor a nerve fibre is, we need to consider what are called its *cable properties*. These depend both on how good its insulation is – the resistance of the axon membrane – and also on how much resistance is offered to currents flowing longitudinally through the axoplasm. If we consider a unit length of axon (Fig. 2.2), we can call the associated transverse resistance of the membrane R_M and the longitudinal resistance of the axoplasm R_L . The whole axon can be thought of as

simply consisting of a large number of these units joined end-to-end. If we now assume that the external medium offers only a negligible resistance to current flow (the justification for this assumption will become apparent later), then we can treat all the outer ends of the individual R_Ms as if they were short-circuited together, producing the ladderlike network of resistors shown in Figure 2.2 that is called the *equivalent circuit* of the nerve fibre.

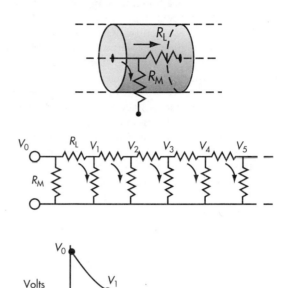

FIG. 2.2 Passive spread of electrical current along an axon. Above, each unit length of fibre can be thought of as having a longitudinal resistance R_L and a transverse or membrane resistance R_M. Then the whole axon may be represented by the ladderlike equivalent shown below. If a voltage V_0 is applied at one end, the voltage measured at different distances x along the axon will fall off exponentially, as shown at bottom, because of leakage through the membrane. The space constant λ is the distance for which the voltage falls by a factor e.

Now imagine a potential V_0 applied to the end of this ladder. In the first compartment, the current it generates has a choice: it can either flow out through R_M or continue through R_L to enter the next compartment. What actually happens is that some fixed fraction of the total current takes the former route and the rest takes the latter: the bigger the resistance of the membrane, R_M, and the smaller that of the axoplasm, R_L, the greater will be the tendency of the current to carry straight on rather than leak away through the membrane. Unless the insulation is perfect or the axoplasm infinitely conductive (in either case R_L/R_M is zero), the current entering the second cell will be smaller than that entering the first by some fixed ratio. In the same way, the current entering the third cell will be smaller than that entering the second, and so on all the way down the chain. The result is that the potential seen at each compartment will fall in a fixed ratio as one goes from compartment to compartment down the line, resulting in an exponential decline in voltage as a function of distance along the axon, at a rate that will depend on the ratio R_M/R_L (Fig. 2.2). Thus V is given by $V_0 e^{-x/\lambda}$, where e is the well-known constant whose value is about 2.718, and λ is a parameter called the *space constant* that describes how quickly the voltage declines as a function of the distance x. λ is in fact the distance you have to go before the voltage has dropped to λ/e (about 37 percent) of its original value V_0. It turns out in fact that λ is actually equal to $\sqrt{(R_M/R_L)}$; as would be expected, the more leaky the axon, the smaller R_M is, and the shorter the space constant.

What does all this mean in practical terms? Consider a large myelinated frog nerve fibre, some 14 μm in diameter, and assume for the moment that the myelin is uninterrupted along its length, without nodes of Ranvier. With 1 mm as our unit of length, it turns out that although the axoplasm is intrinsically a vastly better conductor of electricity than myelin – their specific resistances being of the order of 100 Ω cm and 600 MΩ cm respectively – because the cross-sectional area of the axoplasm is so small, the ratio of R_M to R_L is not very great: R_M comes out as about 250 MΩ and R_L about 14 MΩ, giving a space constant of some 4 mm or so. In other words, a potential generated at one end of such an axon will have dropped to less than half at a distance of 4 mm, to about a tenth of its original value after 1 cm, and by 2 cm will only be some 1 percent of the original stimulus, and probably undetectable in the general background electrical noise. In other words, axons are quite incapable of acting as reliable passive conductors of electricity over distances of more than a centimetre or two at most.

This is not really because nerve fibres are made of unsuitable materials – we have already seen that axoplasm is more than 5 million times better at conducting electricity than myelin – but rather because of their small size. Suppose we were to increase the diameter of our axon by a factor D: R_M would then be reduced by the same factor (since the area of membrane per unit length would be increased by D), while R_L would be reduced not by a factor D but by D^2, since the longitudinal resistance depends on the cross-sectional *area* (Fig. 2.3). Consequently

R_M/R_L would be multiplied by D, and the space constant would be increased by a factor $\sqrt{D}$. Now the longest nerves in the human body are about a metre in length; so to conduct reliably over this distance we would need to increase λ from 4 to about 400 mm; because of the square root relationship, this would mean having a fibre of some 10 000 times its previous diameter, in other words 140 mm instead of 14 μm! (This analysis is not quite fair because we have assumed a constant thickness of myelin: but even if we allow this thickness to increase in proportion with the axon itself, the fibre will still need to be a hundred times bigger. Bearing in mind the fact that many important fibre tracts in the body contain millions of fibres, one must still conclude that passive conduction is not a practical possibility over long distances.)

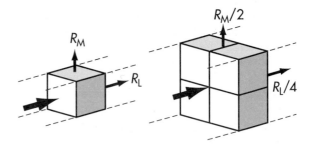

FIG. 2.3 Doubling the diameter of an axon reduces R_M by a factor of 2, but R_L by a factor of 4. (The fact that axons are not usually square does not affect this result.)

The cyclical regeneration of action potentials

In any case, nerve action potentials show a number of properties that demonstrate quite clearly that they are not passive, but actively *regenerated* as they pass along the fibres, amplified in such a way as to overcome the enormous losses that they experience through membrane leakage. If we record the action potential from a single electrical stimulus at different points along a nerve fibre, we find that its amplitude does not in fact decrease at all as a function of distance but stays at a constant value. Even more strikingly, the size of this action potential is not even a function of the size or nature of the stimulus that initiated it in the first place. So long as the strength of the stimulus is above a certain *threshold* value (below which no action potential is seen at all), neither the amplitude nor the shape or speed of the action potential is in any way influenced by the nature of the original stimulus, a property known as the *all-or-*

nothing law. These two features, the all-or-nothing law and the existence of a threshold, are never shown by voltages transmitted through passive conductors. A nerve is very like a burning cigarette: once lit, the temperature and rate of advance of the burning region is not a function of the temperature of the flame which originally ignited it, so long as this was sufficient to light it at all. Here the combustion is continually regenerative: the heat of the burning tip raises the temperature of the next region to the point where it too catches fire, and so on all along its length. In other words, there is a continuous cyclic process in which heat triggers combustion and combustion generates heat, this heat coming of course from the stored chemical energy of the tobacco.

It turns out that this is a surprisingly close analogy to the mechanism of propagation of the action potential. What happens is that the original stimulus to the fibre causes local currents to flow passively through the membrane, causing a spread of potential rather as in Figure 2.2. This voltage is in some way sensed by neighbouring regions of the fibre and triggers a mechanism in the membrane that generates a voltage many times larger (thus introducing an amplification of the original signal) which in turn sets up local currents that cause a potential change still further down the axon ... and so on, until the potential change has been transmitted from the point of stimulation to the end of the axon (Fig. 2.4). This whole cyclical process is known as the *local circuit* mechanism of action potential propagation.

Each cycle consists of three distinct stages: firstly, there is the mechanism by which a potential at one point results in a passive flow of current and thus in depolarization of regions further down the axon; secondly, the mechanism by which this depolarization triggers off some change in the membrane; and thirdly, the mechanism by which this change produces a

new potential that is much larger than what triggered it off. The first of these processes is essentially what has already been described, and can be readily understood in physical terms by means of equivalent circuits like that of Figure 2.2; the second two obviously require identification of this mysterious change in the membrane that is supposed to result in amplification of the voltage that triggers it. It turns out that this consists of a change in the *permeability* of the membrane to certain ions.

Now there are physical mechanisms common to all cells by which changes in ionic permeabilities give rise to changes in potential; what is unique about nerve and muscle cells is that they also possess special mechanisms by which such changes are in turn triggered off by changes in potential, thus completing the cycle of three links by which the action potential is propagated over the membrane surface (Fig. 2.4). Thus to understand how nerves work we need to be able to answer two questions: *How do ionic permeabilities affect membrane potential?* and *How do membrane potentials affect ionic permeabilities?*

THE DEPENDENCE OF POTENTIAL ON IONIC PERMEABILITIES

Imagine that we have a system of two compartments, A and B (Fig. 2.5), and that initially A contains a strong solution of KCl, and B a weak one; and suppose that the membrane separating them, initially impermeable, suddenly becomes permeable to potassium ions. Clearly there will now be a tendency for K^+ to diffuse through the membrane down the concentration

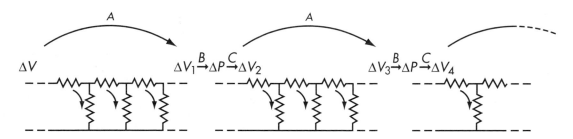

FIG. 2.4 The three components of action potential propagation. A depolarization ΔV at one point on the fibre results, through local current flow *(A)*, in a smaller depolarization ΔV_1 some way down the axon. This triggers off *(B)* a permeability change ΔP in the membrane, which in turn *(C)* produces a voltage ΔV_2 which is larger than ΔV_1. The whole sequence is repeated indefinitely (ΔV_3, ΔV_4 ,etc.). The processes A and C are common to all cells; but B, the conversion of voltage to permeability changes, is found only in nerve and muscle.

gradient between A and B. Since the ions carry a positive charge, compartment B will become more and more positive with respect to A as they migrate in this way, setting up an electrical gradient that will tend to oppose the entry of further ions from A. Eventually there will come a point where the *concentration gradient* from A to B will be exactly equal and opposite to the *electrical gradient* from B to A, and the system will be in equilibrium, since there will be no net flow of ions across the membrane.

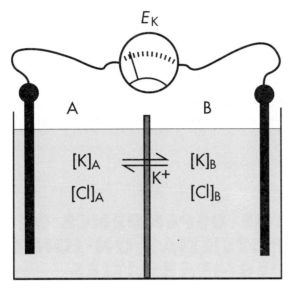

FIG. 2.5 Two compartments each containing potassium chloride, at different concentrations, separated by a barrier permeable only to potassium ions; at equilibrium there will be a potential between them of E_K volts, the equilibrium potential.

The resultant electrical potential between A and B is then called the *equilibrium potential* for potassium, E_K. To work out how big this potential will be, consider the energy involved in moving one potassium ion from A to B. The work done in moving it against the electrical gradient will be given by its charge e multiplied by the potential difference E_K; since the system is in equilibrium, this work must be exactly equal to the energy gained in moving down the concentration gradient, which can be shown to be:

$$\frac{RT}{N}\ln\frac{[K]_A}{[K]_B}$$

where T is the absolute temperature, R the gas constant and N is Avogadro's number. So we can write:

$$eE_K = \frac{RT}{N}\ln\frac{[K]_A}{[K]_B}$$

or

$$E_K = \frac{RT}{F}\ln\frac{[K]_A}{[K]_B}$$

$$\approx 58\log_{10}\frac{[K]_A}{[K]_B} \text{ mV (at } 20°\text{C)}$$

where F is Faraday's constant, equal to Ne. This relationship (the *Nernst equation*) is true for any ion in equilibrium across a membrane to which it is freely (and solely) permeable, with the proviso that if the charge on the ion is not +1 (as for instance in the case of Cl⁻ or Ca⁺⁺) we need to include this ionic charge z as well:

$$E_X = \frac{RT}{zF}\ln\frac{[X]_A}{[X]_B}$$

Only a tiny number of ions need to cross the membrane to set up such an equilibrium, so that the concentrations of the ions on each side remain effectively unchanged, and the equilibrium potential is set up virtually instantaneously after a sudden permeability change of this kind. Thus from the purely electrical point of view, suddenly making the membrane permeable to potassium – perhaps by opening up little channels in it that allow K⁺ through but nothing else – is rather like connecting a battery of voltage E_K across our equivalent circuit in Figure 2.2.

Now suppose we extend the model by imagining a membrane with both potassium and sodium channels, which can be independently opened and closed, and that A and B now contain solutions of NaCl and KCl in different proportions on each side (Fig. 2.6). The potential in mV will then be given by $E_K = 58 \log_{10} [K]_A/[K]_B$ when the potassium channels are open, and $E_{Na} = 58 \log_{10} [Na]_A/[Na]_B$ when the sodium ones are open. So by opening one or other set of channels we can switch the potential from one value to another. But what if *both* are open?

The answer is that the voltage will depend on the relative permeabilities of the two ions, the ratio of the total numbers of each channel that are open. The more freely K⁺ is able to move through the membrane, the nearer the potential will approach E_K; and the greater the permeability to Na⁺, the closer it will approach E_{Na}. The final, compromise, potential is in fact given by an expression called the *constant field equation*, a generalization of the Nernst equation to include cases where more than one ion is present:

$$E = \frac{RT}{F}\ln\frac{P_K[K]_A + P_{Na}[Na]_A}{P_K[K]_B + P_{Na}[Na]_B}$$

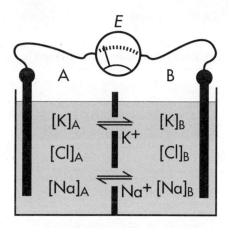

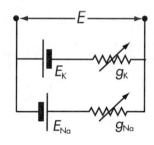

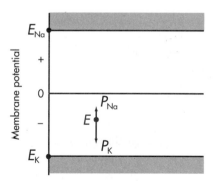

FIG. 2.6 Top, equilibrium potential, E, between two compartments containing sodium and potassium chloride and separated by a barrier having a permeability P_K to potassium and P_{Na} to sodium. Middle, its equivalent circuit: g_K and g_{Na} are the electrical conductances determined by P_K and P_{Na}. Bottom, the membrane potential E can be thought of graphically as being an equilibrium between the pull of P_K towards E_K and P_{Na} towards E_{Na}.

Here P is a measure of the permeability of the membrane to a particular ion. It can be seen at once that the Nernst equation is simply a special case of the constant field equation, for if P_K is very large in comparison to P_{Na}, so that the membrane is in effect only permeable to potassium, much of the equation

shrivels away and E simply becomes E_K; and similarly for sodium. The membrane potential will in fact always lie somewhere between the two extremes of E_K and E_{Na}; since the concentrations of sodium and potassium on each side are effectively fixed – the net flow through the channels is in general exceedingly small – this voltage is only a function of the two permeabilities, in fact of their ratio P_K/P_{Na}. In other words, *changes in permeability cause changes in potential*.

Now nerve cells are ideally suited for converting small permeability changes into large potential changes, since the distribution of Na^+ and K^+ across their membranes is a very lopsided one (Table 2.1). Like all cells in the body, they have a powerful sodium pump in their membranes that transfers Na^+ from inside to outside, exchanging them with K^+ partly by direct reciprocal transport and partly through electrical coupling. In the case of frog muscle fibres, which happen to have been particularly thoroughly investigated, the two equilibrium potentials may be calculated as about –105 mV inside for potassium, and about +65 mV for sodium. If we actually put a microelectrode into the muscle fibre and record its *resting potential*, it is found to be about –100 mV, implying that in the resting state it is much more permeable to potassium than to sodium. We can also try the experiment of bathing the fibre in solutions with different concentrations of potassium: if the membrane were only permeable to K+, it ought to obey the Nernst equation, and we should find that its resting potential is simply proportional to the logarithm of the external potassium concentration. At high external potassium concentrations this turns out to be true, but at lower values the potential is always smaller than what would be expected, because of the added contribution of the sodium ions. The best fit to the experimental points is obtained by using the constant field equation, with a resting sodium permeability about 1 percent of that of the potassium ions (Fig. 2.7). Similar experiments have been done on the giant axons of squids, with the added advantage that because they are so big – often as much as a millimetre across – it is possible to squeeze their axoplasm out with a kind of miniature garden roller, and replace it with fluids of different composition, thus altering the potassium concentration inside as well as outside.

But haven't we forgotten *chloride*? In our simple model, we assumed that chloride ions were unable to diffuse across, so we were justified in omitting them from the constant field equation. But experiments show that real nerve and muscle membranes have significant chloride permeabilities, and it is obvious from the data that have been presented that there is a

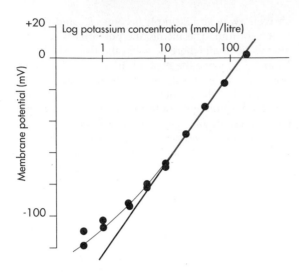

FIG. 2.7 Measurement of membrane potential of frog muscle fibres (data points) in response to different external potassium concentrations. The black line shows what would be expected from the Nernst equation if the membrane were permeable only to K⁺, whereas the red line shows the expectation if it is about 1 percent as permeable to Na⁺ as it is to K⁺. (After Hodgkin and Horowicz, 1959)

TABLE 2.1 Ionic composition of two kinds of electrically active cell

Frog muscle (Resting potential ca. −100 mV)			
	Na⁺	K⁺	Cl⁻
Internal (mM)	10	124	1.5
External (mM)	109	2.3	78
Equilibrium potential (mV)	+65	−105	−100
Squid axon (Resting potential ca. −60 mV)			
	Na⁺	K⁺	Cl⁻
Internal (mM)	50	400	50
External (mM)	440	20	560
Equilibrium potential (mV)	+55	−75	−60

Simplified, after Conway (1957) and Hodgkin (1958)

considerable imbalance in the concentrations of Cl⁻ on each side. Nevertheless, there are two reasons why this ion can, for the moment, be safely neglected. The first is that in practice the Nernst potential for chloride is usually very close to the equilibrium potential of the nerve membrane, so that changes in its permeability have negligible effects on the resting potential. What happens is that potassium and chloride are free to move together as KCl until the Nernst potentials for both chloride and potassium are equal: that is, until $[K]_{out}/[K]_{in} = [Cl]_{in}/[Cl]_{out}$. Because internal [Cl] is so very much smaller than [K], a shift of a given quantity of KCl has an enormously greater effect on the chloride ratio than on the potassium (since the external concentrations remain essentially unchanged). Thus chloride adjusts itself to a resting potential that is essentially determined by potassium. Second, it turns out that during the action potential no significant alterations in chloride permeability occur; as we shall see, this is in sharp contrast to what happens to sodium and potassium. However, when we look at synaptic mechanisms in the next chapter, we shall find that there are certain occasions when chloride cannot be neglected at all, and indeed most inhibitory synapses actually work through changes in chloride permeability.

Now if we put a microelectrode inside a muscle fibre or squid axon, and stimulate it to get an action potential, we find that the potential of the inside relative to the outside suddenly reverses from (in the squid) its resting −50 mV to a peak of some +40 mV, and then rapidly declines back to the resting potential again (Fig. 2.8). This is the *monophasic* action potential: the reason for its shape being different from the diphasic action potential recorded with an external electrode (Fig. 2.1) will be explained later. The size of this reversal during the action potential

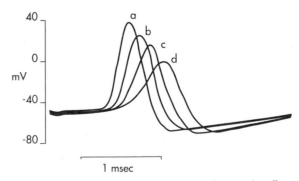

FIG. 2.8 Action potentials in a squid axon, showing the effect of different external sodium concentrations. (a) Sea water; (b) 71 percent sea water; (c) 50 percent; (d) 33 percent; the sea water was diluted with isotonic dextrose. (After Hodgkin and Katz, 1949)

strongly suggests a sudden increase in sodium permeability that pulls the membrane potential temporarily towards E_{Na}. By experimenting with various concentrations of sodium ions inside and outside the axon it is possible to demonstrate directly that the peak of the action potential is indeed dependent on E_{Na}: if the ratio of sodium concentration outside and inside the fibre is reduced, this peak declines in amplitude (Fig. 2.8), and eventually the action potential is abolished altogether.

To anticipate a little, it turns out that the action potential is in fact produced by a characteristic and almost invariant sequence of changes in ionic permeabilities: first a transient increase in sodium permeability, and then – after a short delay – in potassium permeability (Fig. 2.9), and the shape of the action potential can be deduced from the time-course of these permeability changes by using the constant field equation. During the initial phase, when P_{Na} is rising but P_K is still at its resting level, the potential moves rapidly past zero towards E_{Na}. But it never gets there because P_K has meanwhile started to rise, and P_{Na} to fall, and the potential starts to drop back again to the resting level. In some cases it actually undershoots the resting potential because there is a period at the end of the whole cycle in which P_K is still elevated, whereas P_{Na} is back to normal: this pulls the membrane even further towards E_K than it is in the resting state. Thus the voltage changes that occur during the action potential can be explained entirely in terms of the corresponding changes in permeability so the only question that remains is how these changes in permeability are themselves created.

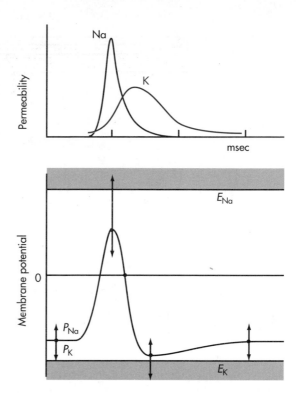

FIG. 2.9 Above, changes in potassium and sodium permeability associated with the action potential. Below, how these changes result in the form of the action potential itself. The arrows above and below the trace indicate roughly by their length the relative sizes of P_{Na} and P_K pulling the potential respectively towards E_{Na} and E_K.

THE DEPENDENCE OF IONIC PERMEABILITY ON POTENTIAL

One might think that it would be a straightforward matter to find out how ionic permeabilities vary with potential: just put a microelectrode into a fibre, pass a current through it in order to set up a particular voltage, and then see what the resultant potassium and sodium permeabilities are. In reality, things are not so simple. In the first place, the movement of ions that results from a change in permeability is exceedingly small, and it is not at all easy to disentangle the effects of sodium and potassium ions from one another, if both permeabilities alter at once. More fundamentally, any changes in permeability that may occur in response to a

potential change that we impose will themselves tend to alter that same potential. So the first experimental requirement is to devise some way of holding the membrane at a particular potential despite whatever permeability changes may be taking place, and this is what the *voltage clamp* technique provides. In essence, this consists of a feedback loop in which the actual membrane potential at every moment is measured with an intracellular electrode and compared with the value at which we want to clamp it, and any difference between the two is sensed and used automatically to increase or decrease a current passed into the fibre through another electrode in such a way as to bring the potential back to where it should be (Fig. 2. 10). Hodgkin and Huxley, whose pioneering use of this technique led to a Nobel prize, used squid axons, which are so large that an electrode can be passed down the middle, increasing the surface area and thus the size of the currents to be measured. If, for example, sodium permeability increases in

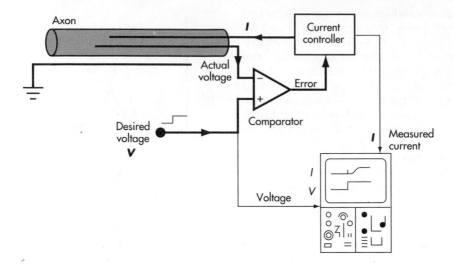

FIG. 2.10 The principle of the voltage clamp. Two electrodes are inserted in the squid axon; the voltage measured by one of them is compared with the 'desired voltage' *V*, and any difference between the two (error) automatically alters the current *I* passed into the axon through the second electrode. The time-courses of *V* and *I* are displayed on an oscilloscope; here the current in response to a step change in *V* is shown (somewhat simplified and schematic).

response to a depolarizing current, thus reducing the membrane potential, the resultant mismatch between the actual value and the desired value of the potential causes the control circuitry to alter the stimulating current until the two are again equal. By designing the control circuits properly, it is possible to make the membrane potential follow the desired value specified by the experimenter as accurately and rapidly as required.

Now the current *I* needed to clamp the membrane at a particular value *V* at any moment is simply equal to the sum of the currents I_{Na} and I_K carried by the movements of sodium and potassium ions respectively, though their contributions will be of opposite sign, since the sodium ions enter the fibre, whereas the potassium ions leave. For any particular voltage, these two currents will be proportional to the conductivities, g_K and g_{Na}, of the two ions. So if we measure the time-course of the current in response to a step-change in voltage, we obtain a curve that is proportional to the combined conductivities of sodium and potassium, though we cannot immediately disentangle one from the other. Such a curve is shown in Figure 2.11(b). After a brief spike of current that is due to charging up the membrane capacitance – to be discussed later – it can be seen that there is first an inward flow of current that rises to a peak but then reverses direction to become an outward flow that lasts as long as the voltage is held: on restoring the original resting potential, this outward current

declines back to zero over the course of a few milliseconds. The direction of these two phases of current flow suggests that the first, inward phase is due to sodium, and the second outward, one to potassium. To separate these two components it is necessary to devise some way of preventing one or other of them from taking place. One way to do this is to replace most of the sodium ions in the external medium with some other cation such as choline that is too large to get through the sodium channels. Under these circumstances the initial phase disappears entirely, leaving only the outward component; by subtracting this from the original record, one can work out what the time-course of both sodium and potassium permeability must have been (Fig. 2.11). These results can be confirmed by other methods, such as blocking the ionic channels with pharmacological agents such as tetrodotoxin (TTX) and tetraethylammonium (TEA) that specifically block sodium and potassium permeability respectively.

Thus the effect of a sudden step of depolarization is qualitatively different for potassium and sodium. Potassium permeability rises quite slowly in response to depolarization, but the increase is maintained for as long as the potential is held, dropping again quite quickly at the end of the step. Sodium permeability rises more quickly, but it is not sustained: even if the potential is held, g_{Na} falls spontaneously back to its resting value. But it is not then in the same state as when the nerve is unstimulated, for a further

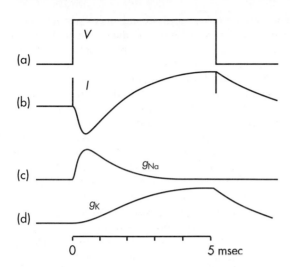

FIG. 2.11 Time-course of current *I* **(b)** in response to a 56 mV depolarization *V* **(a)** in a voltage clamp experiment on a squid axon. Below, **(c)** and **(d)** show the derived time-courses of the changes in sodium and potassium conductivities that give rise to the observed current *I*. (Simplified, after Hodgkin and Huxley, 1952a; Hodgkin, 1958)

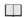

depolarization at this point causes only a very small increase in sodium permeability, if any: the sodium channels are said to be inactivated. When the potential is released, the inactivation rapidly wears off, and the channels revert to their former state. By systematically measuring these permeability changes in response to steps of different size and starting from different initial voltages, Hodgkin and Huxley (1952a, b) were able to derive equations expressing g_K and g_{Na} in terms of membrane potential that summarized their data and made it possible to predict, in general, how the permeabilities would vary in response to any given pattern of depolarization of the membrane.

For once one knows how a system behaves in response to a small step input, then by breaking up any given voltage pattern into a series of small steps and adding the results together one can calculate the response to the whole thing. In particular, starting with the time-course of the intracellular action potential of the squid axon, one can work out in this way what permeability changes would result from it, ending up with the curves already shown in Figure 2.9. We have now come full circle, for these permeability changes are of course precisely those that result, through application of the constant field equation, in the original action potential that we started with: we now have a complete description of the way in which the action potential is able to regenerate itself. More precisely, the action potential represents the solution

of the set of differential equations that embody the results of the voltage clamp experiment, the electrical properties of the membrane, and the constant field equation: the fact that this solution is so nearly identical to the shape of the actual action potential (Fig. 2.12) testifies to the completeness of Hodgkin and Huxley's description of the way in which membrane permeability depends on voltage.

Curves such as these look continuous; but it is important to bear in mind that they are the result of the summation of thousands of single events (the opening and closing of channels) which are themselves quantal or binary: a single channel is either open or shut, and the dynamics of overall permeability changes really reflect the way in which the *probability* of a channel being open varies with time and voltage. This can best be seen by using a refinement of the basic clamp technique called *patch clamping* (Fig. 2.13). Here, rather than deliberately increasing the area of membrane being investigated, as in the squid axon, we deliberately restrict it so that only a handful of channels are involved. Under these conditions the probabilistic behaviour of both voltage activation and spontaneous inactivation become apparent.

A quantitative description such as Hodgkin and Huxley's can also often suggest an underlying mechanism. It turns out that the changes in permeability in response to step depolarizations obey quite simple mathematical laws, with an equally simple mechanistic interpretation. The rise of potassium

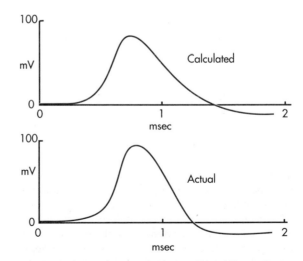

FIG. 2.12 Above, theoretical solution of the differential equations embodying the electrical properties of squid axon, the constant field equation, and the results of voltage clamp experiments. Below, actual action potential in squid axon at 18.5°C. (After Hodgkin and Huxley, 1952b)

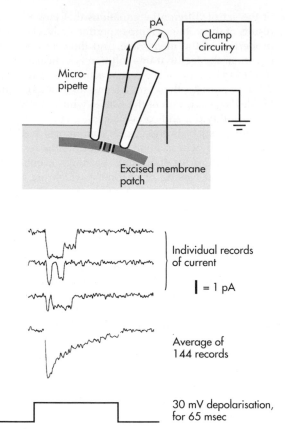

FIG 2.13 Patch clamping. Above, schematic view of the method: an excised patch of membrane is held tightly against a micropipette so that the potential across it can be clamped to various levels by passing current through the pipette. Below, behaviour of individual voltage-gated sodium channels in rat myotube membrane, as revealed by patch clamping. In single trials (three top traces) individual channels can be seen opening in response to depolarization and shutting again spontaneously, their currents adding together when more than one is open (top trace). When many such records are averaged, the probabilistic summation leads to a curve similar to what is seen for whole-fibre preparations. (Data from Pattak and Horn, 1982)

permeability, for instance, obeys the same kind of dynamics as a fourth-order reaction. This is another way of saying that the opening of a potassium channel requires the conjunction of four events whose individual probabilities depend on the potential – for instance, a channel normally blocked by four separate particles that move out of the way under the influence of an electric field. The sodium channel can be modelled in a similar way, but with two important differences: first , it obeys third- rather than fourth-order dynamics (which is why sodium permeability

rises more quickly), and, second, once open it spontaneously closes again, entering the inactivated state. A plausible model is thus of three blocking particles that move aside when the membrane is depolarized, together with a fourth that does the opposite, moving in to inactivate the channel. It is only relatively recently that molecular studies of the channel proteins have broadly confirmed what had been predicted on purely theoretical grounds several decades before. In the electric eel, for example, the sodium channel protein consists of some 2000 amino acids arranged in four linked subunits that are similar to one another but not identical; parts of the sequence, common to other voltage-gated channels, seem likely candidates for the voltage-sensing function.

Thus to summarize what is known of the electrical propagation of the action potential: *a local depolarization of a section of nerve gives rise, at first, to an increase in P_{Na} that causes the membrane to become still more depolarized as the potential moves towards E_{Na}. Meanwhile, however, P_K starts to rise, and the sodium permeability to fall, causing the potential to start to drop back towards the resting value. This in turn tends to shut off both the sodium and potassium channels but because of the delayed response of potassium permeability, there is a period during which P_K is greater than in the resting state, and the membrane is hyperpolarized. Eventually the resting potential is regained. Meanwhile, the currents generated by this process have spread to neighbouring regions of the fibre, causing them to depolarize and thus initiating, at a distance, the same sequence of changes all over again. In this way the whole pattern of potential and permeability changes is propagated down the fibre* (Fig. 2.14).

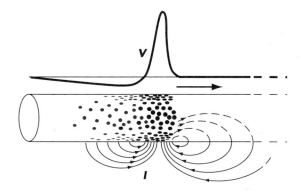

FIG. 2.14 'Snapshot' of a nerve axon with an action potential travelling from left to right. Above, the distribution of potential along its length; below, the associated flow of current. On the axon itself, the black holes represent the approximate relative density of open sodium channels, the red ones of potassium channels.

CONDUCTION VELOCITY

So far, very little has been said about the *speed* at which all these processes occur. We have traced the sequence of events by which one active region of nerve can trigger off a similar pattern of activity in another one at a distance from it by means of local currents: conduction velocity is simply a matter of how *far* and how *soon* these currents are sufficient to reach the fibre's threshold. Thus the factors that will influence this velocity are: how large the currents are, how high the threshold, how far they spread, and how long it takes them to depolarize the membrane.

In Figure 2.2 an equivalent circuit of the nerve membrane was introduced, in order to explain the spread of current from one part of the fibre to another. What was omitted from this circuit was that nerve fibres show not only resistance but also another passive electrical property, *capacitance* – the ability to store charge. Any two conductors separated by a layer of insulation act as a capacitor. The larger the opposed areas of the conductors, and the thinner the insulating layer between them, the larger the capacitance will be. In the case of nerve fibres, the membrane is both a good insulator and extremely thin, and makes a splendid capacitor: it has a capacitance, C_M, of about $1 \, \mu F/cm^2$. So our equivalent circuit

should really be redrawn in the form shown in Figure 2.15.

Now the effect of having capacitance in a circuit of this sort is to make it more sluggish in its responses. If we suddenly pass a current I through a resistor R_M on its own, the voltage across it immediately reaches the value $V = IR_M$; but with a capacitor as well it now takes *time* for the voltage to reach this value, because part of the current must be used to charge up the capacitor to the new level. On injecting a step of current of this kind, the voltage rises only slowly to its final value of IR_M, with a time-course that is exponential and given by $V = IR_M (1 - e^{-t/\tau})$. This is the *time constant* of the circuit (the time taken for the discrepancy $(IR_M - V)$ to fall by a factor e), and is equal in this case to $R_M C_M$. For many nerve fibres, this time constant is of the order of a few milliseconds, setting a limit on the rapidity with which the membrane can generate voltages in response to local currents.

The question of how *far* the local currents spread was considered earlier in this chapter. We saw that a voltage generated at a particular point on the membrane declines exponentially as a function of distance, with a space constant λ. The space constant and time constant together give a measure of the speed with which an electrical disturbance is propagated passively along the axon, regarded as a simple cable. This speed is in fact equal to λ/τ, which has the dimensions of a velocity; other things being equal,

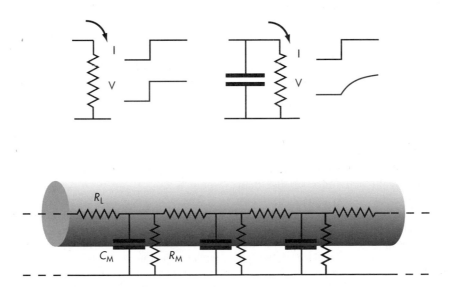

FIG. 2.15 Above, voltage response of a resistor (left) and of a resistor and capacitor in parallel (right) to an applied step of current, showing the slow, exponential rise of voltage in the second case. Below, modification of the equivalent circuit of Figure 2.2 to include membrane capacitance C_M as well as resistance R_M.

the velocity of conduction of action potentials ought also to be proportional to λ/τ. Now we saw earlier that λ is determined entirely by the longitudinal and transverse resistance of the axon ($\lambda = \sqrt{(R_M/R_L)}$), and thus varies with the square root of the fibre's diameter. The time constant $R_M C_M$, on the other hand, does not vary as a function of the diameter: if this is doubled, C_M, being proportional to surface area, is also doubled, but R_M is halved. It follows therefore that the conduction velocity of a fibre ought also to vary with the square root of the diameter, and for unmyelinated fibres this is indeed found to be the case.

However, animals rarely have unmyelinated fibres larger than about 1 μm in diameter: the reason for this is that there is a far better way of increasing the conduction velocity of large fibres than simply increasing their size, and this is *myelination*. As we saw in the previous chapter, the effect of myelination is enormously to thicken the layer of insulation round the fibre (except at the nodes of Ranvier); this has the desirable consequence of greatly increasing R_M and reducing C_M. Although the time constant of the membrane is not influenced very much by myelination, because the effects on R_M and C_M largely cancel out, the space constant is greatly increased. So the external local currents are forced to travel further before they can gain access to the axoplasm through the nodes. Since in myelinated fibres the active, voltage-sensitive sodium and potassium channels are virtually confined to the nodes, the action potential in effect jumps from node to node down the fibre, giving rise to the term *saltatory* conduction. The physics of saltatory conduction is slightly different from that in unmyelinated nerve, and one may calculate that its velocity ought to rise linearly with total fibre diameter (including the myelin) rather than in proportion to its square root. A consequence of this is that if we plot the velocity–diameter relationship for both types of fibre on the same graph (Fig. 2.16), the two curves cross over at a diameter near 1 μm: at this point the benefit of the myelin is exactly offset by the consequent reduction in size of the axon itself. So there is no point in having myelinated fibres smaller than 1 μm in diameter or unmyelinated ones larger than this (squids don't seem to have heard of myelin).

The other factors that govern conduction velocity are those concerned with the mechanisms that generate the local currents in the first place. Although passive conduction velocity is proportional to λ/τ, we need to add to τ a further factor T that represents the time required to restore a threshold potential to full size: thus a more exact representation of velocity is something like $\lambda/(\tau+T)$. Other things being equal,

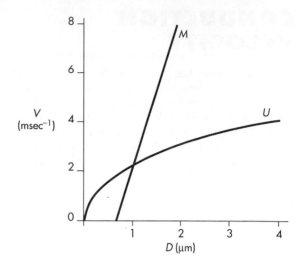

FIG. 2.16 Theoretical dependence of conduction velocity V on axon diameter D, for unmyelinated (U) and myelinated (M) axons. M is extrapolated from observations, U is scaled to fit observations on fast C-fibres. (After Rushton, 1951)

if the currents generated by the sodium channels are increased in size or set up more rapidly in response to voltage changes, then regeneration will be effected sooner than would otherwise be the case, and T will be reduced.

Thus *temperature* has a marked effect on conduction velocity, not because it alters the speed of local currents but because it speeds up the process of amplification by which potential differences cause the ionic channels to open and shut: as these processes are high-order ones, with a marked temperature sensitivity, conduction velocity itself is sharply reduced at low temperatures. The relationship to temperature is an irregular one, because high temperatures appear to affect the potassium mechanism more than the sodium one, so that the action potential actually gets smaller with increasing temperature. In some cold-blooded animals, conduction ceases altogether if the temperature exceeds some 37°C.

The size of the local currents also depends on the ionic concentrations inside and outside the fibre – low external sodium, for instance, reduces the velocity of conduction because it makes the sodium current smaller – and is influenced by local anaesthetics and other pharmacological agents acting on the permeability mechanisms. It is also a function of the density of sodium channels in the membrane; the nodes of Ranvier have a very much higher density of sodium channels than do ordinary unmyelinated

Box 2.1 Factors affecting conduction velocity

Factors that affect conduction velocity either concern the time it takes things to happen or how far the effects spread: *temporal* factors or *spatial* ones. Velocity is given approximately by:

$$\frac{\lambda}{\tau+T}$$

where λ is the space constant, τ the time constant for passive propagation down the axon, and T a measure of how long it takes for a threshold depolarization of the membrane at any point to regenerate itself to full size. These three *primary* factors in turn depend on *secondary* factors, as follows.

The space and time constants depend on the longitudinal and transverse resistances of the axon (R_L, R_M) and the membrane capacitance (C_M):

$$\lambda = \sqrt{\frac{R_M}{R_L}}$$
$$\tau = R_M C_M$$

These in turn are influenced by:

1. Diameter
   ($R_M \propto D^{-1}$, $R_L \propto D^{-2}$, $C_M \propto D$; so $(\lambda/\tau) \propto \sqrt{D}$)
2. Myelination
   (λ is increased but not τ; the effects on R_M and C_M cancel out)
3. The external resistance (Because it contributes to the effective value of R_L)

The effective regeneration time, T, depends on:

1. temperature
2. density of gates
3. ion concentrations
4. anaesthetics, anoxia, etc.

fibres, another factor contributing to the increased conduction velocity of myelinated nerves.

The compound action potential

Most peripheral nerves contain a variety of fibres of different diameters, some myelinated and some not, so that if we use a pair of external electrodes to record the response to a single shock delivered to the whole nerve, we usually obtain a very complex waveform with a number of peaks and troughs, called the *compound action potential*. Some of this complexity is due to the existence of fibres of different velocity, so that action potentials in different fibres arrive at the recording electrodes at different instants. But some is also due to the fact that we are recording with extracellular electrodes rather than an intracellular one. Why does this make a difference?

Consider first just a single axon from the nerve. If we were to insert a microelectrode in it we would record the classic *monophasic* action potential, rising from a resting potential of some –60 mV to become slightly positive, and then returning over the course of a millisecond or two back to rest, as the action

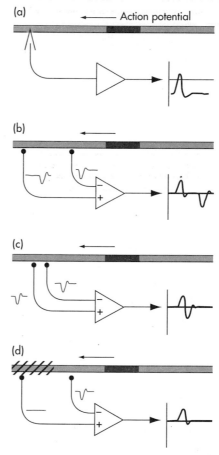

FIG. 2.17 Monophasic and biphasic action potentials. (a) Recording a monophasic action potential with a single microelectrode penetrating the axon. (b, c) A pair of external electrodes produces a biphasic potential whose duration is reduced if the electrodes are brought closer together. (d) If the nerve is crushed between the recording electrodes the action potential never reaches the second electrode: the result is a monophasic recording.

potential passes the point of insertion of the electrode. But if instead we record the same response with a pair of external electrodes some way apart, we shall in effect register the action potential twice over, as it passes each electrode in turn. As it passes the first electrode, it will make it more negative with respect to the other and as it passes over the second, the situation will be reversed, and the first electrode will now be more positive than the second (Fig. 2.17).

Thus although there is of course only one action potential, we will now record a *biphasic* response, with a swing of potential first in one direction and then in the other, about a resting value of zero. If we now bring the two electrodes close together, the two individual responses will begin to overlap, producing a smaller response because of the partial cancellation of the two components: the shape of the whole thing will be peculiarly uninformative. One way to get round this problem – apart from using an intracellular electrode – is to arrange things so that the action potential never actually gets as far as the second electrode, by crushing the nerve between the two recording points. Under these circumstances a monophasic response is obtained that is similar to the intracellular action potential, though a good deal smaller.

Consider now what would be seen if we had not one axon but several. If each of them had the same conduction velocity, and was in good working order, then the situation would not be very different from

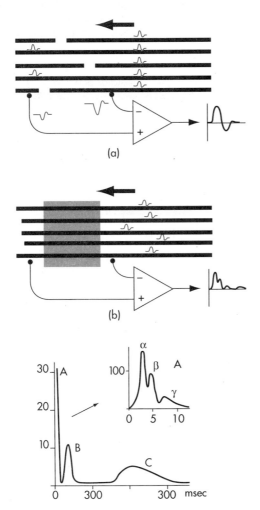

(a)

(b)

FIG. 2.18 The compound action potential. **(a)** Biphasic recording from whole nerve: the fact that some fibres fail to conduct between the electrodes makes the action potential asymmetric. **(b)** As **(a)**, but with the nerve crushed to give monophasic action potentials. Differences between the velocities of individual fibres give rise to a dispersed compound action potential. Below, actual compound action potential from frog sciatic nerve, with the A group shown on an expanded time scale in the inset. (Data from Erlanger and Gasser, 1938)

that of a single axon. But in a real preparation, it is rare for all the fibres in a bundle to be conducting all along their length, and at least some of them are likely to fail to conduct somewhere between the two electrodes. Consequently the biphasic potential from the whole nerve is likely to be a lopsided one, with some of the fibres contributing biphasically and others only monophasically (Fig. 2.18). If in addition they are all conducting at different speeds, then the whole thing will be drawn out into a series of overlapping responses, the peaks of some corresponding to the troughs of others, in a messy and uninformative way. It is then essential to ensure that all the fibres are producing monophasic potentials, by damaging the nerve between the electrodes as before. Under these circumstances, the pattern of peaks in the compound action potential gives a sort of spectrum of the conduction velocities of the fibres in the nerve, though not a very quantitative one, since large peaks may simply be due to large fibres rather than to a large *number* of fibres of a particular velocity. In such a spectrum from a large peripheral nerve, it is often possible to distinguish groups of fibres having roughly similar conduction velocities: the classification of these groups is shown in Table 2.3.

THRESHOLD PROPERTIES

Once we understand the mutual relationship between membrane potential on the one hand and ionic permeabilities on the other, we can easily explain many of the basic properties of nerve that make it behave so differently from a simple passive conductor of electricity, in particular the phenomena of *threshold* and the *all-or-nothing law*.

We have already seen that the relation between potential and permeability is that of a closed cycle or feedback loop, in which potential changes cause changes in permeability, and these in turn cause changes in potential (Fig. 2.19). But if we compare the two cases of sodium and potassium, the functional behaviour of these feedback loops is very different. With potassium, a depolarization causes an increase in P_K, which then tends to oppose the depolarization by bringing the membrane potential nearer to E_K: a good example of a *negative feedback* system that tends to stabilize the membrane near its resting potential. The case of sodium is the exact opposite: here, depolarization again causes an increase in permeability, but this tends to depolarize the membrane still further. Here we have not negative but *positive feedback*.

Positive feedback is a property usually associated with explosive systems. If we light a firework, the initial heat is sufficient to decompose part of the gunpowder, in turn releasing more heat which sets off yet more of the gunpowder, and so on: the positive feedback accelerates the reaction until the whole of the stored chemical energy has been released and converted into a big bang. In the same way, depolarization of the nerve membrane causes an increase in P_{Na}, which depolarizes the membrane still further, causing yet more of an increase in sodium permeability, and so on. If this were all that were happening, the potential would move smartly off to E_{Na} and stay there. (The reason it doesn't is of course

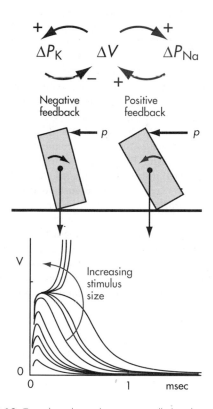

FIG. 2.19 Top, the relation between small depolarizations ΔV and changes in permeability to potassium, ΔP_K, and sodium, ΔP_{Na}, illustrating the existence of negative feedback in the former case, and positive in the latter. Whether the system *as a whole* shows negative or positive feedback depends on the relative size of the two components, as in the domino shown in the middle. For a small push it shows negative feedback, and is stable: for a larger push it shows positive feedback and topples over. Bottom, extracellular voltage response to stimulating currents of increasing size applied to crab nerve near the recording electrode, showing stability for small stimuli and instability (action potential generation) for larger ones: close to the threshold it teeters on the brink. (Partly after Hodgkin, 1938)

both that the increase in P_{Na} is only temporary , and that meanwhile the potassium permeability has also started to rise.) So whether the membrane as a *whole* is stable or unstable depends crucially on the relative contribution of the potassium and sodium feedback loops. If the former predominates, the membrane will tend to resist any potential changes applied to it; if the latter, it will tend to respond with an explosive increase in P_{Na} and a large swing of voltage.

In practice it turns out that the relative contribution of the two mechanisms depends in a non-linear way on the size of the stimulus applied: small stimuli seem to produce more of a potassium response than a sodium one, so that the membrane remains stable, whereas larger stimuli tip the balance in favour of sodium and result in instability – in other words, the regenerative action potential. The situation is very like that of the domino of Figure 2.19, standing on its edge. At rest, it is in a state of negative feedback: a small push tends to raise its centre of gravity, resulting in a turning couple that restores the status quo. A large push, however, that brings the vertical projection of the centre of gravity past the corner on which it rests converts the domino's stable equilibrium into an unstable one: the further it is pushed, the greater the couple acting to topple it over. Like nerve, it thus exhibits a *threshold*; there is a certain size of stimulus that converts its normal condition of negative feedback into one of positive feedback, and it then falls over and releases all its stored potential energy. If one records close to the point of stimulation of a single axon while stimulating with finely graded potentials in the region of the threshold, one can often see the membrane potential teetering on the brink between stability and instability (Fig. 2.19).

In general, therefore, any factor that favours the potassium mechanism rather than the sodium one will tend to raise the membrane threshold. Two important instances of this occur in the *refractory period* and in *accommodation*.

Refractory period

If we try to stimulate a nerve with a pair of shocks, gradually reducing the interval of time between them, we find that there comes a point when the threshold for the second shock begins to rise relative to that for the first. Eventually, as we go on decreasing the interval between the stimuli, we find that we cannot activate the nerve a second time at all, no matter how large the current we use (Fig. 2.20). This period, during which it is impossible to stimulate the nerve for a second time, is known as the *absolute*

refractory period: the period during which it can be stimulated, but only by using a larger current than usual, is called the *relative* refractory period. The latter corresponds quite well with the period just after the peak of the action potential during which P_K is still raised relative to its resting level, thus tending to stabilize the membrane potential.

The absolute refractory period seems to be due mostly to a property of the sodium channels. We saw earlier that in the voltage clamp experiments the sodium permeability rose quickly in response to a step of depolarization, and then declined spontaneously, leaving the channels in an inactivated condition which lasts as long as the voltage is maintained. We noted that even when the voltage is returned to its original value, it takes a certain period of time for the sodium channels to revert from their inactivated state to one in which they can once again respond to changes of voltage. Thus after the peak of the action potential has passed, there is a period of recovery during which the sodium mechanism is unresponsive, making the membrane absolutely stable to stimuli of any size. The existence of the refractory period is of considerable functional importance, since this is what prevents the action potential from being conducted in both directions at once. Because the local currents flow almost equally both ahead of the action potential and behind it (Fig. 2.14) it is essential that the region over which it has just passed should not be reactivated all over again; its refractoriness prevents this happening.

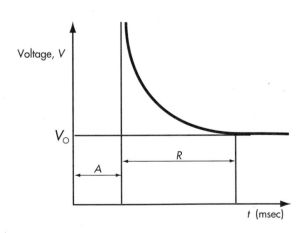

FIG. 2.20 Refractoriness of nerve: the voltage *V* required to stimulate an axon at different times *t* after a previous suprathreshold stimulus, showing the absolute refractory period *A* and the relative refractory period *R*. V_0 is the threshold when a single stimulus is used.

Accommodation

One normally measures a nerve's threshold by using a small voltage step or pulse in which there is a sudden change of potential. If instead we try to depolarize the nerve more slowly, we find that we need to depolarize it further before it will respond with an action potential. Indeed, if the rate of depolarization is sufficiently slow we may find that the nerve never responds at all, however far we depolarize it (Fig. 2.21): the nerve has *accommodated* itself to the changing potential.

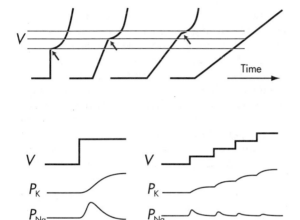

FIG. 2.21 Accommodation. Above, the threshold for generating an action potential (arrows) depends on the *rate* of depolarization: if this is too slow the fibre may never fire at all however much it is depolarized. (After Fabre, 1927) Below, left, the changes in P_K and P_{Na} in response to a clamped step of voltage; right, in response to a series of small steps, approximating a slowly increasing depolarization: potassium permeability increases steadily, while sodium permeability declines through inactivation.

This phenomenon can be readily explained if we think in terms of the balance between the sodium and potassium mechanisms. In the voltage clamp experiments, we saw that a sustained step of depolarization gave rise to an immediate but transient increase in sodium permeability, and a delayed but sustained increase in that of potassium. Thus there is only a short period during which the sodium mechanism dominates: time is on the side of stability. Suppose, for example, we were to stimulate a nerve not with one large step of depolarization but with a staircase-like sequence of little ones (Fig. 2.21). It is clear that whereas P_K increases cumulatively with each new step, P_{Na} does not, since it is only transient; furthermore, the transient increase in P_{Na} will steadily decline with increasing depolarization, because of the steadily increasing degree of sodium inactivation. Thus the more gradually we depolarize a nerve fibre, the more we push the sodium/potassium balance in favour of potassium, and the further we need to depolarize it in order to reach the threshold and if we depolarize it slowly enough, there will come a point where P_{Na} is never great enough relative to P_K for the nerve to fire at all, and the membrane will therefore completely accommodate. We shall see later that the mechanism of accommodation can sometimes be an important determinant of the way in which sensory receptors respond to slowly changing stimuli.

The all-or-nothing law

Any system with positive feedback will tend to behave in a manner approximating to all-or-nothing behaviour. The violence with which a barrel of gunpowder explodes depends very little on the temperature of the flame used to light it, so long as it is big enough to set it off at all. The domino of Figure 2.19 ultimately hits the ground with much the same force, whether the original push was large or small. Much the same, but not *exactly* the same: clearly, if the energy of the push is appreciable in comparison with the domino's stored potential energy, the force with which it strikes the ground will be increased. More exactly, the energy released on falling over will be $P + E$, where E is the stored potential energy, and P the energy imparted by the original push. In the case of nerves, the all-or-nothing law is *not* found to be strictly obeyed if one records close to the point of stimulation – within a space constant or two – since the stimulus energy then contributes in part to what is recorded. But as the action potential is propagated further and further away from its origin, this contribution becomes increasingly negligible, and it eventually settles down to its standard form. What we have, in effect, is not just one domino but a whole line of them (Fig. 2.22): when one falls, it imparts a fraction of its energy to the next, sufficient to knock it over, and so on in turn all the way down the line. Imagine for the sake of argument that one-tenth of a falling domino's energy is used in knocking over the next. Then the first domino imparts an energy $(P + E)/10$ to the second, which in turn imparts $((P + E)/10 + E)/10$ to the third, and so on. It is clear that the contribution of the original push, P, to the energy with which the nth domino hits the ground will get vanishingly small as n gets larger, and that this energy will in fact settle down at a constant level: the system as a whole will then obey the all-or-nothing law exactly.

This law is of fundamental significance in the nervous system, and it is worth reflecting on its

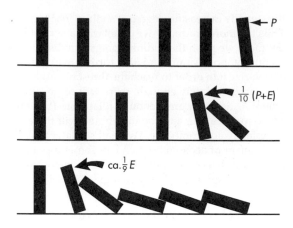

P

$\frac{1}{10}(P+E)$

ca. $\frac{1}{9}E$

FIG. 2.22 All-or-nothing behaviour of a row of falling dominos.

functional implications. Why should it have evolved? It clearly imposes very severe limitations on the kinds of messages that nerves can convey, prohibiting direct transmission of graded quantitative information (of the kind conveyed, for example, by the varying concentration of a hormone in the blood), the only messages permitted being of the binary 'yes/no' variety. The answer certainly lies in the problems of trying to send messages along cables that are so leaky that currents cannot be conveyed passively more than a matter of millimetres. An engineer faced with such a problem – as found on a somewhat larger scale in transatlantic submarine cables – would probably deal with it by introducing a series of booster amplifiers at intervals along the cable, to restore the losses caused by leakage. In the case of nerve axons, we have already seen that the length over which they are required to conduct is so much greater than the space constant that many thousands of such stages of amplification would be required; each node of Ranvier is in effect a booster of this kind.

What are the characteristics of a chain of amplifiers of this sort? All amplifiers, however good their quality, suffer from two defects: they introduce *noise*, and they create *distortion*. Noise includes both the hiss that arises inevitably in any electrical system – including neurones – from the random movements of the electrons or ions in its conductors, and also disturbances picked up from external sources of interference. Now imagine a thousand hi-fi amplifiers connected end to end, so that the output of one forms the input of the next. The noise generated by each one of them will be amplified all the way down the line and added to those of the others, making the final output very much noisier than if there were only

one amplifier. Distortion arises through inaccuracies in the linearity of the amplification. This too becomes exaggerated if a number of amplifiers are connected in series. If, for example, the gain of each amplifier is 1 percent greater than it should be, then the gain of the whole set of a thousand will be too large by a factor of some 2000; and if 1 percent smaller than it should be, then the overall gain will be 1/2000 of the correct value. Thus accurate transmission of quantitative information becomes almost impossible: the system almost automatically becomes all-or-nothing in character, since signals either vanish or become saturatingly huge.

The only solution is to be less ambitious about *what* one is trying to signal. If, for example, one limits oneself to only two possible signals – 'yes' or 'no' – then distortion no longer matters: the signal is either there or not there, and no regard need be paid to how large it is. If we also arrange for each amplifier to have a threshold that is higher than the normal noise level but allows through the signal 'yes', then we can get rid of noise as well. In other words, the only kind of system that is capable of transmitting messages reliably over distances that are much bigger than the space constant is precisely what we have found in the nerve axon itself: a series of regenerative amplifiers (the voltage-sensitive sodium channels) exhibiting a threshold that prevents the fibre from producing spurious signals in response to its own noise. There is no advantage in using such a system for conduction over shorter distances, and in practice it is found that short neurones (as, for example, the bipolar cells of the retina) never use action potentials but rely on the much simpler and more informative method of passively propagated electronic potentials. There is nothing *intrinsically* desirable about action potentials: they are a necessity imposed by the need for nerves to be small, and they severely constrain the way in which information is coded.

NEURAL CODES

So if it is not open to us to use the size of an action potential to convey quantitative information, what possibilities remain? One way is to use the *number* of action potentials. It is very common in the nervous system to find many fibres running in parallel from one location to another, all apparently carrying the same kind of information. In such cases, the magnitude of a stimulus can be coded by how many of the fibres are active at any one moment. A good example of this, as we shall see, is in the nerve from the

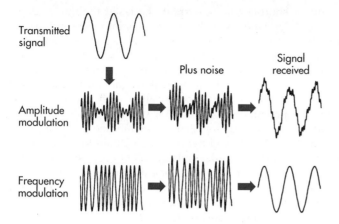

FIG. 2.23 Amplitude and frequency modulation, showing how noise added to the modulated radio wave results in more interference in the decoded audio signal for amplitude modulation (AM) than for frequency modulation (FM).

vestibular apparatus; here the fibres are all found to have different stimulus thresholds, so that increasing stimulation leads to more and more of them firing at once, a phenomenon known as *recruitment*. In the same way, muscular contractions are often controlled by varying the number of active fibres innervating them. One may also use the number of action potentials per unit of time, the *firing frequency*, to convey quantitative information. As we shall see shortly, the normal way in which a neurone responds to stimulation, whether external as in the case of receptors or, in the case of a central neurone, to the synaptic effects of other neurones connected to it, is by firing *repetitively* at a frequency that depends in quite a simple way on the magnitude of the stimulus. Conversely, the degree of tetanic contraction of a muscle depends on the frequency with which it is stimulated.

There is an analogy here with the use of FM (frequency modulation) rather than AM (amplitude modulation) in radio transmission. In amplitude modulation, the amplitude of the radio-frequency carrier wave is a direct copy of the sound wave being transmitted (Fig. 2.23); the radio receiver decodes this signal by converting the envelope of the radio wave back into a sound wave. The disadvantage of such a system is that any variations in the amplitude of the wave caused by transmission itself – fading or noise generated by radio interference – get incorporated in the sound reproduced by the receiver. In FM transmission this is no longer the case: here it is the frequency of the radio wave rather than its amplitude that conveys the sound information, and disturbances that affect its amplitude no longer matter, since it is only the frequency of the received signal that is decoded by the receiver, producing reliable and relatively noise-free transmission.

Frequency modulation is by no means the only way in which quantitative information may be conveyed down a single all-or-nothing or binary channel. A familiar example of a different kind of binary code is the Morse code, where information is carried in the temporal pattern of the only two possible signals – dot and dash. However, coding of such sophistication has never been observed in actual neurones, and we shall see that the mechanism by which neurones are caused to fire repetitively makes it unlikely that information could actually be carried by the nervous system in this form. In computers, quantitative information may be conveyed by a single pulse by varying the time at which it occurs relative to some kind of internal clock within the computer. Again, it is unlikely that this form of coding is used by the brain, both because the slowness of conduction would make it difficult to maintain accurate timing between events, and also because of the apparent absence of anything equivalent to an internal reference clock. Thus in practice we are limited to frequency modulation, and to methods such as recruitment that make use of the spatial patterning of activity across a set of fibres.

The initiation of impulses

How is this frequency code generated? Consider a neurone whose resting potential is E_R with a set of channels which when open tend to short-circuit the membrane and lead to an equilibrium potential around zero. Somewhere between E_R and zero there will be a threshold potential θ for triggering an impulse (though we must bear in mind that the value of θ will depend in general on the *rate* of depolarization, because of accommodation). If we suddenly open these channels and keep them open, the potential will move towards zero, and must at some point cross the threshold, setting off an action potential. The usual stereotyped sequence of changes in permeability will then ensue, terminating in a recovery phase in which P_K will be elevated and the neurone relatively hyperpolarized as its potential is pulled towards E_R. As P_K declines to normal after the impulse, the potential will rise again, not just to the original resting potential but past it (since we suppose that the original channels are still open) towards zero. What happens next will depend on the rate at which this depolarization occurs. If it is sufficiently fast (and θ correspondingly low), the threshold will be crossed once more, and a second action potential will be generated, then a third, a fourth, and so on; impulses will continue to be generated so long as the channels remain open (Fig. 2.24). The greater the

short-circuiting current, the faster the rate of depolarization will be after each impulse, and so the sooner the nerve will fire off again. Thus the frequency of the repetitive firing will depend on the degree of short-circuiting that we have produced: the more channels are open, the higher the frequency. But if the rate of depolarization after the first action potential is too slow, θ may rise so much because of accommodation that the membrane potential never reaches it, and the neurone will fail to fire for a second time. Under suitable conditions, a steady current will imitate the effect of a short-circuiting permeability change, and will elicit repetitive firing: the frequency is often a simple – even linear – function of the applied current (Fig. 2.24).

Even though the current is held constant, one often observes in such a preparation that the frequency of action potentials declines from an initial high value to a lower steady state (Fig. 2.25). A decline of this kind in the response to a steady stimulus is called *adaptation*, and is discussed much more

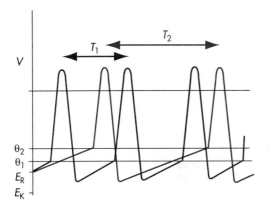

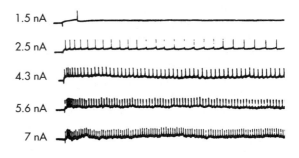

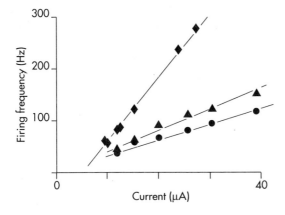

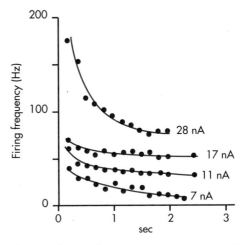

FIG. 2.24 Above, mechanism by which a steady current may initiate repetitive firing. The black line shows schematically the response to a continuous depolarizing current; the red line, to a smaller current. θ_1 and θ_2 are the threshold levels corresponding to the associated rates of depolarization. The frequency in each case is the reciprocal of the interval T between spikes. Below, experimental relation between injected current and resultant steady firing frequency for three motor neurones. (Data from Granit *et al.*, 1963)

FIG. 2.25 Membrane adaptation in motor neurones. Above, spike responses to steadily injected currents of the strengths indicated. (Oshima, 1969) Below, decline in frequency with time in such an experiment. (Data from Granit *et al.*, 1963)

fully in the next chapter (p.48). This particular example of adaptation seems to be a general property of all kinds of neurones, including receptors, and is called *membrane adaptation*. It is sometimes described as accommodation, but this is very misleading since it is not in fact due to the same mechanism as that underlying the true accommodation described earlier.

Membrane adaptation is believed to be caused by the entry of calcium ions during the action potentials. The calcium then acts on a type of potassium channel that opens in response to calcium, as distinct from the voltage-sensitive ones we have come across so far, thus increasing P_K, stabilizing the membrane and raising the threshold for generating action potentials (Fig 2.26). This probably represents a general mechanism for regulating the resting potential, rather than being specifically intended for adaptation.

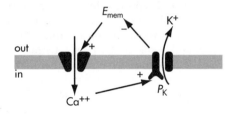

FIG. 2.26 One membrane mechanism that contributes to adaptation. Depolarization increases internal calcium concentration, which in turn activates Ca-dependent potassium channels; the resultant increase in P_K forms a negative feedback loop that tends to restore the original potential.

References

Conway, E. J. (1957) Nature and significance of concentration relations of potassium and sodium ions in skeletal muscle. *Physiological Review* 37, 84–132.

Erlanger, J. and Gasser, H. S. (1938) *Electrical Signs of Nervous Activity*. University of Pennsylvania Press, Philadelphia.

Fabre, P (1927) L'excitation neuro-musculaire par les courants progressifs chez l'homme. *Comptes rendues de l'Academie des Sciences*, Paris 184, 699–701.

Granit, R., Kernell, D. and Shortess, G. K. (1963) Quantitative aspects of firing of mammalian motoneurones, caused by injected currents. *Journal of Physiology* 168, 911-931.

Hodgkin, A.L. (1938) The subthreshold potentials in a crustacean nerve fibre. *Proceedings of the Royal Society B* 126, 87–121.

Hodgkin, A. L. (1939) The relation between conduction velocity and the electrical resistance outside a nerve. *Journal of Physiology* 94, 560–570.

Hodgkin, A. L. (1958) Ionic movements and electrical activity in giant nerve fibres. *Proceedings of the Royal Society B* 148, 1–37.

Hodgkin, A. L. and Horowicz, P. (1959) The influence of potassium and chloride ions on the membrane potential of single muscle fibres. *Journal of Physiology* 148, 127–160.

Hodgkin, A. L. and Huxley, A. F. (1952a) The components of membrane conductance in the giant axon of *Loligo*. *Journal of Physiology* 116, 473–496.

Hodgkin, A. L. and Huxley, A. F. (1952b) A quantitative description of membrane current and its application to conduction and excitation in nerve. *Journal of Physiology* 117, 500–544.

Hodgkin, A. L. and Katz, B. (1949). The effect of sodium ions on the electrical activity of the giant axon of the squid. *Journal of Physiology* 108, 37–77.

Oshima, K. (1969) Studies of pyramidal tract cells. In *Basic Mechanisms of the Epilepsies*, ed. H. H. Jasper, A. A. Ward and A. Pope. Little, Brown, Boston.

Pattak, J. and Horn, R. (1982) Effect of N-bromoacetamide on single sodium channel currents in excised membrane segments. *Journal of General Physiology* 79, 333–351.

Rushton, W. A. H. (1951) A theory of the effects of fibre size in medullated nerve. *Journal of Physiology* 115, 101–122.

NOTES

Page 18 There are many excellent books on electrophysiology. Aidley, D. J. (1989) *The Physiology of Excitable Cells* (Cambridge University Press, Cambridge) is excellent all round, as is Nicholls, J. G., Martin, A. R. and Wallace, B. G. (1992) *From Neuron to Brain* (Sinauer, Massachusetts) (with the added advantage of an appendix on electrical circuits for those who missed out on their physics at school). Matthews, G. (1986) *Cellular Physiology of Nerve and Muscle* (Blackwell, Oxford) is more general in its scope, as is Levitan, I. B. and Kaczmarek, L. K. (1991) *The Neuron: Cell and Membrane Biology* (Oxford University Press, Oxford), a book with remarkably clear text and illustrations. Robertson, R. N. (1983) *The Lively Membranes* (Cambridge University Press, Cambridge) is idiosyncratic and fun.

Page 18 Galvani Galvani's description of his experiments, and his careful reasoning from them, are well worth looking at. His summary of how nerve operates is, in essence, a remarkably percipient description of passive conduction: '*For what pertains to voluntary motions, perhaps the mind, with its marvellous power, might make some impetus either into the cerebrum, as is very easy to believe, or outside the same, into whatever nerve it pleases, wherefrom it will result that neuro-electric fluid will quickly flow from the corresponding muscle to that part of the nerve to which it was recalled by the impetus, and when it has arrived there, the insulating part of the nerve substance being overcome through its then increased strength, as it goes out thence, it will be* *received either by the extrinsic moisture of the nerve, or by the membranes, or by other contiguous parts, and through them, as through an arc, will be restored to the muscle from which, as we are pleased to think, it previously flowed out, from the positively electric part of the same, through impulse in the nerve'.* Luigi Galvani (1791) *De Viribus Electricitatis in Motu Musculari Commentarius*; trans. R.M. Green (Licht, Cambridge, Mass.).

Page 25 Permeability changes causing potential changes A horribly common misconception – actually taught in many schools – is that the potential changes that follow the opening of sodium channels are due to a large increase in sodium concentration: 'Sodium ions rush in, and during recovery they are pumped out again by the sodium pump'. The clearest demonstration of the falsity of such a view is that after blocking the sodium pump with ouabain, a squid axon can carry several thousand action potentials before the internal sodium finally rises to the point where the axon can no longer conduct. The membrane is like a car battery, charged by the dynamo provided by the sodium pump.

Page 27 The voltage clamp technique is well described in Alan Hodgkin's own *Conduction of the Nervous Impulse* (Liverpool University Press, Liverpool) (1964). Something of the atmosphere in the lab in the exciting time that led up to these findings can be felt in Hodgkin, A. (1992) *Chance and Design: Reminiscences of Science in Peace and War* (Cambridge University Press, Cambridge).

Page 28 Voltage-driven permeability changes One additional factor, however: it turns out that in many cell bodies, terminals and dendrites (though less so in axons) calcium as well as sodium may enter during action potentials. Since calcium concentrations outside cells are normally very much larger than those inside, this calcium entry can also contribute substantially to membrane depolarization (an important example of this is cardiac muscle). But calcium entry is also important in another way, for in many situations it also acts as a *chemical messenger*, triggering other kinds of responses from the cell apart from changes in potential. A good example of this is in synaptic transmission, discussed in the next chapter; another is of course muscular contraction. In addition, when calcium enters it may indirectly contribute to membrane potential by altering the permeability to potassium, through more than one type of channel: these channels are distinct from the purely voltage-sensitive ones discussed so far. For the most part, these mechanisms tend to stabilize the resting potential (see p. 39).

Page 29 Time constant One might wonder why R_L does not contribute to the time constant. The reason is that just as the space constant is defined in terms of what happens when we disregard time (by considering what happens when everything reaches equilibrium), so the time constant is defined in terms of what happens when space is entirely neglected: that is, when a current is applied uniformly along the fibre. Since there is then no spatial variation, no current flows through R_L so it cannot contribute.

Page 30 Saltatory conduction Students sometimes get the impression that saltatory conduction is fast *because* the action potential jumps in this way. This is really to think of it back-to-front: each node causes the action potential to be delayed while it is regenerated, like pit stops in a motor race. The nerve would conduct faster if there were no nodes, but not very far.

Page 30 Conduction velocity and diameter Apart from Rushton's classic paper mentioned above, you may care also to look at Arbuthnott, E. R., Boyd, I. A. and Kalu, K. U. (1980) Ultrastructural dimensions of myelinated peripheral nerve fibres in the cat and their relation to conduction velocity. *Journal of Physiology* 368, 125–157. One might wonder why the myelinated curve doesn't go through the origin: is there really a certain size at which the fibre stops conducting altogether? The answer is that in the model it is assumed that one can alter the thickness of the myelin for optimum conduction velocity; as the diameter goes down, this optimum thickness gets relatively bigger. There comes a point where the model says that one does best with solid myelin and no axoplasm at all! You can investigate this yourself with the NeuroLab Conduction Velocity exhibit.

Page 30 37° causing nerve block Good news for oysters, anaesthetized as they are swallowed. And possibly for lobsters, traditionally brought slowly to the boil whilst still alive.

Page 36 Better not to use action potentials An antidote to the common misconception that all nervous communication has to be through action potentials is Roberts, A. and Bush, B. M. H. (1981) *Neurons without Impulses* (Cambridge University Press, Cambridge).

NEUROLAB

General instructions for running NeuroLab may be found on page vii.

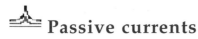 Passive currents

Page 20

This models a stretch of cable with longitudinal resistance and transverse resistance and capacitance. The two sliders enable you to alter the space and time constants. You can choose either to apply a steady current or a pulse of current (a charge, in other words) with the radio buttons on the right. Pressing Start shows a series of snapshots of voltage as a function of distance on each side of the point of stimulation, at equal intervals of time after application of the stimulus. In the case of a steady current, you will see the voltage gradually reach an equilibrium in which it falls off exponentially on each side. If you have chosen Charge, you can see how it gradually spreads itself out over the cable, collapsing away to nothing as it is dissipated through the membrane resistance. See for yourself the effect of altering the space and time constants.

Ionic equilibria

Page 23

This enables you to play around with a simplified model cell, altering ion permeabilities and pumps and seeing the effects on membrane potential and cell composition (on the left) and volume (the cell is shown in the box on the right: its colour (and that of the extracellular fluid) reflect its ionic composition – red is sodium and blue potassium). You can select the cell to be either a red blood cell or a squid axon with the radio buttons at middle left; you can also use the check box to turn the sodium pump on or off.

Select squid axon, make sure the sodium pump is on, and press the Start button. The membrane potential will settle around −64 mV. Use the up and down buttons next to the displayed numbers in the table at top left to alter external sodium and potassium, and note the effect on membrane potential and cell volume. Alter some of the permeabilities in the same way. Try turning the sodium pump off. You can reset the original values with the Reset button, halt the simulation temporarily and resume with Halt and Continue, and quit (as in all the NeuroLab exhibits) with Quit.

⌐⌐ Action potentials

Page 27

This exhibit provides a model of some aspects of action potential generation under normal and clamped conditions. The model is a highly simplified one, and as a result the time-courses of the action potentials are not like those in any particular preparation or species, but they do illustrate many of the principles involved.

The main window shows a display of potential, g_{Na}, g_K, total membrane current and stimulus size as a function of time: a sweep is initiated by clicking on the Sweep button at bottom right. The stimulus controls are at top right: you can choose either a current stimulus under natural conditions or a clamped voltage stimulus, varying the size with the slider and the polarity with the radio buttons. Normally the stimulus is applied when you click on the Stimulate panel and stops when you release it; alternatively you can click once on the On panel and then once on the Off. If you select Ramp, the stimulus changes gradually, at a constant rate: use this to look at accommodation, for instance. Below, two check boxes enable you to apply TTX (blocking sodium channels) or TEA (potassium).

In Current mode, short or small stimuli cause a disturbance that settles back to equilibrium; if larger than a certain threshold, an 'action potential' of fairly fixed time-course is generated. See what factors affect the threshold. You can also investigate refractoriness and accommodation. Then select Voltage Clamp mode, and simulate a Hodgkin–Huxley experiment. Note that small stimuli have more effect on potassium than on sodium permeability; you can also look at inactivation of the sodium channels.

⊏⊒⊐ Time constants

Page 29

This exhibit shows an electrical circuit, together with a hydraulic analogue of it, and provides a graphic display of how it responds to different kinds of stimuli. The values of the two resistances and the capacitor can be altered with the sliders at right. The radio buttons at top right select one of three operating modes: for the moment, select Voltage. The circuit then consists of a capacitor and resistor in parallel (as in an axon membrane): when the switch is closed (click on the panel below the sliders) the capacitor is charged up by a fixed voltage source through another resistor. The hydraulic analogy is a tank of a certain capacity with a leaky outlet, being filled through a tap from another source of constant pressure. Press Sweep, and a trace will start to appear in the window, showing the voltage across the capacitor as a function of time. Then open and close the switch and see for yourself how the voltage is affected.

Selecting the Current option replaces the battery and resistor with a constant current source, equivalent to water flowing into the tank through a tap at a constant rate. Notice that closing the switch now makes the potential move towards a constant equilibrium value at which the rate of current coming in is equal to the rate of its leaking out again.

The third option, R_2, will be more relevant when we consider synaptic and receptor mechanisms in Chapter 3, and it is described there (p. 70).

Conduction velocity

Page 30

Here you can design your own nerve fibre by altering its diameter and the degree of myelination: the display at right shows you the resultant electrical properties, and at bottom left you can read off the conduction velocity. You can see for yourself how diameter affects conduction velocity for unmyelinated fibres. In the case of myelinated ones, you need to adjust the myelin thickness for each diameter to create the maximum possible speed. If you are feeling keen, plot graphs of all these things, including optimum myelin thickness. This model is a very simple one, taking into account only general physical principles, but it generates surprisingly realistic results.

Compound action potentials

Page 31

A simple demonstration of the complications introduced when recording from multifibre nerve trunks, especially when they are partly damaged and when extracellular electrodes are used. A set of fibres is shown symbolically in the window. They are stimulated at the black line at left when the Stimulate button is clicked. The recording electrodes are the red and blue lines crossing the fibres to the right. You can move them with the sliders called Electrode Position at top right, and you can also select either monophasic or diphasic recording. When you stimulate, action potentials (yellow) start to move along the fibres at different rates, and in the window below you can see the resultant potential that is recorded, as a function of time. You can alter the dispersion of the fibres (i.e. the range of velocities they show) and also introduce some damage, blocking the action potentials at random points as they pass along.

3 COMMUNICATION BETWEEN NEURONES

Common features of all neurones 43
Sensory receptors 47

Synaptic transmission 54

COMMON FEATURES OF ALL NEURONES

In the last chapter we saw how information may be carried from one part of an excitable cell to another: by passive conduction when the distances are short enough to permit it, and otherwise by means of action potentials. We need now to consider how these signals are generated in the first place, by stimuli in the outside world, and by the action of other neurones.

Electrical transmission

The simplest of all kinds of intercellular communication is when currents pass directly from one cell to another. The best known example is perhaps that of conduction between the muscle fibres of the heart, where the currents pass through gap junctions (Fig. 3.1) forming part of the intercalated discs. But electrical transmission can also occur between neurones, either informally through casual sets of gap junctions (as, for example, between photoreceptors in the retina) or at more organized regions of contact called *electrical synapses*. But rather stringent structural conditions have to be met before this mode of synaptic transmission will work. Figure 3.2 shows an idealized electrical synapse and its equivalent circuit. It is clear that the currents generated by the presynaptic bouton have two alternative routes: they can either cross the gap and enter the postsynaptic cell, or they can simply leak out sideways through the synaptic cleft. The greater the fraction of current that takes the former route, the greater will be the degree of electrical coupling between the two neurones, since by

entering the postsynaptic cell the currents will cause potential changes that may, if large enough, trigger a new action potential. The degree to which the current chooses one route rather than the other will in turn depend rather critically on the width of the synaptic gap. The smaller it is, the lower will be the impedance to current passing into the postsynaptic cell, and the higher the impedance to current escaping sideways. Those synapses that are known to operate electrically are invariably found to include intercellular contacts in the form of gap or tight junctions, reducing or preventing this sideways leakage of current.

But even if no leakage at all occurs, and the transmembrane impedance at the junction is reduced to zero, there is *still* no guarantee that an action potential will be able to pass successfully from one cell to

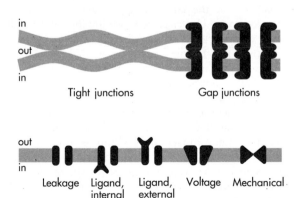

FIG. 3.1 Membrane structures that help neurones communicate. Above, direct intercellular contacts. Tight junctions prevent sideways leakage of currents or solutes; gap junctions permit them to flow directly from cell to cell. Below, types of membrane channel, shown in the symbolic form used throughout this book.

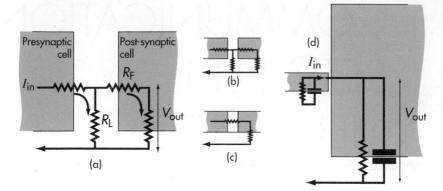

FIG. 3.2 The requirements for electrical transmission. **(a)** If a presynaptic current I_{in} is to create a sufficiently large depolarization V_{out} of the postsynaptic cell, sideways leakage through R_L must be small: thus the forward resistance R_F needs to be much less than R_L. This can be achieved if the gap is reduced **(b)** or with a gap junction or tight junction **(c)**. Even if loss through R_L is negligible, if the postsynaptic area is large in comparison with the presynaptic ending **(d)**, its large capacitance and small resistance result in a low impedance, and I_{in} may still be insufficient to cause a threshold change in V_{out}. This would be the case for an ordinary neuromuscular junction.

another. The size of the local currents that flow during the passage of an action potential along an axon is strongly dependent on the size of the axon itself. The larger it is, the greater the number of sodium channels per unit length and so the larger the active currents that can be generated. But equally, larger axons have greater capacitance and smaller transverse resistance per unit length; consequently the currents have to be that much larger to achieve a particular threshold level of depolarization. In other words, the currents automatically keep up with the increased requirements as the fibre's diameter is increased. But if we imagine a small axon whose diameter suddenly gets bigger at a particular point or – as comes to the same thing – a small axon with a low-resistance electrical synapse joining it to a cell body of larger size, this is obviously no longer the case (Fig. 3.2). To trigger action potentials, the larger cell requires larger currents which the small axon may well be unable to provide; if a burning thread is attached to a rope, the heat the thread generates may be insufficient to ignite the rope. One can calculate, for example, that electrical transmission across the ordinary neuromuscular junction is in principle impossible even if the junction were a low-resistance one (which it is not): the impedance ratio on the two sides is much too large for the axonal currents to make any significant impression on the potential of the muscle cell. It is clear, therefore, that in such cases an *extra* source of amplification in addition to that provided by the action potential mechanism is needed: the knot between thread and rope must be soaked in petrol.

Channels

This amplification – the petrol – is provided by membrane channels sensitive not to voltage but to chemical transmitters – *ligand-gated* channels. In the case of sensory receptors, amplification is often also required, and when in later chapters we go through the senses one by one, we may be struck by the extraordinary sensitivity that is shown by many sensory receptors: to single photons in the eye, to subatomic movement in the ear, to single odorant molecules in the nose. As a result, there is a very great similarity between the way channels in sensory receptors respond to stimuli, and the way those in interneurones respond to transmitter, and it is convenient to start by considering both at once.

There are essentially two ways in which a transmitter or stimulus may open (or close) a channel. Some channels look outwards, with processes on the extracellular side that respond to specific stimuli or transmitters. One example of such *direct* gating mechanisms is the nicotinic acetylcholine receptor of skeletal muscle, where recognition of the transmitter causes opening of an unselective, short-circuiting channel, with depolarization and the generation of an action potential in the muscle; it is discussed in more detail later in this chapter (p. 55). All mechanoreceptors work – as far as we know – by a direct mechanism of this kind, with the mechanical stimulus acting immediately to cause opening of the channel. The other possibility is *indirect* gating; here the channel is inward-looking, responding only to chemical messages from inside the cell. The link with the outside world is provided by a second protein that straddles the membrane and responds to transmitters or stimuli in the outside world by triggering off a chemical response on the other side of the membrane, which then results in the required message being sent to the channel. This intracellular communication may involve just one intermediate or a cascade of several of them; very often the first link in the chain is formed by a *G-protein* (GTP-binding protein). An example of short indirect coupling is the M_2-muscarinic acetylcholine receptor, where the G-protein, activated by an acetylcholine receptor, then acts directly on a potassium channel to cause hyperpolarization (Fig. 3.3). The transduction mechanism in retinal rod receptors is a good example of a cascade: here a photolabile pigment molecule,

rhodopsin, is coupled to a G-protein that activates a phosphodiesterase that in turn results in the conversion of cGMP to GMP; since cGMP opens sodium channels on the surface of the receptor cell, the effect of light is to close them, and thus to cause hyperpolarization. A similar cascade, but with cAMP instead of cGMP, appears to operate in olfactory receptors.

These two general methods of generating permeability changes each have their advantages. Direct activation is fast and secure. Indirect activation provides for *amplification* (in rods, one photon can trigger the breakdown of a million or so cGMP molecules), for *prolongation* of effects, for *control* by the cell (which can intervene in the link between receptor and channel), and for *intracellular effects*. An example of cellular control is again in photoreceptors, where intracellular calcium modifies the sensitivity and time-course of the cGMP changes. An obvious example of intracellular effects is the β-adrenergic response to noradrenaline, where cAMP production is again coupled via a G-protein to the receptor itself, the cAMP then having metabolic effects within the cell (Fig. 3.3).

In neurones of all kinds, these permeability changes give rise to currents and potentials that may spread passively to the terminal or may induce repetitive action potentials as described in Chapter 2 (p. 38). In the latter case, the area of membrane that is specialized for transduction cannot actually carry action potentials because it lacks voltage-sensitive channels. Thus in the pressure-sensitive Pacinian corpuscle, described in detail below, the currents generated by the deformation-sensitive ending only cause action potentials because they flow to the portion of axon where the myelination begins, and depolarize it; and it is likely that impulses are in fact normally generated at the first node of Ranvier. Similarly, in many central neurones action potentials are normally initiated only in the region where the cell body merges with the axon, the axon hillock. Often – for example, in the hair cell receptors of the ear – the receptor and the nerve axon that joins it to the central nervous system are quite separate, the receptor cell acting on the axon by means of a chemical transmitter whose release depends on the amount of depolarization of the ending. One sometimes needs to remind oneself that the purpose of a neurone is not to generate action potentials – or any other kind of potential – but to *release transmitter*; whether it does in fact use action potentials is not actually of huge significance.

The mechanism at the *terminal end* appears remarkably similar in all neurones and receptors: depolarization opens voltage-sensitive calcium

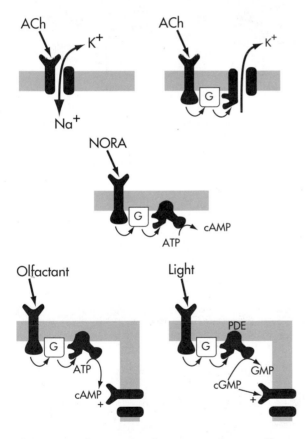

FIG. 3.3 Specific examples of receptor mechanisms. Above, two cholinergic receptors: nicotinic (direct ligand-gated channel) at left, and muscarinic, causing increased P_K (indirect, via G-protein) at right. Middle, a ß-adrenergic receptor also using a G-protein, in this case resulting in cAMP. Bottom, two sensory receptor mechanisms, both using a G-protein, in one case (olfaction) to increase membrane permeability, and in the other (light) to decrease it.

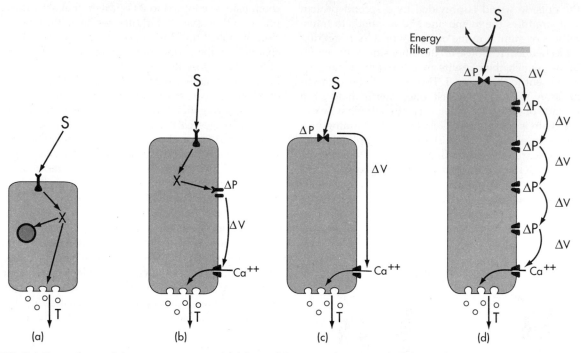

FIG. 3.4 Types of intercellular communication. At left **(a)**, a cell that responds to a stimulus S by producing a secondary messenger X, that may cause the release of a transmitter (or hormone) T in addition to purely internal effects. Then two examples of short neurones without action potentials: in each case a depolarization of the terminal opens voltage-sensitive calcium channels that trigger the release of T; in one case **(b)** this depolarization is the result of the opening of membrane channels by X (indirect transduction), while in **(c)** the membrane receptor that responds to the stimulus also opens the channels (direct transduction). In **(d)**, a longer neurone, the initial depolarization results in the propagation of repetitive action potentials, which again result in calcium entry at the terminal. S may be a transmitter or hormone rather than an external stimulus, as in interneurones.

TABLE 3.1 Theme and variations: some types of chemical transmission

	Striated muscle	Smooth muscle	Photo-receptor	Olfactory receptor	Hair cell	Pacinian corpuscle
Stimulus	ACh	ACh	Light	Chemical	Mechanical	Mechanical
Indirect?	no	yes	yes: cGMP	yes: cAMP	no	no
ΔPNa?	+		−	+	+	+
ΔPK?	+	+		+	+	+
APs?	yes	(no)	no	yes	no	yes
Result	Mechanical	Mechanical	Glutamate	Glutamate?	Glutamate?	Glutamate?

channels, and the resultant rise in intracellular calcium causes exocytosis of *vesicles* about 50 nm across, containing the transmitter substance that is to act on the next cell along (Fig. 3.4). These vesicles are normally created by the pinching off of parts of the transmitter-filled Golgi apparatus in the cell body, and are then transported down microtubules in the axon to the terminal.

Once this basic neuronal ground plan is understood, differences between particular neurones and receptors become a matter of filling in the blanks in a rather simple table (Table 3.1). We need to know only the type of stimulus, whether direct or indirect (and if the latter, what intermediate), what permeability change occurs, whether action potentials are used, and what the final result is, for example the transmitter released. What could be simpler?

SENSORY RECEPTORS

Types of transduction

The general term for a process by which energy of one form is converted into energy of another is *transduction.* The energy incident on a receptor cell, whether thermal, electromagnetic, mechanical or chemical, must be turned into electrical energy in the form of potentials across the cell membrane that eventually cause release of transmitter. As we have seen, in general the effect of the stimulus energy is to alter the *permeability* of the cell membrane to certain ions, resulting in a flow of current and a movement of the potential towards some new equilibrium value.

But not all kinds of energy are able to do this in any particular receptor. It is clearly important, if the brain is to make any sense of the outside world, that receptors respond specifically to certain *kinds* of stimulus, perhaps light or heat. For this reason, transduction is in effect preceded by a specialized *energy filter* that allows certain types of energy through to cause electrical effects, and not others (Box 3.1). This filtering is seldom absolute: the receptors of the eye, for example, though exquisitely sensitive to light, will also respond to mechanical deformation if it is severe enough. If in the dark you shut your eye and press on the side of it with your finger, you will see a faint blue patch of light called a phosphene: the receptors respond to mechanical stimulation by sending the brain exactly the same

message that they would have sent if a real blue light had been present. Specificity of receptors is in fact a relative matter, and many receptors are actually surprisingly unspecific in what they respond to. Fine discriminations between one type of stimulus and another are to a large extent the work of the central nervous system rather than of the receptors themselves.

Box 3.1 Classification of sensory receptors	
Mechanoreceptors	
Special sense:	Cochlear hair cells
	Vestibular hair cells
Muscle:	Spindles
	Tendon organs
Skin and visceral:	Pacinian corpuscle
	Ruffini endings
	Merkel discs
	Meissner corpuscles
	Lanceolate endings
	Free endings
	Nociceptors
Vascular:	Arterial baroceptors
	Venous and atrial stretch receptors
Thermoreceptors	Skin (warm and cold, nociceptors)
	Hypothalamic
Photoreceptors	Retina
Chemoreceptors	Olfactory
	Gustatory
	Hypothalamic
	Vascular
	Visceral
	Nociceptors

Transduction in the Pacinian corpuscle

One receptor that because of its peculiar anatomical structure happens to be very specialized indeed has been studied in great detail, and that is the *Pacinian corpuscle* (Fig. 3.5), a mechanoreceptor found in the skin and mesentery. Here the naked tip of an otherwise myelinated axon is sheathed in concentric onion-like layers called *lamellae* that shield it from virtually every type of stimulus except that of mechanical deformation. It is a good preparation for studying the transduction process in general, since one can easily isolate individual corpuscles and record their electrical responses to precise mechanical stimuli applied to the capsule's surface. A convenient means of stimulation is to hold against it a probe mounted on a small piezoelectric crystal: when a voltage is applied across the crystal, it changes its shape slightly and causes a controlled deformation of the capsule, and a change in membrane permeability. Now a complicating factor when trying to measure the relation between a stimulus and the permeability changes that result from it is that if the permeability changes are big enough they will trigger off action potentials that will in turn interfere with the very permeabilities one is trying to measure. Consequently it is helpful to disable the active properties of the axon by poisoning it with a substance like tetrodotoxin that blocks the voltage-dependent sodium channels. If this is done, we find that mechanical stimulation of the ending results in a depolarization of the axon – the *generator potential* – whose magnitude depends on the size of the stimulus.

We can show that this change in potential is indeed due to a change in permeability of the receptor membrane by measuring something called the *reversal potential*. This is a fundamental technique that forms the basic way of finding out what permeability changes are going on in receptors and in postsynaptic membranes. The principle is a simple one: since every combination of permeabilities results in some corresponding equilibrium potential E_s (from the constant-field equation, p. 22), then a change in equilibrium potential implies some change in permeability. The problem is that most sensory and synaptic events are shortlived, so that there is no time for the membrane potential actually to settle down at its new value of E_s. But the *direction* of its movement tells us whether the new equilibrium is above or below the resting potential; and if we have some way of setting the resting potential artificially to different levels, we can see how this influences the direction of the response. As the resting potential is made to approach E_s, the response will get smaller and smaller, then reversing in sign as the resting potential passes through E_s. The reversal potential, defined as the value of the resting potential at which stimulation has no effect, is simply equal to E_s. Once we know E_s we can make an informed guess as to what permeability change must be causing it.

In the case of the Pacinian corpuscle, we can create different artificial resting potentials simply by passing a steady current into its axon, and the reversal potential turns out to be very close to zero. The simplest kind of permeability change that would generate an equilibrium potential around zero would be an increase in both sodium and potassium permeability. So when we deform the cell membrane it seems that we open up ionic channels in it which are indiscriminately permeable and so act as a sort of short-circuit: perhaps distorting the membrane simply increases its leakiness.

Adaptation

A striking feature of the response that is obvious in Figure 3.5b is that its time-course is very different from that of the stimulus itself. If we apply a prolonged but constant deformation to the surface, we find that the generator potential rises quite rapidly to a peak, and then spontaneously falls back again to the resting potential; when the stimulus is removed a second peak is generated. The cell seems, in fact, to

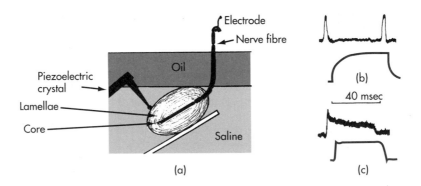

FIG. 3.5 **(a)** A Pacinian corpuscle dissected out, and arranged for electrical recording and mechanical stimulation by means of a piezoelectric crystal. Right, generator potentials recorded from a Pacinian corpuscle before **(b)** and after **(c)** removal of the outer lamellae, in response to a brief maintained deformation. (After Loewenstein and Mendelsohn, 1965)

respond to *changes* in the degree of stimulation rather than to its steady level, a very common type of receptor response that is called *adaptation*. It turns out that much of this adaptation is due to the mechanical properties of the lamellae that surround the ending that act as an energy filter. If we strip them off, and apply the stimulating probe directly to the surface of the axon, we find that although the generator potential still falls off after its initial rise, it remains depolarized so long as the stimulus is maintained, with no hint of a second peak of depolarization when the stimulus is removed (Fig. 3.5c). This kind of response is known as *incomplete* adaptation, as opposed to the complete adaptation seen when the lamellae are intact, and the response falls to zero.

There is a simple mechanical model of the Pacinian corpuscle that explains how it filters out steady levels of stimulation (Fig. 3.6). We can think of the end of the axon itself as behaving in a simple elastic manner, so that any force applied to it results in a corresponding deformation, and hence in a change in permeability. The lamellae, on the other hand, behave very differently because they are separated from one another by layers of viscous fluid: when a steady pressure is applied to a particular part of the capsule, the lamellae in that region slowly collapse as the fluid between them oozes sideways to neighbouring regions. The lamellae thus act very like the oil-filled cylinders or dashpots that make up part of the shock absorbers fitted to car suspensions or to the tops of swing doors, whose function is to resist sudden movement; they are what are known to engineers as *viscous elements* (represented in the figure by the conventional symbol of a dashpot), while the axon tip acts as a purely *elastic* element (the spring symbol). In the case of the Pacinian corpuscle, both these elements are connected in series: if we apply a sudden steady displacement to the outer end of the viscous element, at first there is no time for it to collapse, and the displacement is taken up by the elastic element, which is thus compressed. But in being compressed (B, Fig. 3.6), it exerts a force on the viscous element which then tends to collapse (C,D), through the sideways oozing of fluid described above. The elastic element, the axon itself, therefore gradually resumes its original shape, and the potential returns to its resting value. But if the stimulus is removed (E), the whole process is reversed: at first the elastic element must stretch to take up the new displacement but in doing so it pulls on the viscous

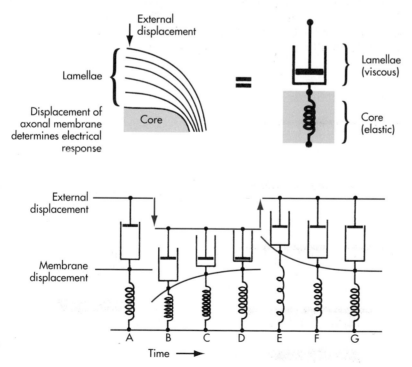

FIG. 3.6 Above, highly schematic representation of the mechanical elements of the Pacinian corpuscle, and their mechanical equivalent 'circuit' in the form of a viscous element (dashpot) and elastic element (spring). Below, response of such a model to steady displacement applied just before B and removed just before E, showing adaptation of the degree of distortion of the elastic element, and hence of the electrical response of the receptor.

element, expanding it again (F,G), so that in the end all is as it was originally.

It is clear that deformation of the axonal ending only occurs in association with change in the stimulus that is applied, and that in the case of a steady stimulus it will be deformed both at the onset and cessation of the stimulus. If we suppose that inward and outward deformations of the cell membrane are equally good at causing changes in permeability, then we can see how the biphasic generator potential of Figure 3.5 comes about. This indifference to the sign of a stimulus is quite exceptional amongst receptors, however, and is one of several respects in which the Pacinian corpuscle – though a popular example of adaptation – is not at all typical of receptors in general.

This kind of mechanical filtering is a common one in the body, and we shall meet it again in discussing the stretch receptors that are found in muscles. It is sometimes called a *high-pass filter* because it passes high-frequency vibratory stimuli much better than low-frequency vibrations of the same amplitude, since for a given amplitude of vibration the *rate* of movement is higher at high frequencies than at low. This is precisely what does happen in the Pacinian corpuscle, where a steady deformation normally produces only one action potential when the stimulus is applied, and another when it is removed: the accommodation of the ending is too great for the rate of depolarization after the action potential. But this is far from typical of sensory receptors, which generally respond to a steady stimulus with a continuous train of impulses. Under these conditions, adaptation will manifest itself as a steady decline in firing frequency after application of the stimulus, as may be seen in the responses from various receptors shown in Figure 3.7. If the receptor is of the completely adapting sort, it will eventually stop firing altogether; otherwise the frequency will decline to some steady level. Receptors vary a great deal in the speed with which this decline occurs. Some, like the Pacinian corpuscle, are very fast; others, like the receptors in the semicircular canals that adapt over some 20 seconds, are very slow. It is important not to confuse speed with *degree* of adaptation: fast-adapting receptors may be completely or incompletely adapting, and so may those that adapt only slowly (Fig. 3.8)

There are many receptors in which adaptation is at least partly due to energy filtering of a kind analogous to what is done by the lamellae of the Pacinian corpuscle. The muscle spindle stretch receptor, for example, has a mechanical high-pass filter that behaves in a very similar way. Adaptation in the Pacinian corpuscle cannot be *entirely* due to the lamellae, since we have seen that there is still a decline in response at the beginning of a period of constant stimulation even when they have been stripped away. In most cases at least some adaptation

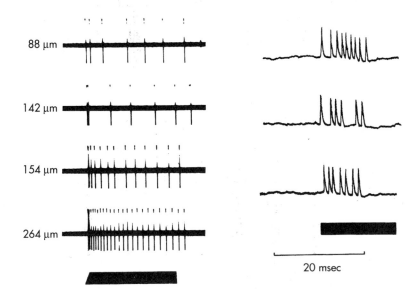

FIG. 3.7 Examples of adaptation in different receptors. Left, tactile receptor in the skin of a cat's paw, responding to different indentations maintained for the duration shown by the bar below (after Mountcastle, 1966). Right, hair receptor, cat skin, showing complete adaptation after a few impulses (Hunt and McIntyre, 1960).

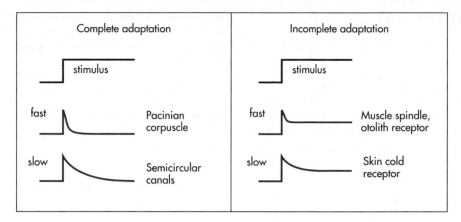

FIG. 3.8 Types of adaptation. Adaptation may be complete or incomplete, depending on whether during a steady stimulus the response declines to the unstimulated level; and fast or slow, depending on how long it takes to reach an equilibrium response.

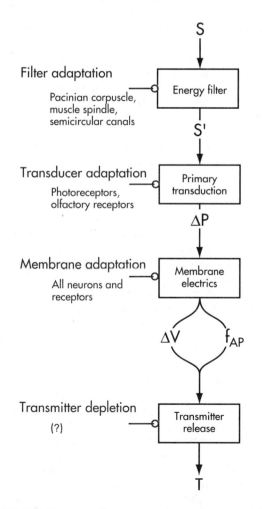

FIG. 3.9 The stages of sensory transduction showing, at left, the various ways in which adaptation may occur.

is also the result of the *membrane adaptation* that was described in Chapter 2 (p. 39), which is a universal feature of neurones of all kinds. One way to demonstrate this is to bypass the transduction stage altogether and send currents directly into the cell through a microelectrode. A third way in which adaptation may occur is by *cellular modification* of an indirect transducer mechanism. In the eye, for example, incident light causes intracellular calcium to fall, which lowers the receptor's sensitivity during steady illumination.

Figure 3.9 may help to summarize the whole sequence of events in sensory receptors, and the stages at which adaptation may occur. The energy impinging on a receptor is first *filtered*, possibly by virtue of surrounding structures, as in the Pacinian corpuscle or in the visual receptors of some birds where little coloured oil droplets contribute to their colour selectivity. This filtering may incorporate an element of adaptation. It then brings about – by mechanisms that are yet unknown – *a change in the permeability* of the neuronal membrane, which if indirect may also be subject to adaptation. This in turn produces a *generator current* causing depolarization. In 'long' receptors, if conditions are right, this may be followed by *repetitive* firing at a frequency dependent on the degree of stimulation, although this frequency will in general decline because of membrane adaptation. Otherwise, if the degree of accommodation is too great in relation to the rate of depolarization after the first impulse, only a single action potential will occur. Either way, the final stage is depolarization of the terminal calcium entry, and transmitter release.

Efferent control

Another way in which this chain of events may be modified is through *efferent control*. Here, signals from the central nervous system are sent back to the receptor, and may act either on the energy filter or on the coupling between terminal depolarization and transmitter release (Fig. 3.10). If these efferent signals are driven by the signals coming from the receptor, and they are such as to reduce the receptor's sensitivity, then they will effectively function as negative feedback, a further source of adaptation. A well-known example of central control over energy filtering is the iris of the eye, which shrinks as the ambient light level increases. But very often the control is exerted quite independently of the afferent signals. As we shall see in Chapter 5 (p. 92), muscle spindles receive efferent fibres that affect their sensitivity to stretch, essentially specifying the range over which the receptor should be working. Efferent control over transmitter release, typically through inhibitory efferent synaptic terminals, is often found on mechanoreceptors in particular, for instance on hair cells in the inner ear and on terminals of afferents from the skin, in the dorsal horn of the spinal cord (see below, p. 63), but they do not seem to be essentially for adaptation.

Functions of adaptation

It may perhaps seem strange that the pattern of impulses generated by what is supposed to be a deformation receptor should be so very different from the time-course of the stimulus that it actually experiences (Fig. 3.5); it looks as though the receptor is throwing away useful information. Is there any advantage in signalling changes rather than steady levels?

In the first place, it is not quite true to say that information has been thrown away. So long as the brain 'knows' how an adapting receptor responds to different patterns of deformation, it can in principle reconstruct the time-course of the original stimulus from the coded signals that it receives from the receptors, so that no information is really lost. But we have certainly lost a lot of action potentials, and one advantage of adaptation may be that it makes for economy of nervous impulses. If a stimulus is such that it tends to remain constant for long periods of time, with only occasional shifts to some new value – for example, the pressure sensed by Pacinian corpuscles in one's buttocks during a long lecture – then there is little point in sending a stream of information to the brain which only tells it, in effect, that nothing has happened. Since the same information could have been carried by many fewer impulses, by sending a message only when something new occurs that might call for a response, one general function of adaptation could be said to be to get rid of unnecessary action potentials – it reduces the *redundancy* of the messages that are conveyed. Similar mechanisms are used in computers when storing data on disk: since computer data often contain long strings of repeated bytes, by storing only information about *changes* files can be considerably compressed.

A second possible reason for the widespread existence of adaptation in sensory systems is that it may improve sensitivity by increasing the *signal-to-noise ratio* of the receptor. This is a concept that is fundamental to understanding the coding of sensory information, and is well worth the little investment of

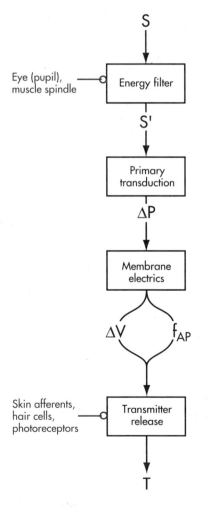

FIG. 3.10 The two points at which efferent control of sense organs may occur (cf. Fig. 3.9).

intellectual effort needed to master it. Any signal, whether it consists of frequencies of action potentials or simply of varying voltages as in a telephone wire, is inevitably subject to a certain degree of uncertainty on account of the all-pervasive random *noise* that is an inescapable feature of the physical world. For example, if we measure the frequency of firing of a sensory fibre under conditions that are as constant as we can make them, we shall find nevertheless that the frequency we observe is not fixed but undergoes continual random perturbations (Fig. 3.11). This noise may be due to small changes in the temperature or chemical environment of the receptor, to slowly acting properties such as fatigue that are not under our control or, ultimately, to the fact that the ions whose movement generates the potentials we measure are themselves in continuous random thermal motion, so that the currents they carry must equally be subject to a certain degree of unpredictability. Thus we can never say that a nerve is firing exactly 70 times a second: the best we can do is to estimate with more or less confidence that its frequency lies somewhere between 69 and 71 Hz. This in turn puts a limit on the amount of information that a fibre can carry.

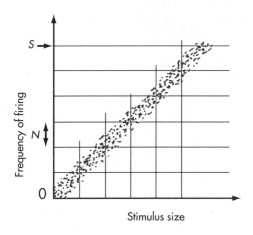

FIG. 3.11 Signal-to-noise ratio. Schematic relationship between stimulus size and firing frequency for a hypothetical sensory fibre, measured on a large number of occasions (single data points), showing the band of frequency scatter of width N associated with any particular value of the stimulus. As a result, frequencies must be separated by N before they can be discriminated reliably from one another. Thus the number of significantly different frequencies, and hence of discriminable stimuli, is given by the *signal-to-noise ratio S/N*, where S is the maximum firing frequency of the fibre. In this case, S/N is only about 6.

Now the function of a nerve axon is to convey messages from one place to another: in the jargon of information theory, it is a communication channel. The most fundamental thing we need to know about any communication channel, whether it is a telephone wire or the cable that joins a computer to its printer, is what its *capacity* is. How many different messages can it convey in a given time? In the case of nerves, this amounts to asking how many distinguishably different frequencies it can fire at. Clearly, the refractory period sets an upper limit to firing frequency, perhaps around 500 Hz or so. One might think that since it could fire at any frequency below this limit, the number of possible frequencies (and thus the number of different messages it could send) must be infinite. But this is not so, for the existence of the noise that has just been described means that the brain may not be able to *discriminate* between frequencies that lie close together, because of the impossibility of determining exactly what the frequency actually is at any moment. More specifically, if we call the size of the largest signal that a nerve fibre can carry S, and the amplitude of the ever-present noise N, then the number of different frequencies that can be discriminated reliably from each other is only of the order of S/N (Fig. 3.11). For example, if the noise in a fibre leads to an uncertainty of about 1 Hz in determining its frequency, the ratio S/N – the signal-to-noise ratio – will be 500: in other words, at any moment the nerve can only convey one of 500 distinguishably different messages. Now if one thinks of this as being equivalent to an accuracy of one part in 500, or 0. 2 percent, this may not seem too bad a performance. But the problem is that the dynamic *range* – the ratio of the largest stimulus normally encountered to the smallest – over which most receptors have to operate is exceedingly large. In the case of the eye, for example, the dynamic range corresponds to the ratio between the brightness of the sun and the visual threshold in the dark, and is of the order of 10^{15}. If there were no adaptation in the eye, and each receptor coded a particular level of light intensity directly as a particular steady frequency of firing, its 500 possible output levels would have to be spread – pretty thinly – over the entire 10^{15} range of possible inputs. Clearly, a just-discernible difference in receptor firing would correspond in general to a very large difference in light intensity, and our power of perceiving small differences in intensity would be very much worse than it actually is.

But in practice the whole of this 10^{15} range is never present in our field of view at the same time, and – for reasons that are explained in Chapter 7 – the ratio between the darkest and lightest parts of our field of view at any particular instant is typically only about 1:100. It is true that in the course of the day the absolute level on which this range of brightnesses is centred may fluctuate very widely indeed, as the sun rises and sets, and night follows day. But these shifts of *absolute* level, as well as being of little interest to us, are comparatively slow. Adaptation, acting as a high-pass filter, will tend to get rid of them, leaving behind the significant and relatively rapid changes of intensity that are generated by our eye movements as we look around, and which lie in a dynamic range that is not so very different from that of the nerve fibres themselves. Adaptation, in other words, provides a kind of automatic *sliding scale* by which the limited signal-to-noise ratio of our neurones can be shifted to match the range of inputs we are interested in, ignoring slower and larger changes of the baseline that could only be accommodated by sacrificing overall sensitivity (Fig. 3.12). This argument assumes, of course, that the slow changes really are unwanted: one man's noise is another's signal. One may find a separate population of cells that are relatively insensitive but which do provide information about static levels acting parallel with adapting channels: in the

eye, there are a very few cells that do not adapt, and are used to signal time of day and to control the pupil. But as a general rule, things that don't change don't demand a response and need not be coded.

Adaptation thus acts like the automatic level control sometimes fitted to tape recorders, which automatically adjusts the amplification to compensate for the average level of sound that is being recorded, but lets through the more rapid fluctuations that constitute the sound itself. In the case of the Pacinian corpuscle, for example, it means that we can be made aware of very small changes even when superimposed on large steady background pressures – for example, in the soles of the feet when standing – because adaptation has again shifted the scale of the receptor to allow for the steady background. Finally, for proprioceptors such as joint receptors and muscle spindles that essentially give information about position of the limbs, the fact that adaptation implies response to *rate of change* rather than to steady levels means that such receptors, if completely adapting, will essentially signal *velocity* of the limbs rather than position, which may be more relevant in the control of certain kinds of movement such as throwing.

SYNAPTIC TRANSMISSION

We now need to consider the initiation of activity in neurones other than receptors, driven not by the outside world but by the activity of other neurones that make contact with them at specialized regions, the *synapses*. At a typical synapse, a branch of the afferent axon forms a swelling, the terminal *bouton*, the further side of which forms an enlarged area of intimate contact with the postsynaptic cell body: in the case of the neuromuscular synapse, the *muscle endplate*, this area is much increased by the presence of invaginating folds (Fig. 3.13). In most cases there is a clear *synaptic cleft* between pre- and postsynaptic membranes, typically of the order of 20 nm wide. Transmitter is released from the presynaptic side and diffuses to the postsynaptic side, where it causes permeability changes through the various mechanisms already outlined. Anatomically, many variations on this basic pattern of *axosomatic* contact can be found. Most neurones have an elaborately branched dendritic tree which is smothered in *axodendritic* synapses; dendrites may also make contact with each other in *dendro-dendritic* contacts; and in *axoaxonic* contacts one axon may terminate on the terminal of

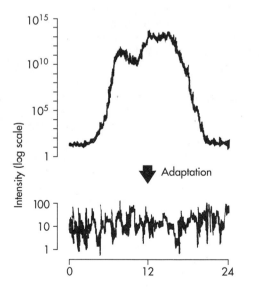

FIG. 3.12 Adaptation reducing low-frequency noise. Above, a plot of the intensity of light falling on a typical retinal receptor throughout one day, showing that the rapid fluctuations that convey visual information are dwarfed by changes that are much slower. A receptor capable of responding to the entire range of steady intensities would necessarily be insensitive to the smaller but more important variation. Below, adaptation has the effect of filtering out the slow changes of intensity level: the receptor now need only cope with some two log units of intensity rather than 10, and can thus respond better to the important details.

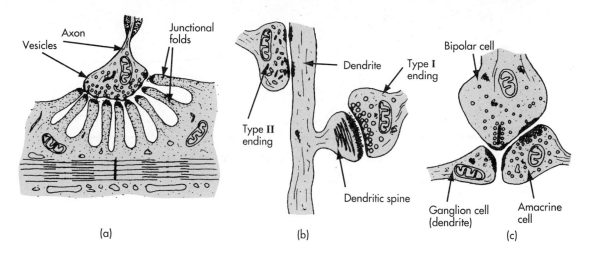

FIG. 3.13 Somewhat stylized representations of some synaptic types. **(a)** Neuromuscular junction. **(b)** Two types of presynaptic axonal endings synapsing with a dendrite; the synapse on the right is with a dendritic spine. **(c)** A three-way synapse from the retina; the junction between bipolar and amacrine cell permits the transfer of information in both directions.

another and modify its transmitter release. But it is convenient to begin with the most familiar type of synapse of all, whose working is most thoroughly understood: the neuromuscular junction between motor axon and striated muscle fibre.

Transmission at the neuromuscular junction

The transmitter at the neuromuscular junction is acetylcholine; each vesicle contains some 10^5 molecules of ACh, and when an action potential arrives at the endplate it triggers the release of the contents of some 200–300 vesicles: each vesicle appears to obey a kind of all-or-nothing law in that it either empties completely into the synaptic cleft or not at all. The transmitter thus released must diffuse across the synaptic cleft – a process that takes a millisecond at most – before it can act on the muscle cell. To see what it does there when it arrives, it is best to work backwards from the electrical changes that are observed in the muscle cell when the axon is stimulated.

If we put a microelectrode close to the endplate, and poison the muscle with tetrodotoxin so that our observations of the primary electrical events are not obscured by any subsequent action potentials that may be generated, we see that a single action potential in the afferent nerve is associated with a characteristic electrical response in the muscle cell, called the *endplate potential* (Fig. 3.14). Although the original action potential only lasts a millisecond or

so, the endplate potential or EPP is relatively prolonged. Most of this prolongation is due to the capacitance of the membrane, and knowing the value of the appropriate time constant, we can estimate the duration of the current flow that must have produced the potential change. It turns out to have a timecourse not very different from that of the original action potential, though delayed in time by the millisecond or so of synaptic delay that is the result of diffusion across the synaptic cleft. This brief current discharges the membrane capacitance, which subsequently must recharge relatively slowly through the resting membrane resistance (Fig. 3.14). The fact that the current hardly lasts longer than the afferent impulse is largely due to the presence at the ending of high concentrations of the enzyme *cholinesterase* that mops up the acetylcholine almost as soon as it arrives. If this enzyme is blocked by an anticholinesterase such as eserine, one finds that the current flow, and hence the endplate potential, is enormously prolonged, leading to a depolarization block of the muscle fibre.

The first clue as to the source of the current produced by the arrival of acetylcholine comes from measuring the reversal potential of the response, in exactly the same way as was described in the case of the Pacinian corpuscle. A steady current is passed into the muscle cell in order to set the resting potential at a new artificial level, and the size of the EPP is then observed. Just as with the corpuscle, it is found that the EPP gets smaller and smaller as the resting potential is reduced to near zero, and that if the membrane is hyperpolarized, the EPP is reversed. The

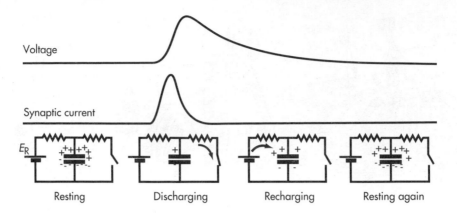

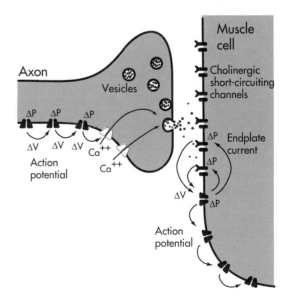

FIG. 3.14 Above, relation between endplate potential and synaptic current (somewhat idealized); below is a schematic equivalent circuit of the postsynaptic membrane showing: membrane capacitance charged to resting potential E_R, rapid discharge through opening of unselective channels, channels closed, capacitance recharging relatively slowly, until equilibrium is finally restored when the capacitor is fully charged.

conclusion is therefore that the effect of acetylcholine is to open channels that allow sodium as well as potassium to pass through the postsynaptic membrane, and thus produce something like a short-circuit. Since the number of ACh molecules released by each impulse, and hence the number of channels opened, is very large, it is clear that this is the mechanism whereby the relatively small currents in the axon can trigger off the relatively enormous currents needed to initiate an action potential in the muscle cell: the source of these currents is the muscle cell itself.

If one records from the endplate with very high sensitivity, one finds that even when the afferent fibre is not stimulated there are continual spontaneous potential changes taking the form of a random succession of *miniature endplate potentials* having roughly the same shape as a normal evoked EPP, but about 0.2–0.3 percent of its size. These miniature potentials have been shown to be due to the fact that the presynaptic ending, even at rest, releases individual vesicles randomly at a very low rate. This rate of spontaneous release is strongly dependent on the resting potential across the presynaptic terminal, and if this is artificially reduced – for example, by changing the external potassium concentration – the average rate of vesicle release increases sharply. By extrapolation, one can show that the size of a normal EPP is about what would be expected if the action potential simply had the effect of temporarily increasing the rate of spontaneous release of vesicles. It is also strongly influenced by the concentration of calcium ions at the ending: if it is increased, one again finds that the rate of vesicle release goes up. In other

words, when the action potential invades the terminal, channels in the presynaptic ending are opened that permit the entry of calcium, and this in turn stimulates the emptying of the vesicles into the synaptic cleft (Fig. 3.15). As in the case of the Pacinian corpuscle, it is found that the subsynaptic membrane, being specialized in having short-circuiting channels

FIG. 3.15 Schematic representation of the sequence by which nerve action potentials (left) lead to muscle action potentials (right) at the neuromuscular junction. Channels sensitive to voltage are shown in black; channels sensitive to the transmitter acetylcholine which is represented by the red dots, are shown in white.

that are opened by acetylcholine, does not have enough of the voltage-sensitive sodium channels to be able to propagate an action potential, and is therefore electrically inexcitable: it initiates impulses only by generating local currents which pass through the surrounding region that is excitable. In some muscle fibres – for example, the slow fibres of the frog – no action potential is generated at all: here there is not just one endplate on the cell but a large number of synapses distributed all over its surface. Activation of the afferent fibres thus causes a widespread passively summated EPP over the whole cell, leading to a relatively slow contraction of the muscle fibre.

Central excitatory synapses

Once the principles of operation of the neuromuscular junction are understood, those of excitatory synapses between one neurone and another present little extra difficulty. The most frequently studied synapse of this kind is one forming part of the *monosynaptic reflex arc* in the spinal cord that generates the tendon jerk response. This reflex pathway, whose functions will be discussed in Chapter 10, consists of exactly two neurones: a primary (Ia) afferent fibre carrying impulses from stretch receptors in a muscle synapses excitatorily with a motor neurone in the ventral horn of the spinal cord, whose axon returns to innervate the same muscle from which the afferent fibre came (Fig. 3.16). Tapping the tendon of the muscle causes a brief stretch of the sensory ending, firing the Ia fibre, which then excites the motor neurone and causes a reflex twitch of the muscle – the familiar knee-jerk response, if we use the patellar tendon.

The advantage of this reflex pathway from the experimenter's point of view is that the afferent fibres are readily accessible in the dorsal root for controlled stimulation, while the postsynaptic cell bodies are large enough to be punctured easily by a microelectrode. If we apply a single brief shock to the Ia fibres whilst recording from the motor neurone, we find that the postsynaptic response consists of a small depolarization rather similar in shape to the EPP, called the *excitatory postsynaptic potential* or EPSP; if it is large enough, it may trigger off an impulse in the motor neurone. By measuring the reversal potential in exactly the same way as in the case of the neuromuscular junction (Fig. 3.17), it is possible to show that the EPSP is the result of a transient increase in permeability to sodium and potassium ions. Although this increase lasts only about as long as the action potential, just as in the case of the endplate, the EPSP itself is relatively prolonged because of the long time constant of the cell membrane (Fig. 3.14). One may therefore assume that the arrival of an impulse releases some transmitter substance from the vesicles visible in the presynaptic endings and that this substance diffuses across the synaptic cleft and causes the opening of short-circuiting channels. Could this transmitter also be acetylcholine?

It would be nice if we could simply extract the vesicles from the ending and see what was in them; but this is seldom a practical procedure. However, there are histological stains (and most recently and usefully, *immunohistochemical* stains) that are selective for particular transmitters or their metabolic precursors, or for enzymes that are associated with them, which can help to identify transmitter substances. In the case of acetycholine, which is widely found as a

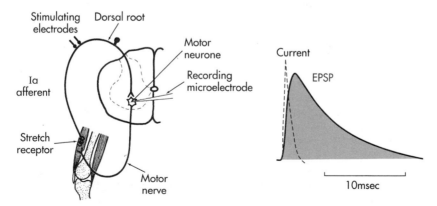

FIG. 3.16 Excitatory synaptic action in the monosynaptic stretch reflex. Left, the neural circuit: Ia afferents from stretch receptors in a muscle enter the dorsal root and then synapse excitatorily with motor neurones in the ventral horn which innervate the same muscle. Right, EPSP (shaded) recorded with a microelectrode in a motor neurone after a single stimulating shock to the afferent fibres. The dotted line shows the time-course of the synaptic current.

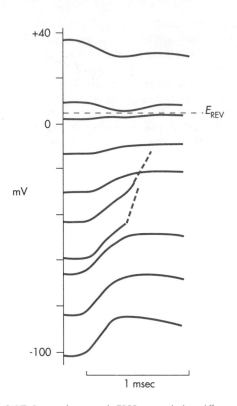

FIG. 3.17 Reversal potential. EPSPs recorded at different initial resting potentials produced by passing current steadily in or out of the neurone by means of a double-barrelled microelectrode. The response reverses at E_{rev}, not far from zero potential. (Partly after Curtis and Eccles, 1959, and Coombes *et al.*, 1955)

prolong its action, do so for the other. Ideally, one should also be able to show that afferent action potentials really do release the supposed transmitter, but this also is often technically extremely difficult to establish adequately. In fact it is only at a relatively small proportion of the synapses in the central nervous system that we are certain of the identity of the transmitter in the sense that all these criteria have been met. But if one is satisfied with circumstantial evidence, then one can generate quite long lists of putative transmitters (Box 3.2) and create maps indicating their distribution throughout the brain. It would be nice to think that such maps would reveal some deep pattern of meaning as regards which transmitter does what, but disappointingly this is not really so. Knowing what the transmitter is at a particular synapse does not really help us to understand what the synapse *does*, not least because that is a function of what the receptor site is linked to: the same transmitter may do many quite different things that bear no obvious functional relation to each other. In addition, some synaptic terminals are known to release more than one chemical, often a conventional transmitter in conjunction with one or more small peptides such as substance P, CCK, etc., called *cotransmitters*.

In the case of the afferent terminals of the monosynaptic reflex arc, we have no certain knowledge of the nature of the transmitter, except that it is certainly not acetylcholine. It may well be *glutamate*, a very common excitatory transmitter both in receptors and in the central nervous system; it has three main classes of receptor, whose properties and mechanisms are very different. But whatever the transmitter released by the Ia fibres, it is clear that it opens unselective channels in the motor neurone, which in turn cause depolarizing currents to flow. How do the effects of these channels, operating at different times all over a neurone, combine to determine its final output?

transmitter within the brain as well as at the neuromuscular junction, one may stain for the enzyme cholinesterase, whose presence suggests strongly the use of acetylcholine itself. But the mere presence of a possible transmitter in the presynaptic endings is not sufficient evidence by itself that it is actually being used as a transmitter. There are a number of further criteria that have to be met. We need to confirm, for example, that application of the supposed transmitter actually causes the *same effects* as the real transmitter. It is not enough simply to note that both are excitatory: they must both open the same channels, and so have the same reversal potential. Ideally it should also do so in plausibly small concentrations, but this is a difficult criterion to meet because the postsynaptic membrane is very much less accessible from outside than it is to transmitter released in the proper way from the terminal. We must also demonstrate that the real and supposed transmitter have the *same pharmacology*: that they are blocked by the same pharmacological agents, and that substances that inhibit the inactivating enzyme for one, and hence

Synaptic integration

The situation in central neurones is not quite the same as at the neuromuscular junction: there, in striated fibres at least, each muscle fibre receives only one endplate and it is usually the case that a single afferent action potential will trigger off a single impulse in the muscle. But things are very different at a typical central neurone: here there is not one afferent synapse but an enormous number – typically some 10 000. The last thing we want is for a single action potential arriving at any one of them to fire off the whole cell: the whole point of neurones is that

---

Box 3.2 Examples of types of synaptic transmitter

Neuropeptides (size in brackets)
β-Endorphin* (31)
Enkephalins* (5)
Oxytocin* (9)
Glucagon* (29)
Somatostatin* (14)
Substance P (11)
VIP (vasoactive intestinal polypeptide)* (28)
(and many others)

Amino acids
Aspartate
Glutamate
GABA (gamma-amino butyric acid)
Glycine

Monoamines
Dopamine
Noradrenaline*
5-HT (5-hydroxytryptamine, serotonin)*

Other
Acetylcholine
Nitric oxide?

* also used as a hormone

---

they act as miniature computers, responding to certain spatiotemporal patterns of afferent activity and not others. Post-synaptic activity is a function of the *integrated* discharge of all its afferent terminals. Neurones thus exhibit what is called *spatial and temporal summation*. The classic experimental set-up, with huge synchronized volleys in the dorsal root followed by just one action potential in a motor neurone, is a good way to find out the basic mechanism of synaptic action but a ludicrous travesty of how neurones actually go about their daily business. Bear in mind that in ordinary life, most neurones fire most of the time.

Neurones also show *temporal* summation: because the potential produced by a brief synaptic current falls off relatively slowly, it is possible to get summation of the effects of repeated stimulation of a single ending if the frequency of firing of the afferent fibre is high enough. In fact, because of both this smoothing effect of the membrane time constant and the very large number of endings synapsing with each neurone, most of which will probably be tonically active at any moment, it is probably more helpful to forget about the quantized nature of the action

potentials at afferent synapses. Indeed, it is misleading to think in terms of individual EPSPs at all – they are essentially artefacts. Rather, one should think of the way in which all of them together provide a combined inward *current* that is continually varying as the result of changing patterns of afferent discharge: a trickle in the furthest dendrites, the brooks and streams that flow together into the larger and larger dendrites, that finally empty themselves into the lake formed by the cell body. This river system receives a continual patter of rain from the afferent synapses, with local cloudbursts and deluges from time to time; and at the end of the lake is a waterwheel (the axon hillock) which turns repetitively to generate action potentials in response to the total flow of water. It is possible to show that whenever a motor neurone is excited to fire by its afferent connections, the action potential actually starts not in the region near the excitatory synapses themselves but rather at the axon hillock, from which it spreads both forwards down the axon, and also backwards over the cell body and also possibly the dendrites (a phenomenon that fits less easily into the watery metaphor!).

This summation is not in general linear unless the synapses are sufficiently separated from one another for no interaction to occur *between* them. If a particular point on the cell surface is short-circuited by an excitatory synapse, short-circuiting another point very close to the first will have little additional effect; because the membrane is already depolarized, the second synapse will contribute less additional current than it would do if it were acting on its own (Fig. 3.18). Thus although sometimes the effect of stimulating two separate afferents to a motor neurone is the sum of the effect of stimulating each separately, more often it is substantially less, a phenomenon known as *occlusion*. Other things being equal, the nearer an excitatory ending is to the axon hillock the greater will be its influence on the firing of the cell. Synapses on distant dendrites will be relatively less effective: like real riverbeds, the dendrites are leaky, so that much of the current generated at distant sites is lost. Finally, there are systems of sluices that modify the local flow: these are the *inhibitory* synapses.

Inhibitory synapses

Now a nervous system in which the only connections were excitatory would not be a very useful one: clearly there are occasions on which the proper response to a stimulus is inhibition rather than excitation, withdrawal rather than attack, relaxation rather than activation. In particular, the way in which our muscles

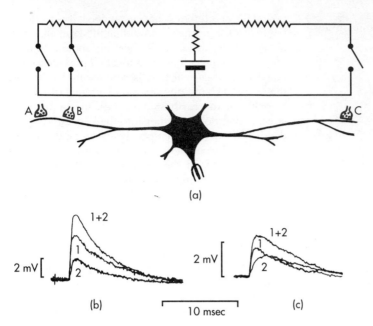

(a)

(b)   10 msec   (c)

FIG. 3.18 Linear and non-linear addition of EPSPs and spatial summation. **(a)** Schematic neurone with its electrical analogue, showing three excitatory synapses. If A is active, activation of B as well will have little additional effect; but the excitation produced by C will add linearly to either A or B. Below, actual records of linear (**b**; equivalent to A+C) and non-linear (**c**; equivalent to A+B) addition of EPSPs obtained by stimulating different afferent nerve bundles. (Partly from Burke, 1967)

are generally arranged in pairs that oppose one another implies that excitation of one muscle is usually associated with inhibition of the other, by a process of *reciprocal innervation*. In the tendon jerk, for example, the reflex contraction of the muscle that is stretched is accompanied by a relaxation of its antagonist. In this case, the inhibition of the corresponding motor neurones is brought about by branches of the afferent fibres from the stretch receptors that, after entering the dorsal cord, send excitatory branches to interneurones which in turn form *inhibitory synapses* with the motor neurones in the ventral horn (Fig. 3.19). One might wonder why a seemingly unnecessary interneurone is interpolated in this pathway. The reason may lie in a general rule that seems to be true of the transmitters used by cells in the central nervous system, namely that a neurone always releases the same transmitter, acting in the same way, at all its terminals (Dale's hypothesis). Since the stretch receptor fibres are excitatory to the motor

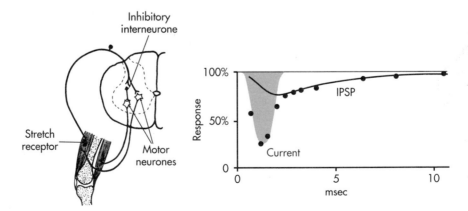

FIG. 3.19 Left, schematic neural circuit for reciprocal innervation of flexor and extensor muscles by reflex afferents. The inhibitory interneurone is shown in black, excitatory cells in white. Right, inhibition of the monosynaptic reflex and its electrical correlates. Data points show the size of reflex evoked at different times after a shock that stimulates inhibitory afferents. The line shows, on the same time scale, the time-course of the IPSP associated with the inhibition and the shaded area is the approximate time-course of the inhibitory synaptic current. The degree of inhibition in this case appears to be related to both current and potential. (Data from Araki *et al.*, 1960)

neurones of the agonist muscle, they cannot also be inhibitory to the motor neurones of the antagonist: thus they must first excite an interneurone, by opening the same kind of short-circuiting channels that they open in the motor neurones, and this interneurone must then inhibit the antagonist motor neurones.

The existence of reciprocal inhibition in the tendon jerk reflex is convenient from the experiment's point of view, since it is possible first to insert an electrode in a motor neurone, and then stimulate various dorsal root fibres until some can be found that produce either excitation or inhibition of the motor neurone. If we then give a single shock to the inhibitory fibres, and follow it with an excitatory stimulus delivered after different time delays, we can measure the time-course of the inhibitory effect by measuring the size of the subsequent response to the excitatory stimulus: some results of this kind are shown in Figure 3.19. Here, an inhibitory shock clearly leads to a depression of the excitatory response that lasts for many milliseconds. One may also, of course, simply see what happens to the motor neurone's potential when the inhibitory shock is delivered in the absence of any excitation. One then finds that the stimulus is followed by a potential change in the neurone, of rather similar time-course to an EPSP but of opposite polarity: this hyperpolarization is called the *inhibitory postsynaptic potential* or IPSP.

To find the origin of the IPSP, we can follow our usual procedure of passing various steady currents in or out of the cell by means of one half of a double-barrelled electrode, and using the other half to measure the resultant size of the IPSP, and hence determine its reversal potential. What we find then is that the IPSP, unlike the EPSP, gets larger and larger instead of smaller as the resting potential is reduced to zero; but that if we artificially hyperpolarize the membrane, the potential is reduced in size and eventually reverses at about -80 mV, the reversal potential for the IPSP (Fig. 3.20). This voltage lies somewhere between the equilibrium potentials for potassium and chloride ions, so our guess might be that the increase in permeability caused by the inhibitory transmitter here is not unselective as in the case of the EPP, EPSP and generator potential, but specifically only of chloride and potassium (in many central sites, inhibition occurs through changes in chloride permeability alone).

As in the case of excitation from Ia fibres, the transmitter here is not known for certain but elsewhere in the central nervous system both GABA (gamma aminobutyric acid) and glycine have been

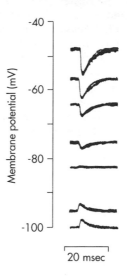

FIG. 3.20 Reversal potential of the IPSP. IPSPs were recorded at different initial levels of depolarization as in Fig. 3.17. They show a reversal potential of about -80 mV .(After Eccles *et al.*, 1964)

confirmed as inhibitory transmitters. At this site in the spinal cord, however, GABA fails to meet the pharmacological criterion mentioned earlier, for although the inhibition here is blocked by the convulsant poison strychnine, as is the action of glycine, that of GABA is not. Where GABA is known to be an inhibitory transmitter it is blocked by another convulsant, picrotoxin, which is ineffective at this site in the spinal cord. Incidentally, the convulsant effect of these inhibitory blockers illustrates another general function for inhibition in the brain: if we have a large network of cells that are connected together in highly convergent and divergent pathways that are entirely excitatory, we have a situation that is potentially explosive. Stimulation of any one cell is likely to lead to a chain reaction involving the progressive spread of activity over a large area, and this is precisely what is observed with convulsants like strychnine and picrotoxin. At least as much inhibition as excitation is required if this sort of explosive response is to be avoided, and we shall see later, in Chapter 14, that special systems exist in the brain to regulate the general level of neural activity through diffuse inhibition – very like the damping rods in a nuclear reactor – and thus prevent fits of this kind from occurring.

There is another site in the spinal cord where inhibition is relatively easy to study. The axons that leave the motor neurones of the ventral horn on their way to the muscles also send off branches that turn back into the cord and innervate – excitatorily – small interneurones called *Renshaw cells* (Fig. 3.21). From Dale's hypothesis we would expect the transmitter at this synapse to be acetylcholine, and this is found to be the case; it acts in the usual way, by causing an unselective increase in membrane permeability, though here the response is much more prolonged than at the neuromuscular junction, the response to a single shock being a burst of firing at high frequency. But these Renshaw cells themselves send off short axons that in turn synapse with the pool of motor neurones by which they are stimulated, and their synapses are inhibitory. They are relatively easy to study because one can activate the Renshaw cells by stimulating the motor neurones antidromically in the ventral root. (This kind of feedback inhibition is a common one in sensory systems as well, as we shall see, and really embodies yet another kind of adaptation. During a period of constant afferent stimulation, the efferent discharge will be large at first but then reduced as the inhibitory pathway comes into play, producing a transient response that is essentially the same as incomplete adaptation (Fig. 3.21). However it is not clear that this is actually the primary function of Renshaw cells; rather, they probably serve to discourage synchronized firing that would lead to unwanted clonus in the muscle.)

Voltage and current inhibition

We have now completed the chain of events by which stimulation of inhibitory afferents leads to release of a transmitter that then opens up hyperpolarizing channels in the postsynaptic membrane. But how

does this result in actual inhibition? The answer is not quite as simple as might appear at first sight. In some cases, the time-course of the inhibition mirrors quite accurately the time-course of the IPSP itself. Other things being equal, a hyperpolarization means that the potential has to be driven further than would otherwise be the case in order to reach threshold, and so one might well expect to find a substantial correlation between the degree of hyperpolarization at any moment and the degree of inhibition. But in many instances, as can be seen in Figure 3.19, there is an extra peak of inhibition at the beginning that cannot be explained in this way, and in some cases one may find this short-term component even in the absence of the IPSP-like slow component. It turns out that the shape of this peak is very similar to the time-course of the burst of current that generates the IPSP: this current is shorter in duration than the IPSP, being roughly the same as that of the action potential, because as usual the decline of potential back to its resting level is prolonged by the membrane capacitance. Thus there appear to be two separate components of the inhibition that may be observed: one that is closely related to the *potential* at any moment (voltage inhibition), and is relatively easily explained, and one that seems to be associated with the *current* (current inhibition).

To see how current inhibition arises, consider two synaptic endings, one excitatory and one inhibitory, lying close to one another on the postsynaptic cell membrane. It is clear that if both happen to be active simultaneously, they will to some extent cancel each other out, since one is a current source and the other a current sink. The currents that would otherwise be generated by the excitatory ending, and might eventually initiate impulses at the axon hillock, are

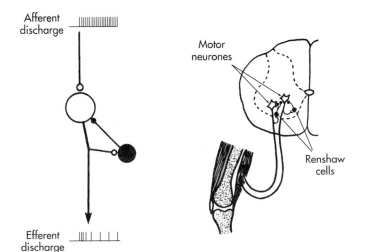

FIG. 3.21 Feedback inhibition. Left, schematic representation, showing how a sudden maintained onset of afferent activity is converted into an adapting efferent response. Right, Renshaw cells in the spinal cord, showing feedback inhibition of motor neurones (inhibitory cells and endings shown in black).

mopped up before they have got any distance at all. But this inhibitory effect would clearly only operate while the inhibitory channels are actually open: as soon as they close the excitatory current would be free to exert its effects at a distance as before. This kind of inhibition is quite distinct from the effect of hyperpolarization, and may indeed produce inhibition in the absence of an IPSP. Imagine, for example, a hypothetical channel whose associated reversal potential happened to be exactly the same as the resting potential. Clearly such a mechanism could not generate an IPSP but it would still be inhibitory because while it was open it would tend to clamp the membrane potential firmly at the resting level by draining away current generated by any nearby excitatory synapses that happened to be active. In a sense, the increase in P_{Cl} during the IPSP does just this. Because E_{Cl} is normally close to the cell's resting potential, this increase contributes nothing to the hyperpolarization: in fact, it actually makes the amplitude of the IPSP less than it would be if there were only an increase in P_K. The importance of Cl⁻ lies in its current effect in *clamping* the membrane potential close to its resting level.

We can now perhaps see why it is that some inhibitory effects seem to be of the current type and some of the voltage type or a mixture of the two. If the excitatory and inhibitory synapses involved happen to be close to one another, the inhibition will be predominantly of the current type, and of short duration. If they are separated, for example on different dendrites, they will not interact directly with one another but their effects will simply summate at the site of initiation of action potentials, producing the voltage effect. Spatial summation of excitation and inhibition is thus rather complex and – as in the case of summation of EPSPs – not just a matter of simple linear addition. Again, inhibitory endings that are very close to the axon hillock region will be particularly good at preventing the cell from firing, because they will ambush the excitatory currents just before they reach the detonator region. Indeed, it is frequently found in the central nervous system that powerful inhibitory synapses are seen clustering near the axon hillock and acting as a sort of guard ring around it: a sluice-gate next to the waterwheel.

It is important not to underestimate the complexity of the processes of spatial and temporal summation in central neurones. Each individual neurone in the brain is a little microcomputer that calculates the size of its output on the basis of the whole spatiotemporal *pattern* of excitation and inhibition that it receives from the enormous number of afferent fibres that drive it. When we look at the varying dendritic shapes of different kinds of neurones – sometimes of extraordinary complexity (Fig. 1.6) – we are in a sense looking at something like a diagram of the rules that determine the neurone's behaviour. Furthermore, although we have been treating the production of action potentials in the axon as the final output of the cell, it is important also to remember that the intermediate slow changes in potential that occur in remote dendrites as the result of local synaptic activity may, in some cases, generate other outputs as well. There are many sites in the brain (notably the retina and olfactory bulb) where dendrodendritic synapses occur, and transmitter is released locally by dendrites in response to the potential changes caused by nearby synaptic currents, rather than to action potentials. Indeed, neurones of this kind need not possess axons at all.

Presynaptic inhibition

A phenomenon that puzzled early investigators was that sometimes one could find clear evidence of inhibition of a cell – in the sense that stimulation of certain fibres resulted in a reduction of the usual response to stimulating other afferents – *without* any corresponding change in its potential or permeability. In some cases this could be explained as 'remote inhibition': in other words, an interaction between neighbouring inhibitory and excitatory endings of the type just described, on a dendrite so far from the recording site that although the inhibitory synapse was capable of cancelling the effect of the excitatory one through current inhibition, it could not generate currents large enough to be measurable at the cell body. But when histologists first noticed that not all the synaptic endings that could be seen in the cord were between axon and cell body or dendrite but that, on the contrary, there were many occasions when an ending appeared to terminate against another ending that in turn synapsed in the conventional way (an *axoaxonic* synapse: Fig. 3.22a), it became clear that another explanation of inhibition in the absence of any detectable change in the postsynaptic cell was possible: that of *presynaptic inhibition*. The notion here is that the ending on the second terminal may somehow hinder the latter's excitatory action, and so cause inhibition of its effects without influencing the postsynaptic cell in any way.

Further evidence of such a mechanism came to light in the phenomenon known as *primary afferent depolarization* or PAD. Selective stimulation of the small fibres of the dorsal root tends to cause a somewhat long-lasting inhibition of the monosynaptic

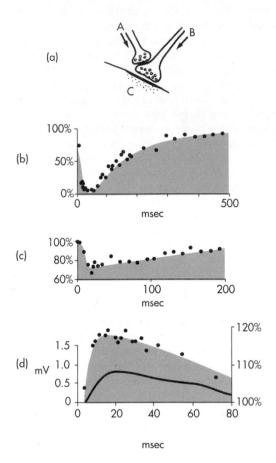

been almost entirely confirmed: the presynaptic transmitter (which is possibly GABA) causes an unselective increase in the permeability of the excitatory ending, leading to depolarization. This action is blocked by the convulsant picrotoxin but prolonged by such CNS depressants as chloralose and the barbiturates.

One might well wonder why this should lead to inhibition: surely an increase in the excitability of the ending ought to cause an increase in the amount of transmitter released by each impulse? The answer seems to lie in the relationship that is thought to hold between terminal depolarization and rate of release of transmitter. For those synapses where it is possible to study this relationship quantitatively, it is found that there is a very sharply rising increase in the rate of release of transmitter as a function of the potential across the ending: in other words, during the entry of the action potential it is really only the *peak* of the impulse that contributes significantly to the number of vesicles that are released. Now if we open up short-circuiting channels in the terminal itself, although admittedly the consequent depolarization of the resting potential should increase the steady rate of transmitter release, equally it will reduce the peak potential of any afferent impulses, by pulling the membrane potential towards zero (Fig. 3.23), and also through the reduction in excitability caused by

FIG. 3.22 Presynaptic inhibition. **(a)** Schematic representation of a terminal A that presynaptically inhibits the excitation of C by B, by synapsing with B's terminal. **(b)** Time-course of depression of monosynaptic reflex after brief stimulation of afferents producing presynaptic inhibition, and **(c)** the time-course of the EPSP size in the same experiment. **(d)** Time-course of primary afferent depolarization: the solid line shows the potential measured across a Ia afferent fibre after a stimulus generating presynaptic inhibition: the shaded area and data points show the corresponding increase in excitability due to the depolarization. (Data from Eccles, 1963; Eccles *et al.*, 1961, 1962b)

response to stimulation of the Ia afferents. If one records from Ia fibres themselves close to the cord, one finds that stimulation of these smaller fibres also leads to a depolarization of similar time-course (Fig. 3.22d). Since one can also observe that the primary afferents are among those that receive synapses on their terminal boutons from interneurones in the dorsal horn, it seemed likely that the PAD was simply the result of the action of these axoaxonal contacts on the terminals, and a side effect of the mechanism by which they were inhibited from releasing as much transmitter as they normally would. This has now

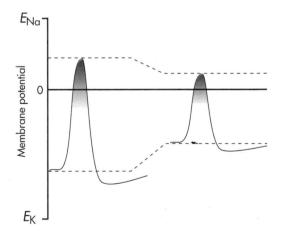

FIG. 3.23 Effect of depolarization of terminal on size of peak of action potential (schematic). Left, a normal action potential. Because the rate of transmitter release depends steeply on depolarization, only the peak of the action potential (shaded) contributes significantly to the amount of transmitter released. Right, partial short-circuiting causes a tonic depolarization, but also reduces the peak of the action potential since the effect is to pull the voltage at every moment towards zero (dashed lines). Consequently there is a relatively large reduction in the amount of transmitter released.

steady depolarization (see Chapter 2, p. 35). Since the peak is what counts, this latter effect will more than compensate for the resting depolarization, and the consequence will be a *reduction* in the amount of transmitter released by the terminal, and hence in the size of the ensuing EPSP.

However, it must be said that not all investigators believe that such a mechanism will explain every kind of presynaptic inhibition. In particular, the extremely long time-course of presynaptic inhibition is puzzling (though it could simply be due to a particularly prolonged indirect cascade), and other explanations for presynaptic inhibition are possible. For example, in considering the way in which the neural elements of the central nervous system are densely packed together with apparently rather little extracellular space, we ought not to neglect the possibility that ionic concentration changes, of a kind that we can usually neglect when considering transmission in peripheral axons, may cause long-term changes in permeability and excitability. In particular, the role of the ubiquitous *glial cells*, that occupy most of the space not taken up by the neurones themselves, is far from clear. Although they do not carry impulses, microelectrode recording shows that they act very like 'potassium electrodes', and show potential changes that reflect the local concentration of potassium in their environment. Since this in turn depends on the average degree of activity in the neurones around them, they are well placed to mediate some kind of long-term regulatory action that could be spatially integrated through the gap junctions that they make with one another. For all we know, glial cells may play some more active role than merely acting as a kind of ionic buffering system for central neurones, conceivably being responsible for certain types of presynaptic inhibition or even possibly the longer term changes associated with memory (Chapter 14), and this will certainly be an area of interest in the future. Finally, in some invertebrates an analogous process of presynaptic *facilitation* may be seen. Here the mechanism is much better understood: the presynaptic ending releases a transmitter, serotonin, that enhances transmission by increasing the level of cAMP within the ending. This in turn increases the size of the presynaptic action potential by reducing potassium permeability.

Functionally, presynaptic inhibition has the advantage of being rather more precise and specific in its actions than postsynaptic inhibition. In the latter case, an inhibitory ending acts on the postsynaptic cell as a whole, regardless of what the source of excitation may be (although it will affect some excitatory afferents more than others because of the spatial

effects outlined earlier). But presynaptic inhibition provides a mechanism whereby certain inputs may be disabled while others are left unhindered: a gating function, which implies control over *which* of the many types of input to a cell may or may not be allowed to influence it. In the case of a motor neurone, we shall see that many different neuronal pathways converge to form synapses on it: tendon jerk reflex afferents, inhibitory afferents for reciprocal inhibition, descending fibres from the higher levels of the brain, afferents controlled by pain and other receptors in the skin, Renshaw cells, and many others. It would clearly be an advantage to be able to alter the strength of some of these inputs independently of the others, and presynaptic inhibition provides a mechanism for doing this.

Long-term changes in excitability

All the phenomena described so far in this chapter are really rather brief in duration, and fall into the category of what has been described as 'millisecond physiology'; but some other synaptic phenomena are of a rather longer time scale. The first of these concerns the effects of *repetitive* stimulation, effects most easily seen at the neuromuscular junction or at autonomic ganglia. If we stimulate a frog neuromuscular junction with a short train of action potentials, under suitable conditions we may find that the size of the evoked EPPs gradually increases throughout the period of stimulation, a phenomenon often called *facilitation* though of course it is distinct from the serotonergic facilitation described earlier. One can show that it is a presynaptic rather than postsynaptic phenomenon, and due to an increase in the amount of transmitter released by each action potential. The reason for it seems to be that not all the calcium that enters in one action potential is pumped out again before the next, so that its concentration within the ending steadily rises, resulting in increasing numbers of vesicles being released. Confirmation for this explanation comes from the fact that the rate of miniature endplate potentials is raised after the end of the pulse-train. If, however, we stimulate for a long period at a rather high frequency, we find a reduction rather than increase in the size of the synaptic potential: this reduction is called *post-tetanic depression*, and is thought to be due simply to a depletion of the amount of transmitter in the ending that is available to be released. If the vesicle release is blocked by lowering the calcium content of the medium, it is found that instead of declining, the size of the evoked potentials actually increases (*post-tetanic potentiation*). A possible explanation for this phenomenon is that the arrival of an action potential at the ending not only causes the release of transmitter, but also in some way promotes the mobilization of stored transmitter so that it is more readily available. Normally, this mobilization is insufficient to keep up with the rate at which transmitter is being used up when the nerve is tetanically stimulated, and post-tetanic depression is observed; but if the rate of release is artificially reduced the transmitter begins to accumulate, resulting in a gradual increase in the amount of transmitter which is released by each action potential.

The mechanism by which neural activity stimulates transmitter mobilization as well as release is at present unknown. In this context it is worth remembering that in many neurones the transmitter is synthesized in the cell body rather than in the endings. It is transported there by means of a specialized system that is probably associated with the activity of neurotubules and neurofibrils within the axon, at rates that may be as high as 15 mm/hour, and it is quite possible that this transport mechanism may also be stimulated by the electrical activity of the axon. Another way in which the effectiveness of a synapse may undergo slow modification, that has been demonstrated in some invertebrate neurones, is by gradual inactivation of the calcium channels in the presynaptic ending as a result of its activity: this will reduce the calcium entry and so cause a reduction in transmitter release.

Of course, the most interesting long-term alterations in synaptic activity are those which are the result of *learning*. We shall see later that it appears to be possible to explain all of the different kinds of memory and learning that the brain is capable of by postulating changes in synaptic effectiveness that are a function of the patterns of activity that the pre- and postsynaptic cells have experienced, and synaptic receptors with exactly these postulated properties are now well established (NMDA receptors); but consideration of this area must be postponed until Chapter 13. A rather simpler phenomenon that is more appropriately discussed here because of its obvious relation to adaptation is *habituation*. Like adaptation, habituation is a decline in response to a constant stimulus; but whereas adaptation means a decline during the application of a continuous stimulus, habituation implies a decline in the successive responses to a stimulus that is *repeatedly* applied. It is essentially a high-level phenomenon, seen not in the responses of sensory receptors but rather in behavioural responses to stimuli and in the parts of the brain that control behaviour. As a consequence, it is typically very specific to one particular pattern of stimulation – in a way that cannot be explained by simple adaptation of peripheral receptors. For instance, when one reads for the fourth time in a month of some appalling plane crash one is rather less shocked than the first time: but this is evidently not because of adaptation in the eye. Again, the fact that one is not continually aware of the somatic sensations produced by one's own clothes is often attributed to adaptation by touch receptors in the skin. But this is clearly wrong, for the stimulus here is repeated rather than continuous, and sensitivity to other patterns of stimulation is not affected: it is actually due to habituation.

The development of synaptic connections

Finally, there is the interesting and really rather basic question of how synaptic connections are set up in the first place. The human brain is perhaps the most complex structure known and if we understood the rules that govern the way in which its innumerable and intricate synaptic connections are specified and formed, we would have come a long way in our understanding of its function. Bearing in mind that there are some 10^{11} neurones in the brain, and that each one receives and gives on average some 10^4 synaptic connections, it is quite inconceivable for these patterns to be specified in *detail* by the instructions for building the brain embodied in our DNA. Though the broader structure of the brain – in terms of tracts that connect nuclei and other subpopulations that are relatively homogeneous within themselves – might be genetically specified, one must conclude that the connections between individual neurones are either essentially random or, more probably, that they are in some way governed by our own sensory experience. The latter is an attractive hypothesis, since it implies that the structure of the brain may in a sense be capable of *self-organization*, of adapting itself to the particular tasks and the particular types of sensory stimulation it has to cope with. In this sense the brain may be thought of as rather like a telephone exchange, in which, when first built, only the broad outlines of the connections between its various elements are specified by its designer, and up to a point almost every unit in it is potentially capable of connection with every other. Once in use, the actual pattern of links at any moment is clearly a function of the patterns of impulses that subscribers have sent to it from their telephone dials. It is also clear that something of this sort must be present to explain the modification of synaptic connections as a result of experience that is implied by the existence of memory, a topic that will be pursued further in Chapter 13. This is a very active area of research, and it is becoming clear that in particular cases there do exist mechanisms by which the brain can in effect build its own connections so as to adapt itself to a particular task, and that the instructions given it by the genetic code are essentially rather vague. Neural development is an area rather beyond the scope of this book, and there is not room here to do more than mention a few underlying principles and simple examples.

Let us consider first a question that may already have occurred to the reader. Clearly a synapse will only function properly if on the postsynaptic membrane there exist receptors that match the transmitter released by the presynaptic terminal. Often one finds nuclei containing a mixture of cell types, and groups of incoming fibres that connect specifically with one cell type or another. Is there then some mechanism that guides the tip of a developing axon towards only those cells that have receptors corresponding to its own transmitter? Or is it rather that when a nerve fibre approaches another neurone, in some way it stimulates the manufacture of the appropriate kind of receptor site? One piece of evidence on this point comes from the study of the formation of the neuromuscular junction. If acetylcholine is applied locally to different parts of a muscle cell's surface, it is found that only the region underlying the neuromuscular junction will respond with depolarization: presumably the cholinergic receptors are confined to the postsynaptic membrane. If we now cut the nerve fibre to the muscle we find that progressively more and more of the muscle cell's surface becomes sensitive to the transmitter, a phenomenon called *denervation hypersensitivity*. But if a new axon starts to grow towards the muscle cell, this process is reversed, and once again we find that the response to acetylcholine becomes limited to the region where the new junction is developing. It seems therefore that the presence of the nerve ending, presumably by the release of some substance, either attracts the receptors or at least encourages their formation while suppressing those that are present elsewhere. We saw in Chapter 1 that damage to an axon not only causes degenerative changes in the parent neurone but may also produce transneuronal degeneration in the neurones with which it is in contact. The implication is that synapses are not merely for communication but are also *trophic:* they not only transmit messages, they also contribute to the maintenance of the cells they contact.

Furthermore, it appears that the development of hypersensitivity is itself in turn a stimulus that attracts nearby axons and leads them to form new synaptic junctions. A normal frog muscle fibre has only one neuromuscular junction, and if a severed motor nerve is placed in its vicinity it will not form additional endplates to it. But if the original innervation is cut, it is found that the resulting hypersensitivity is also accompanied by the acceptance of a synaptic junction from a fibre that previously was ignored. In the same way, transplanting an extra limb at an inappropriate site in many amphibia leads to new fibres growing out from the central nervous system to innervate it, through the release of a small protein, *nerve growth factor*, that attracts potential axons.

Similar work on the regeneration of neural connections in amphibia (regeneration is not observed – at least not over such large distances – in the mammalian central nervous system) has shown that this guidance of neurones on to their targets can sometimes be even more specific; not just on to the correct type of cell, as defined by its receptor properties, but even on to the correct part of an extended mass of such cells. In the frog, there is an orderly projection of the fibres of the optic nerve to the frog's 'visual brain' (the tectum) that preserves the topology of the retinal image. If the optic nerve is cut, it is found that the fibres not only regenerate back to the tectum but do so in such a way as to retain, at least approximately, their correct spatial arrangement. The mechanism by which this specificity of connection arises is not yet understood. It is perhaps worth emphasizing that in these experiments the guidance is anatomical rather than functional: if, after cutting the optic nerve, the frog's eye is rotated in its orbit through 180°, the pattern of the regenerating fibres is not also rotated through 180°. As a result, the animal's subsequent visual behaviour is inverted, with upward movements in response to objects in the lower visual field, and so on. In other words, there is no suggestion in these experiments that the pattern of activity in the incoming fibres can influence the pattern of their connections.

But other recent experiments in mammals have shown that connections can in certain circumstances be altered by the pattern of neural activity, in such a way that only useful connections are formed or useless ones are lost. For example, the cells of a cat's visual cortex (Chapter 7) are usually found to be driven in almost equal numbers by each eye, and many by both. But if one eye of a kitten about 5 weeks old is kept closed, even if only for a few days, one finds when it has grown up that the number of its cortical cells that are driven by the eye that had been closed is very greatly diminished. There has been no anatomical interference here: the only difference between the two eyes was the degree of their neural activity during the period of closure, so it must follow in this case that the synaptic connections have been influenced by the pattern of neural activity experienced. What seems to happen in the course of development is that initially there is an excess of synaptic contacts that form randomly in a somewhat promiscuous way. But at a certain critical period in development, perhaps because of a fall in the general level of trophic factor, there is intense competition between endings and neurones, and those which are in some sense less successful than others simply degenerate or die.

An even clearer example of degeneration of useless connections and the growth of useful ones has been demonstrated in the spinal cord of the kitten. If part of the innervation of unrelated pairs of synergic muscles is cut, and the cut ends crossed and reunited as in Figure 3.24, regeneration will occur both of the motor nerves and of the sensory fibres coming from the muscle stretch receptors. In the normal animal, the afferent fibres form monosynaptic excitatory connections with the motor neurones both of the parent and its synergist but after the cross-union, part of this excitatory projection will at first – quite inappropriately – be to motor neurones of the unrelated muscle

pair. If, after 6 months or so, one records the electrical responses of the motor neurones to stimulation of the various possible afferent pathways, one finds that the inappropriate synaptic connections have weakened, and that conversely some new and appropriate monosynaptic connections have developed that were previously non-functional. As can be seen in the figure, growth of new connections appears to be limited to those motor neurones whose axons were severed in the course of the experiment, suggesting some mechanism akin to denervation sensitivity by which the injured neurone becomes more receptive to the formation of new synapses. Here again, the pattern of connections seems to be determined by the pattern of activity in the nerve fibres themselves, and synapses are maintained only between afferent and efferent neurones whose activities are mutually correlated because they are connected to synergistic muscles. One can see how such a mechanism might well – in principle – determine the correct wiring of the monosynaptic pathways in the first place, whereby the stretch receptor afferents only maintain contact with the properly corresponding motor neurones. It is not too wild an extrapolation to imagine how similar processes might lead to the development of specific and appropriate neural connections in the central nervous system in general, and thus contribute to the brain's ability to *learn* (Chapter 13): but our knowledge of such processes is still in its infancy.

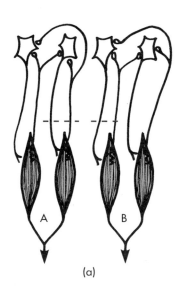
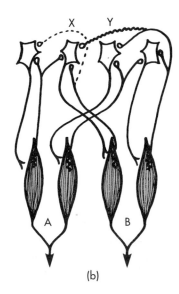

(a)   (b)

FIG. 3.24 Plasticity of neural circuits. **(a)** The connections existing before the experiment between stretch receptors in two independent pairs of synergistic muscles, A and B, and their motor neurones. After cutting the nerves at the level indicated by the dashed lines, they were reunited as shown on the right **(b)**. After recovery, certain inappropriate connections (dashed line X) were found to have weakened while new appropriate ones (wavy line Y) were found to have appeared. (After Eccles *et al.*, 1962a)

References

Araki, T., Eccles, J. C. and Ito, M. (1960) Correlation of the inhibitory postsynaptic potential of motoneurons with the latency and time course of inhibition of monosynaptic reflexes. *Journal of Physiology* 154, 354–377.

Burke, R. E. (1967) Composite nature of monosynaptic excitatory postsynaptic potential. *Journal of Neurophysiology* 30, 1114–1137.

Coombs, J. S., Eccles, J. C. and Fatt, P. (1955) Excitatory synaptic action in motoneurones. *Journal of Physiology* 130, 374–395.

Curtis, D. R. and Eccles, J. C. (1959) The time courses of excitatory and inhibitory synaptic actions. *Journal of Physiology* 145, 529–546.

Eccles, J. C. (1963) Presynaptic and postsynaptic inhibitory actions in the spinal cord. In *Brain Mechanisms*, ed. G. Moruzzi. Elsevier, Amsterdam.

Eccles, J. C., Eccles, R. M. and Magni, F. (1961) Central inhibitory action attributable to presynaptic depolarization produced by muscle afferent volleys. *Journal of Physiology* 159, 147–166.

Eccles, J. C., Eccles, R. M., Shealy, C. N. and Willis, W. D. (1962a) Experiments utilizing monosynaptic excitatory action on motoneurones for testing hypotheses relating to specificity of neuronal connection. *Journal of Neurophysiology* 25, 559–579.

Eccles, J. C., Schmidt, R. F. and Willis, W. D. (1962b) Presynaptic inhibition of the spinal monosynaptic reflex pathway. *Journal of Physiology* 161, 282–297.

Hubbard, S. J. (1963) Repetitive stimulation of the mammalian neuromuscular junction, and the mobilisation of transmitter. *Journal of Physiology* 169, 641–662.

Hunt, C. C. and McIntyre, A. K. (1960) An analysis of fibre diameter and receptor characteristics of myelinated cutaneous afferents in the cat. *Journal of Physiology* 153, 99–112.

Ito, M., Kostyuk, P. G. and Oshima, T. (1962) Further study on anion permeability in cat spinal motoneurons. *Journal of Physiology* 164, 15–156.

Loewenstein, W. R. and Mendelsohn, M. (1965) Components of adaptation in a Pacinian corpuscle. *Journal of Physiology* 177, 377–397.

Lundberg, A. and Quilisch, H. (1953) On the effect of calcium on presynaptic potentiation and depression at the neuromuscular junction. *Acta Physiologica Scandinavica* 111, 121–129.

Mountcastle, V. B. (1966) The neural replication of sensory events. In *Brain and Conscious Experience*, ed. J. C. Eccles. Springer, Berlin.

NOTES

Neurones in general Excellent general coverage of this area is provided by Bradford, H. F. (1986) *Chemical Neurobiology.* (W. H. Freeman, New York); Hall, Z. W. (1992) *An Introduction to Molecular Neurobiology* (Sinauer, Sunderland, Mass); and Shepherd, G. (1994) *Neurobiology* (Oxford University Press, Oxford); a particularly clear account of the basics is given by Levitan, I. B. and Kaczmarek, L. K. (1991) *The Neurone: Cell and Membrane Biology* (Oxford University Press, Oxford).

Page 45 Similarities between channels The evolutionary relationships between these various types of channel have been discussed in Hille, B. (1989) Ionic channels: evolutionary origins and modern roles. *Quarterly Journal of Experimental Physiology* 74, 785–804.

Page 52 Signal-to-noise ratio An excellent account of this area for the general reader, but sadly long out of print, is Pierce, J. R. (1962) *Symbols, Signals and Noise* (Hutchinson, London).

Page 57 Spinal synaptology The classic account of the pioneering experiments in this area is Eccles, J. C. (1964) *The Physiology of Synapses* (Cambridge University Press, Cambridge).

Page 58 Diversity of transmitters Nieuwenhuys, R. (1985) *Chemoarchitecture of the Brain* (Springer Verlag, Berlin) provides a comprehensive survey of the location of transmitters in different parts of the brain.

Page 60 Dale's hypothesis It is not clear that Dale's hypothesis is actually true, at least as far as 'acting in the same way' is concerned. The glutamate released by retinal receptors, for instance, causes inhibition of some bipolar cells and excitation of others. What is probably true is that a cell of a certain class, A, cannot have two different effects on cells of another class B (or any effect at all on cells of class A). Such a rule would prevent certain difficulties in the way the brain wires itself up.

NEUROLAB

 Photoreceptors

Page 45

This exhibit embodies the cascade of events between absorption of light by photoreceptors (toad rods), the activation of PDE, reduction in cGMP, and closing of sodium channels. If you press Sweep, a trace is initiated showing the stimulus (a brief pulse of light) in red, and the resultant photocurrent in green. You can set different background levels as well as different sizes of stimulus (radio buttons at right). Observe saturation with large stimuli, and also the way in which a steady background reduces sensitivity mostly by affecting calcium levels, which mediate adaptation by altering the rate at which cGMP is recycled. The Auto-zero check button makes every response start at the same level; if you want to examine steady states, turn it off. For easier comparison, sweeps are superimposed until the Clear button is activated.

Pacinian corpuscle

Page 49

This is a simple model of the mechanical properties of the Pacinian corpuscle, considered as an elastic element (spring) representing the core, acted on by a viscous element (dashpot) representing the fluid-filled outer layers. Sweep starts a sweep showing the input displacement (green) and degree of compression of the core (response, yellow) as a function of time. On the right, there are controls for the stimulus: you can alter the waveform and the frequency. Notice how high frequencies are in general transmitted better than low; and observe the phase relation at low frequencies between input and output.

Adaptation

Page 50

This exhibit allows you to explore various aspects of sensory adaptation. As usual, clicking on Sweep starts a sweep in the window, showing a stimulus (green) and the corresponding response (yellow) as a function of time. Radio buttons on the left allow you to choose various repetitive stimuli: step (square wave), ramp (triangle wave) or sinusoidal; the slider bar alters the frequency. In the middle, slider bars alter two crucial parameters of the adaptation itself: how complete it is (i.e. the extent to which the response to a maintained stimulus falls to zero) and the time constant (determining whether it is fast or slow). Experiment for yourself with various combinations of these settings. Note in particular with sinusoidal stimulation how the effect of complete adaptation is to increase the response at high frequencies and reduce it at low – it acts as a *high-pass filter*. There is a button called Waterfall illusion that relates to something dealt with in Chapter 7 and is described there.

Time constants

Page 55

This exhibit was introduced in Chapter 1, and general instructions for it can be found on page 41. Selecting the third of the three options, R_2, simulates a situation found at many excitatory synapses and sensory receptors, where the membrane is normally at the resting potential but the arrival of a stimulus opens short-circuiting channels that lower the membrane resistance. Note that while the transmitter is present (switch closed) the membrane depolarizes rapidly; afterwards the exponential recovery is quite slow.

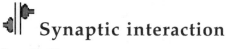 # Synaptic interaction

Page 59, 63

A highly stylized neurone – soma and dendrites – is shown at left with excitatory (red) and inhibitory (black) synapses. Start a sweep (showing the membrane potential at the axon hillock) by pressing Sweep. Then click on synapses to activate them, and see for yourself how they interact both spatially and temporally. Note the particularly devastating effect of the inhibitory synapse near the axon hillock itself, and see if you can demonstrate temporal and spatial summation, current and voltage inhibition.

PART

2

SENSORY FUNCTIONS

4

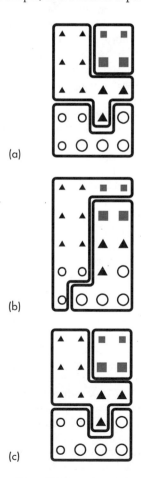

SKIN SENSE

Sensory modalities 73
Types of receptor 74
Central projections 77

Neural responses 79
Central responses 84
Pain 84

This chapter is concerned with the information that comes from sensory receptors in the skin, and from the very similar ones of the gut and other visceral organs. The whole system is often loosely termed the *somatosensory system*, but this strictly also includes receptors from muscles and joints, which as proprioceptors are considered in Chapter 5.

SENSORY MODALITIES

Many types of stimulus can produce sensations from the skin and to a large extent the receptors and pathways of cutaneous sensation are modality-specific, responding preferentially to such specialized categories as pressure, cold, warmth and so on. But the concept of 'modality specificity' is not quite as straightforward as might be thought at first sight, and requires some preliminary discussion.

The concept of modalities comes about through our natural urge to classify the objects around us; the reason that difficulties arise in its use is that there are many *criteria* by which objects may be classified, and unless one is clear about which type of classification is referred to, misunderstandings become inevitable. If we consider all the kinds of things that may come in contact with the skin, we might group them according to their *physical effects* (as mechanical, thermal, etc.) or according to the *sensations* they produce (pain, tickle, softness) or even in terms of the types of peripheral *nerve fibres* they stimulate. Each of these classifications will in general divide the whole set of stimuli into different patterns of subsets (Fig. 4.1) which may or may not correspond with one another. Now if it happened that in each system of classification

the boundaries were identical, as in (a) and (c) of the figure, then no difficulties would arise, and we could say with certainty that the fibres were modality-specific. For example, if we found a particular type of

FIG. 4.1 A set of miscellaneous objects classified according to shape (a), size (b), and colour (c).

fibre that responded only to heating of the skin, and that this in turn was also a clear and distinct class of sensation, then one could say that the fibres in question were specific for that particular stimulus or sensory modality. But in practice, things are seldom so simple, and there is no uniquely valid way of classifying either the physical attributes of objects or the sensations they evoke. In particular, there is a danger of introducing a degree of tautology: one may be influenced by one's knowledge of one of three levels of classification when drawing up the boundaries for the others.

If just for a moment you forget all you have been taught and ask yourself what you really *feel* to be the categories of cutaneous sensation, your list is likely to include not just the familiar stereotypes of pain, warmth, pressure and so forth but also other sensations that are just as immediate and apparently 'primary': tickle, itch, softness, roughness, hardness, stickiness, wetness, sharpness, and many others. It is doubtful whether someone who had never read a physiology book would naturally consider the classic modalities to be more 'primary' than the others. Our classification of the physical classes of stimuli is almost equally biased. Some physical attributes are left out: for instance, the all-important factor of local curvature of the skin, that gives rise to the sense of sharpness and roughness, is usually wholly ignored. Other, mythical, physical stimuli are simply invented. In an effort to try to produce some physical quality that could be said to correspond with the obvious sensation of pain, it is customary to invent a special class of physical stimulus, whether mechanical, thermal or even chemical, that causes tissue damage of some kind and may therefore be called 'noxious', and sensed by 'nociceptors'. Yet many kinds of pain are not associated with tissue damage at all.

In other words, there is a danger of unconsciously falsifying what might be called 'natural' classifications of sensations or physical types of stimulus; and if our modalities are thus defined by what is observed in sensory fibres, then it must follow tautologically that one fibre responds only to one modality. A discussion about whether a particular system is modality-specific or whether on the contrary a particular mode of stimulation gives rise to a characteristic *pattern of activity* amongst a set of afferent fibres that is indicative of that class of stimulus (as, for example, seeing the letter 'A' does to our retinal fibres) amounts in the end simply to an argument about how we happen to name what we perceive.

A further, insidious, bias that may creep into investigations of sensory systems – this applies with equal if not greater force to other special senses such as vision and audition – is that by having preconceived notions as to what the categories of stimulus are, based on categories of primary fibres rather than on what might be important to the organism in controlling its behaviour, one may tend to limit oneself to those categories when trying experimentally to evoke responses from higher levels of the brain. This error may become self-perpetuating: if one explores the neurones of the somatosensory cortex using only stimuli of light touch, warmth, cold or one of the other traditional modalities, then naturally all the cells that respond at all must fall into one of these categories. If there were cells responding to more useful things like stickiness or wetness, one would never discover them: and so the myth would be perpetuated. So it is very important to bear in mind these reservations about over-simple categorizations of stimuli into modalities when considering the specificity of receptors and of central neurones to cutaneous and other kinds of stimulation. Our cutaneous sensory world is vastly richer than the pathetic number of 'modalities' derived from studies of skin fibres.

TYPES OF RECEPTOR

The afferent fibres from cutaneous receptors are bipolar cells: their bodies lie in the *dorsal root ganglia* near the spinal cord, and axons run all the way from the sensory endings in the skin to their terminals within the central nervous system (Fig. 4.2). The dorsal roots are connected in an orderly way to different areas of the skin, and one may draw maps of the body surface showing the *dermatomes* or regions projecting to each dorsal root (Fig. 4.3). The demarcation of the different zones is not actually as sharp as such idealized representations suggest, and because of overlap between adjacent dermatomes, each point on the body surface is connected to at least two dorsal roots; overlap is more marked for touch than it is for pain or temperature. Sensory fibres from the *viscera* are found in both the sympathetic and parasympathetic divisions of the autonomic nervous system. The former pass in peripheral sympathetic nerves to the sympathetic chain, and thence via the dorsal root ganglia (where their cell bodies are) to the dorsal root; parasympathetic afferents of the sacral region travel with the corresponding efferents and again have their cell bodies in the dorsal root ganglion, while the cell bodies of afferents in the vagus are in the inferior (nodose) ganglion.

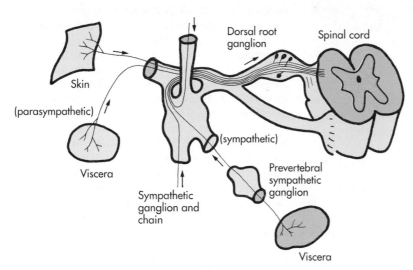

FIG. 4.2 Afferent pathways from the skin and viscera (schematic).

At the peripheral end, the fibres branch and terminate either as naked endings or in terminal *encapsulations*, of which many varieties have been described One such is the *Pacinian corpuscle*, whose responses to deformation were discussed in the previous chapter. Others include *Meissner's corpuscle, Merkel's discs,* and the *Ruffini endings* (Fig. 4.4). Encapsulated endings are found mainly in hairless or *glabrous* skin: the palms of the hands and soles of the feet, the lips, eyelids, mucosal surfaces and parts of the external genitalia. Some, notably the Pacinian corpuscles, are distributed in visceral structures and in joints and ligaments and deep connective tissue. Free or naked endings are abundant in hairy skin, some innervating the hair follicles themselves and sensing hair movement, and are also to be found in both glabrous skin and in deep fascia and visceral organs. Their afferent fibres are small and sometimes unmyelinated, falling into group C and group Aδ (or III and IV, with a few in II): the fibres from encapsulated endings are mainly of group Aβ (or II) (Box 4.1).

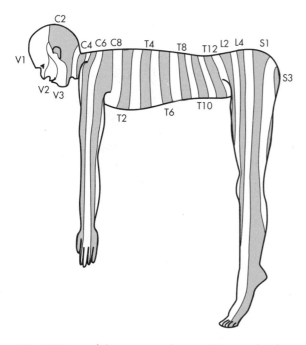

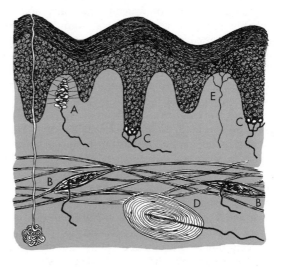

FIG. 4.3 Pattern of dermatomes in humans: C, cervical; L, lumbar; S, sacral; T, thoracic; V, trigeminal.

FIG. 4.4 Representative types of endings in glabrous skin (somewhat schematic). A, Meissner's corpuscle; B, Ruffini endings; C, Merkel's discs; D, Pacinian corpuscle; E, free endings.

Box 4.1 Types of skin receptors

Meissner	Complete	Aβ
Merkel	Incomplete	Aβ
Pacinian	Complete	Aβ
Ruffini	Incomplete	Aβ
Krause	Complete	Aβ
Free endings	?	C?
(Warm)	Incomplete	C
(Cold)	Incomplete	Aδ, C
(Nociceptive)	Prob. None	Aδ, C

In addition, there are specialized sensory structures associated with *sinus hairs* (the eyelashes, for example, or the whiskers of a cat: Fig. 4.5). The hair is surrounded at its base by pressure-sensitive Pacinian corpuscles; in the middle it is encircled by a ring of Merkel's discs; and along part of its length the hair is linked by thin filaments to a palisade of fast-adapting lanceolate endings. The result of this battery of mechanoreceptors is to provide the brain with exquisitely sensitive and highly directional information about displacements of the hair brought about by contact with external objects.

It is only recently that we have begun to form a clear picture of what this great variety of receptor types in the skin is actually *for*. One might perhaps have expected each type of ending to correspond to one of the classic modalities, but this turns out not to be the case. The naked or free endings seem to serve the modalities both of warmth and pain, and are probably sensitive to mechanical stimuli as well. Specific encapsulated endings for cold have recently been described, but do not yet have a name: unusually for encapsulated endings, their axons fall into the Aδ category. All the other endings that are known are mechanoreceptors of one kind or another, and it is clear that the classic descriptions of 'light touch' or 'pressure' are inadequate for classifying just what it is that they respond to. In most cases the structure of the endings makes it pretty clear what they do. The concentric layers of the Pacinian corpuscle, apart from making it a complete and rapid adapter, also imply a rather non-directional sensitivity to local deformation, and hence *pressure*. Ruffini organs consist of branched naked nerve endings twisted in between collagen fibres that leave the capsule and are anchored to nearby muscle cells and other structures. *Tension* in these fibres appears to distort the nerve endings and thus stimulates them; they adapt incompletely. (Similar endings are found in the tendons of

muscles, called *Golgi tendon organs*: as proprioceptors they are considered in Chapter 5.) Merkel's discs lie much closer to the outside world, at the bottom of the epidermis, to which they are attached by desmosomes: they are extremely sensitive to deformation of the skin, and show incomplete adaptation. In classic terms, they might be regarded as light touch receptors; more functionally, they may serve to indicate *contact*. Finally, Meissner's corpuscles, like Ruffini endings, have nerve endings that are associated with collagen fibres. The corpuscles are found in the dermal folds beneath the epidermal ridges, and the collagen fibres are connected sideways with the epidermal cells on each side. Thus they are ideally placed to register sideways *shearing* of the skin, of the kind that is experienced, for example, when holding an object in the fingers and then lifting it (they are in fact most commonly found in the fingertips). A curious feature is

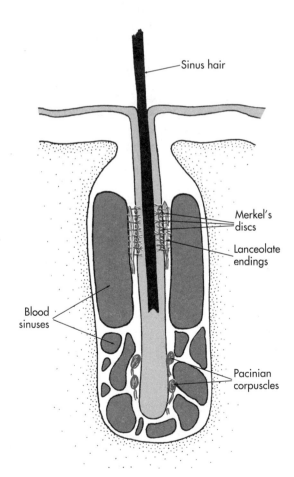

FIG. 4.5 Stylized longitudinal section of base of a sinus hair showing the mechanoreceptors with which it is associated. (After Halata, 1975)

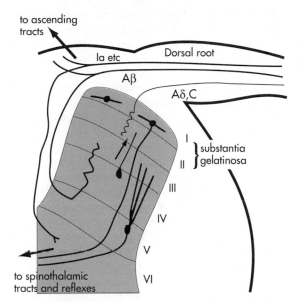

FIG. 4.6 Schematic representation of laminae in the dorsal horn of the spinal cord, showing the approximate sites of termination of different kinds of sensory afferent, and the cells of origin of the spinothalamic tracts. Also shown are lateral inhibitory interneurones found in layers I and II, and interneurones relaying information from large (mechanical) afferents from layer IV to layer II. There are also descending fibres (not shown) that enter layer II and inhibit the transmission of pain signals.

that their density declines dramatically with age, from some 50 per square mm at 10 years to about 10 at 50 years.

The fact that many of these receptors show complete adaptation means that it is only when the pattern of stimulation to the skin is changing that we perceive very much. Shut your eyes, and run your hand over some nearby object, perhaps the table-top: your hand gives you a vivid impression of its texture, of its cracks and dents and all its other surface properties. Now keep your hand still: at once this perception vanishes, and it is hard to be sure that one is sensing anything at all except its temperature. It is evidently the *temporal patterns* of firing of mechanoreceptors from the skin, combined with knowledge of the movements we make, that determine what we feel when we touch something.

The broad division of afferent fibres into two groups (small, mostly from free endings; large, from encapsulated endings) is reflected in their mode of termination within the central nervous system. In the spinal cord, they both terminate in the dorsal horn but in different parts of it. The dorsal horn is conventionally divided into a set of six roughly parallel laminae (*Rexed's laminae*: Fig. 4.6). Smaller fibres enter directly from the dorsal root and terminate in layers

I and II; the largest fibres sweep round dorsally to terminate in layers III–V, where amongst other cells they make contact with short interneurones conveying mechanical information back to layer II, a fact of some importance in the processing of pain signals (p. 86). The neurones of the dorsal horn are also under firm control from the brain: if the descending pathways are experimentally blocked the receptive fields of dorsal horn cells undergo radical alteration. We shall see that this too is of very great significance in the case of pain.

CENTRAL PROJECTIONS

The mode of projection to higher levels is also distinctive. Branches of the larger fibres, from encapsulated mechanoreceptors, turn upwards soon after entering the dorsal horn of the spinal cord to form a pair of large ascending tracts called the posterior or *dorsal columns* (Figs 4.6, 4.7). These continue ipsilaterally up to the level of the medulla and terminate in the *dorsal column nuclei (gracile* and *cuneate)*; the gracile receives afferents from sacral, lumbar, and lower thoracic segments, and the cuneate from higher regions. From these nuclei, second-order fibres cross to the other side and continue up as the *medial lemniscus* to the ventral posterolateral (VPL) and other posterior nuclei of the thalamus, and thence relay through the *internal capsule* to a region of cerebral cortex called the *somatosensory cortical area* or SI (areas 3, 2 and 1 in Brodmann's classification, based on the different histological appearance of different cortical regions). Throughout this system – often called the *lemniscal system* – the general topological relationship between the representations of different areas of the skin is preserved, so that the somatosensory cortex itself embodies a map of the opposite side of the skin surface. This map, the sensory homunculus, is topologically correct in the sense that neighbouring parts of the body surface are on the whole represented by neighbouring regions of cortex, but very much distorted in shape (Fig. 4.7); those areas such as the hands and lips with the greatest cutaneous sensitivity and acuity have a much larger area devoted to them than regions like the trunk and back.

A second somatosensory area, SII, is found in primates which differs from SI in receiving somatosensory information from both sides, and to some extent in the modalities to which it responds.

The smaller afferents, derived from free endings and also from some of the encapsulated ones and concerned with temperature, pain and light touch, do not immediately ascend on entering the cord: instead, either directly or via an interneurone, they activate neurones in layers I and V whose axons cross to the other side and proceed upwards as part of the *spinothalamic* projection (Fig. 4.8). There are two of these spinothalamic pathways, the *anterior spinothalamic* tract and the *lateral spinothalamic* (the whole system is called the *anterolateral system*). Though they are both evolutionarily older than the more recent lemniscal system, the anterior tract is more highly developed in higher animals than the lateral, and for this reason they are also known as the neo- and palaeospinothalamic pathways. However, more recent work suggests that one should not exaggerate the difference between them. The former projects only to the border of VPL, and to nearby regions that are not wholly somatosensory, terminating in large bushy arborizations (in contrast to the more compact lemniscal endings). The palaeospinothalamic afferents project to central and intralaminar regions of the thalamus, and also rather diffusely to the reticular formation of the medulla and pons: they are concerned more with pain and temperature than with touch.

Thus on the one hand we have the new, fast lemniscal system with its precise and orderly projection of accurate mechanical information directly up to the cortex; and on the other, the older, slower, and more diffuse projection of less precise but in a sense more immediately important information – often with an affective or emotional quality to it – by the anterolateral system, which scarcely projects to the cortex at all. One provides objective information which we can take or leave; the other demands a response. One goes straight up the brain with hardly a nod to the spinal cord; the other terminates in the spinal cord, which may or may not bother to inform the brain about it.

The differences between the two systems can be of diagnostic value in certain kinds of disorders of the spinal cord. Thus a hemisection of the cord, that interrupts all ascending fibres on one side, will result in a loss of deep pressure and vibration sense below the level of the section on one side, and loss of pain, temperature and light touch on the other (cf. *Clinical Neurology*, Ch. 3). Deliberate anterolateral cordotomy is in fact sometimes performed to deal with otherwise intractable pain of peripheral origin; it has little effect on tactile sensibility. Finally, some cutaneous fibres ascend to the cerebellum in the *posterior spinocerebellar* tract (see p. 93).

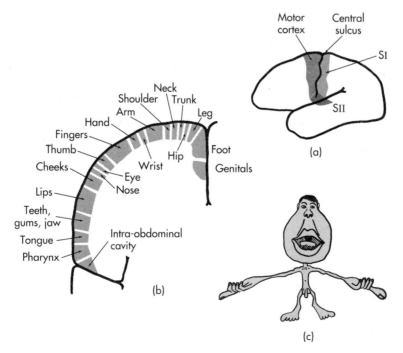

FIG. 4.7 (a) Lateral view of human cerebral cortex, showing approximate positions of somatosensory areas SI and SII. **(b)** Frontal section through the primary somatosensory cortex in humans, showing the approximate areas associated with different parts of the body. **(c)** Sensory homunculus, distorted so as to indicate by the relative size of different parts of the body the relative areas devoted to each in somatosensory cortex. (After Penfield and Rasmussen, 1950)

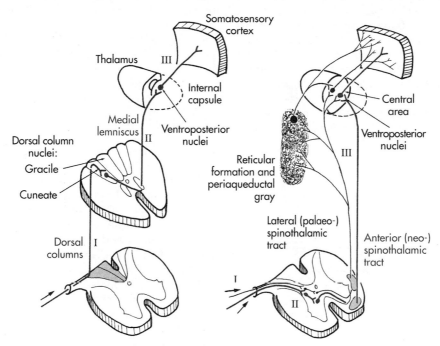

FIG. 4.8 The main ascending somatosensory pathways. Left, the lemniscal system; right, the neo- and palaeospinothalamic divisions of the anterolateral system. (The thalamus is shown in section to make the position of the central and ventroposterior nuclei clearer.)

NEURAL RESPONSES

The larger Aβ or group II fibres from the skin all respond specifically to mechanical stimuli. As we have seen, some are completely adapting, and thus only respond to changes in the deformation of the skin: they originate from the Pacinian and Meissner corpuscles and from some of the endings in hair follicles. Because of their adapting properties, they are particularly sensitive to vibration, and thus are well suited to contribute to the sense of roughness when the hand is passed over a textured surface. They are also extraordinarily sensitive: the threshold of a Pacinian corpuscle is of the order of 10 μm of skin displacement, provided this is rapidly applied. They may well help one to sense when an object being lifted between the fingers begins to slip, and thus assist in regulating the pressure with which such an object is grasped. One can show this by comparing the strength used to grip and lift an object covered with surfaces of different slipperiness: normally grip force is modified with short latency to take account of the nature of the surface, but if the skin of the fingers is anaesthetized these rapid responses to slip do not

occur. Other fibres show only incomplete adaptation and can therefore signal static deformation as well: they come mostly from Merkel's discs and Ruffini endings. Useful information has come from microelectrode recording from afferents from the hand running in the medial nerve in conscious human subjects, the particular advantage being that one can also perform microstimulation and see what the subject feels. One can demonstrate, for instance, that a single action potential in some of the fastest-adapting fibres is sufficient to evoke a sensation.

Responses from smaller afferents

The cutaneous fibres of groups Aδ and C that are associated with light touch, pain and temperature show response patterns that are a little more complex than those of the larger fibres. *Warm and cold fibres*, of Aδ size, fire tonically at a rate that is a function of temperature, with a peak for warm fibres around 45°C and for cold receptors around 30°C (Fig. 4.9). Both also show incomplete adaptation: sudden warming of the skin results in a transient increased discharge of warm fibres, whose activity then settles down to a new level, while sudden cooling has the same effect on cold fibres. However, it appears that the cold receptors also respond transiently to warming above some 45°C, giving rise to the familiar sensation of *paradoxical cold*: a hot object, when briefly touched, may often give the immediate impression of being intensely cold. These adapting properties of the thermoreceptors dominate one's sense of skin temperature. Thus a swimming pool that seems

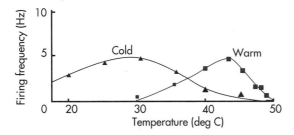

FIG. 4.9 Tonic firing frequencies of cold and warm fibres from monkey skin in response to different temperatures. (Data from Kenshalo, 1976)

appallingly cold when one first dives in soon seems quite comfortable, and a bowl of warm water may feel simultaneously cold to one hand and hot to the other, if previously the two hands had been held respectively in hot and cold water. The receptive fields of thermoreceptors are very small and, far from overlapping, are actually separated from one another by large areas of skin that do not respond at all. Thus one may find warm and cold *spots* on the skin; on the hand the cold spots are about 5–10 mm apart and the warm spots some 15 mm. (Temperature is not of course a cutaneous sense for which accurate localization is particularly important, and as a consequence the spatial resolution of these small-fibre afferent systems is poor: this is reflected in the very small number of fibres that ascend in the spinothalamic tract – in humans perhaps as few as a thousand.)

Thermoreceptive properties similar to what is described above are also found amongst C fibres, more of them responding to cooling than to warming; other C fibres respond to light touch in the same general way as A fibres. The remaining Aδ and C fibres serve the sense of pain, produced by noxious stimuli, and are discussed later in this chapter.

Receptive fields

In order to be effective in stimulating a fibre, a stimulus must lie within a particular area of the skin called the *receptive field*. The size of this field is partly a consequence of the unavoidable spread of the stimulus itself – any indentation of the skin, however localized, will cause deformation of the layers of the skin over a much wider area – but is also the result of the branching of the afferent fibre and consequent distribution of its endings over an extended region. In the case of the fibres innervating hair follicles, for example, one finds that each fibre may innervate as many as 100 follicles, and each follicle in turn receives branches from several fibres. Thus the receptive fields of the individual fibres are quite large, and also show a considerable degree of *overlap* (Fig. 4.10). Such a pattern of overlapping receptive fields is a common one in all kinds of sensory systems. What is the point of it? Surely, one would think, it would be better to avoid this duplication by making the receptive fields smaller, resulting in an improvement of the precision with which a stimulus can be localized. Yet it turns out, on closer analysis, that a system in which the receptive fields overlap is not only just as good as one in which they are discrete, but in many ways actually much better.

Consider first the question of *accuracy of localization* of a stimulus. If the fields were discrete, then all the brain could tell about the position of a stimulus is that it must lie somewhere inside a particular receptive field: there is no way in which it could find out where it lies within that field. But consider the case of two overlapping fields: if a stimulus lies within the

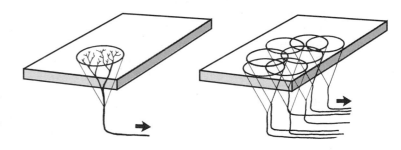

FIG. 4.10 Left, the receptive field of a single idealized cutaneous afferent fibre; right, showing the overlap between neighbouring fields.

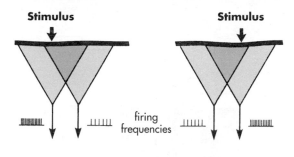

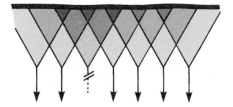

FIG. 4.11 Advantages of overlap. Above, the brain can determine the exact position of a stimulus within an area of overlap by analysing the relative activities of the corresponding fibres. Below, overlap means that damage to any one fibre does not necessarily produce an area of anaesthesia.

area of overlap, then it will stimulate the two fibres in different proportions, depending on its exact position. So by analysing the pattern of discharge of the two neurones – by comparing the frequency of firing of one with that of the other – the central nervous system could determine the position of the stimulus much more accurately than if the fields were discrete (Fig. 4.11). Overlap has the further advantage that it makes the system much less vulnerable to damage: destruction of any one fibre will still leave each area of skin with the innervation of its neighbours.

Now it is perfectly true that if one thinks of the receptors as converting the spatial pattern of the stimulus into a kind of 'neural image' – a corresponding pattern of firing amongst the array of afferent fibres – then it must follow that the effect of having large receptive fields will be to blur this neural image. Sharp stimulus boundaries will be converted into a rather fuzzy gradation between those fibres that are firing maximally and those that are not firing at all. However, there is a simple way in which the brain can mitigate the effects of this kind of neural blur, called *lateral inhibition*.

Lateral inhibition

Imagine that at the level at which the incoming fibres first relay on to ascending, second-order neurones – in this case, in the gracile and cuneate nuclei – they excite local interneurones as well; and suppose that the interneurones in turn send inhibitory connections to neighbouring second-order cells (Fig. 4.12). What will happen now is that each incoming fibre will stimulate its own second-order cell but inhibit the ones that surround it: the cells will, in effect, be pushing on each others' shoulders. Thus a cell that is

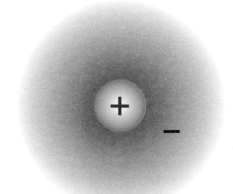

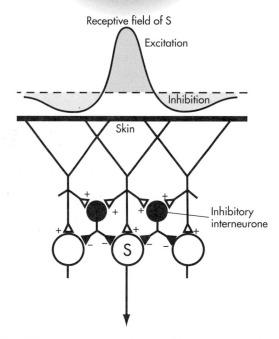

FIG. 4.12 Lateral inhibition. If a second-order neurone, S, is excited by one receptor but inhibited by interneurones driven by its neighbours, the result will be to reduce the size of the excitatory receptive field, and to surround it with an area in which stimulation will give rise to *inhibition*.

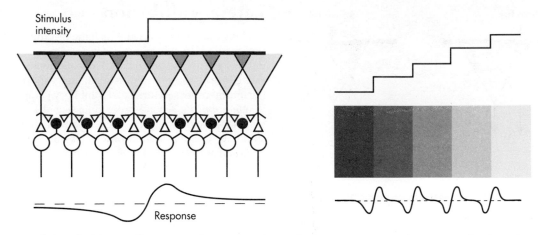

FIG. 4.13 Left, lateral inhibition will exaggerate the response of second-order neurones to an edge, compared to the uniform areas on each side. A similar effect can be perceived directly as an illusion when viewing a series of steps of intensity (right).

stimulated more than average will have a larger effect on its neighbours than they will in turn have on it. The result will be to exaggerate changes in intensity, compensating to some extent for the blurring effect of the original overlap of the receptive fields. This mechanism of *lateral inhibition* is of fundamental importance in understanding the processing of neural information, and occurs in every kind of sensory system. It is also found universally within the central nervous system itself, since blurring can occur not only through having large receptive fields but also whenever there is convergence and divergence in the projection from one neuronal level to another.

Lateral inhibition also tends to enhance edges. A cell lying just within the edge of an extended uniform stimulus will receive less lateral inhibition than one further in (Fig. 4.13), resulting in a pattern of neural activity that is maximal around the border of the stimulus. In many ways, lateral inhibition is analogous to adaptation but in the spatial rather than in the temporal domain: it makes neurones sensitive to a change in activity across a *pattern* of neural activity, as opposed to a change in any one neurone as a function of time. Just as adaptation causes a burst of activity at the onset of a steady stimulus, so lateral inhibition emphasizes those regions where an area of stimulation begins or ends.

One can sense this quite easily in one's own skin: stepping into a bath when the water is almost too hot to bear, the maximum discomfort is localized not so much in the foot but rather at the line formed by the surface of the water around the leg, where the spatial rate of change of temperature is greatest. Or if you put your finger into a beaker of mercury (since mercury is poisonous you need to wear a light rubber glove), what you feel is a tight constriction round the meniscus, even though the pressure is of course greatest at the fingertip. And like adaptation, lateral inhibition helps reduce the redundancy of neural signals. An analogy may help to make clear why this is.

Imagine a central weather bureau whose function is to gather information from a network of weather stations to compile up-to-the-minute charts of the changing patterns of weather in the region as a whole. One way of obtaining the necessary information would be to get the local weather stations to ring up every 5 minutes and describe local conditions. But this would not be a very economical arrangement; quite apart from the cost of the enormous number of telephone calls that would be required, the central office would have to employ a very large staff simply in order to receive them. Clearly the weather at any one place does not in practice vary much from one 5-minute period to the next, so that most of the phone calls in such a system would be redundant, consisting simply of the message 'same as before'. The first rationalizing step would be to instruct the local stations to ring only when a *change* in the weather has occurred; to act, in fact, like completely adapting sense organs. The next improvement would be to recognize the existence of *spatial* redundancy in their reports; in general, the weather experienced by any one station is likely to be much the same as that experienced by its neighbours. So by telling the local stations to call only when they are aware that they are on the *edge* of a particular condition (a cold front, for instance), the number of calls, and the staff required to process them, could be reduced still further. We

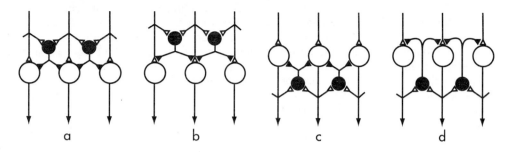

FIG. 4.14 Four possible varieties of lateral inhibition. **(a)** Feedforward, postsynaptic; **(b)** feedforward, presynaptic; **(c)** feedback, postsynaptic; **(d)** feedback, presynaptic.

shall see later that this process is particularly prominent in the visual system. It helps to explain why outline drawings are as effective as they are in evoking the appearance of what they represent, even though topologically they are so different: since the visual system in effect converts everything it sees into an outline drawing anyway, it doesn't mind if what it normally throws away isn't there.

However, the one thing that lateral inhibition cannot do – contrary to a popular misconception – is to improve *acuity*. Acuity is a measure of how well a sensory system can transmit in its neural images the spatial detail that is presented to it. A common test of cutaneous acuity is the *two-point discrimination test*: the skin is stimulated at two points simultaneously – a pair of dividers does this very well – and the distance between the points is gradually increased until the subject has the sensation that there are two points and not one. Cutaneous acuity varies greatly from one part of the body to another, almost in proportion to the size of its representation in the somatosensory cortex, from a few millimetres on the fingers to nearly 50 on the calves. This variation essentially reflects the size of the cutaneous receptive fields, for if two points of stimulation are separated by less than the receptive field size, no amount of subsequent neural processing in the form of lateral inhibition or anything else will enable one to distinguish the neural image from that produced by a single point. *Localization*, on the other hand, is in general more accurate than acuity, because of the extra information provided by the overlap of receptive fields. Consequently, one finds the apparently paradoxical situation that with the dividers set to a distance less than the local acuity, so that we cannot tell whether

there is one point or two, one can nevertheless still tell, when only one of the points is applied, which one it was.

Finally, it is worth mentioning that the neural circuit for lateral inhibition presented in Figure 4.12 is only one of several possible arrangements that have broadly similar effects. The one that is shown there is a feedforward system – the source of the inhibition is the incoming fibres, and the inhibition itself is of the postsynaptic type. In fact, it appears that the lateral inhibition actually observed in the dorsal column nuclei is presynaptic in nature (Fig. 4.14b), and results in depolarization of the afferent terminals. At higher levels of the somatosensory system, in the thalamus and cortex, lateral inhibition appears to be mainly postsynaptic. A further possibility is that it may be not the incoming fibres but collaterals of the outgoing ones that excite the inhibitory interneurones: this is called *feedback* lateral inhibition, and is found, for instance, at the level of the thalamic relay of ascending somatosensory pathways; its functional properties are slightly different. Finally, feedback inhibition may originate not from the outgoing fibres themselves but from the higher levels to which they project; the cortex can be shown to inhibit both thalamic and dorsal column relays in this way, as well as the spinothalamic pathways at the level of the cord itself.

We shall see later (Chapter 13, p. 268) that the idea of lateral inhibition can be extended considerably, particularly to cases in which the 'laterality' is not literally spatial, and inhibition extends to neurones which are adjacent in a more abstract sense (for example, responding to stimuli that are similar in terms of modality).

CENTRAL RESPONSES

Thalamic responses to lemniscal and anterolateral afferents are not particularly interesting: they show the modality specificity that would be expected from the fibres that project to them, in contralateral receptive fields that may sometimes be larger than those of neurones at lower levels in the somatosensory system. In somatosensory area SI of the cortex, responses are again not qualitatively different from those in the thalamus. One striking feature of the distribution of responses over the cortical surface, apart from its large-scale organization in the form of the sensory homunculus already described, is the fact that the cortical organization appears to be in the form of a mosaic of *columns* a few hundred micrometres in diameter, such that responses from cells at any depth within a particular column are confined both to a particular modality and also to a localized region of the skin. In general, each column is surrounded by neighbours of different modality but similar location, and there are mutually inhibitory connections between columns that presumably accentuate differences in their activity by a kind of lateral inhibition. There also appear to be differences between the Brodmann areas 1, 2 and 3 in the predominance of the different classic modalities, at least as regards deep versus superficial receptors. What is also striking is the extent to which these maps are labile and dynamic: simply bandaging a monkey's hand is sufficient to cause a reduction within a matter of hours in the hand's representation in the cortical map, and after amputation or severing of peripheral nerves the cortical representation is lost altogether, taken over by other parts that are more functional.

In the second sensory area, SII, we begin to find evidence of more complex kinds of analysis of afferent information. Units here are on the whole bilaterally activated, and the receptive field for one side of the body is approximately the mirror image of that for the other. Many of the cells show specific responses to stimuli that move across the skin in particular directions. As one examines more and more outlying regions of the somatosensory cortex, one begins to find cells that may respond to more than one stimulus modality, and also to painful stimuli, a property not usually reported in the main part of SI and SII.

Electrical stimulation of the somatosensory cortex in conscious human subjects tends to produce tingling, 'electrical' sensations rather than the illusion of actual tactile stimulation; pain is only rarely reported. Lesions here result in raised tactile thresholds, in reduced two-point discrimination, and a general impairment in the finer somatosensory judgements such as estimating weights. In humans, lesions affecting the further, posterior parietal regions of the somatosensory cortex are sometimes associated with *astereognosis*, an inability to 'put together' somatosensory information in judging such things as the shape of an object held in the hand, even though primary somatic sensibility – as measured by tests such as the two-point acuity threshold – may be relatively unimpaired. Posterior parietal cortex is further considered in Chapter 13.

PAIN

It is a common experience that there are two qualities of pain sensation, often called pricking pain or first pain and burning pain or second pain. If one stubs one's toe against something, the feeling is a sort of immediate 'Ow!' followed by a more drawn-out 'Ooooh!', and these two kinds of pain are thought to be the result of stimulating the Aδ and C fibres respectively. The main evidence for this comes from experiments in humans in which the conduction of peripheral nerves is partially blocked either by anoxia or by local anaesthetics. Anoxia, which can most easily be produced by inflating a cuff round the arm, affects the largest fibres first and the C fibres only after a considerable delay. The subject loses pressure and position sense first; then, as the Aδ fibres begin to be affected, temperature sense and pricking pain; and lastly burning pain and itch. The sequence of block for local anaesthetics is different: the C fibres are the first to suffer, and the largest A fibres the last; as a result it is then burning pain and itch that are the first to go, followed by temperature and pricking pain, and lastly pressure. Recordings from single afferents have shown that the Aδ pain fibres are specifically sensitive to mechanical deformation of the skin and that although their receptive fields are quite large, *within* each field the sensitivity is limited to specific 'pain spots' similar to those found in the case of thermoreception. The C fibres, on the other hand, are of various types: some show a response to mechanical stimulation while others respond specifically to extreme cold or heat. Both these and the Aδ fibres responding to noxious stimuli are thought to originate in the free endings of the skin.

One might wonder what purpose is served by having both fast and slow fibres signalling pain. It is often helpful, when faced with peculiarities in sensory coding, to think not so much of the sensations they produce but rather what *use* they are to the body – what behaviour they are meant to control. Pain elicits two very different kinds of response. One is reflex *withdrawal,* as when touching a hot object; the other is *immobilization,* protecting the affected part from being further injured by movement (particularly obvious after a back injury). Withdrawal demands a rapid response and fast-conducting fibres; immobilization is a long-term response where slow fibres will do perfectly well. (The question of why we have warm and cold endings rather than a single temperature receptor may be answered in an analogous way.) It is significant that visceral pain is mediated by C fibres only, since withdrawal here is not an option.

Pain may also be experienced by certain kinds of stimulation of the viscera, particularly severe distension or constriction; yet the digestive tract is said to be quite insensitive to some stimuli – notably cutting and burning, and some chemical stimuli – that are painful when applied to the skin. Visceral pain is often felt not in its 'true' position but *referred* to the region of body surface that shares the same dorsal root: thus pain is felt in the groin in response to a stone in the ureter, and in the left arm in angina pectoris. A corresponding observation is that all cells in the spinal cord that respond to stimulation of visceral afferents also have a somatic receptive field. *Itch* is not well understood. The blocking experiments described above indicate that the information generating the sense of itching is carried in C fibres but specific itch fibres have never been found. It may, like tickle, simply represent the sensation produced by a particular pattern of stimulation of the C fibres, perhaps as the result of the release of histamine from damaged tissue, an extremely powerful stimulus for itch when injected locally. Both stimuli, as always with C fibres, *demand* a response.

The central pathways for pain start with the anterolateral system, a section of which causes a complete peripheral analgesia for both pricking and burning pain. At higher levels the two types of pain show slightly differing distributions; ascending fibres concerned with pricking pain go to the somatosensory thalamus and from thence to the cortex, particularly area SII, while the pathways for burning pain appear to be both older and more diffuse, involving the more central thalamic regions, with their rather general projections to the cortex, the ascending reticular formation, periaqueductal grey and hypothalamus. In humans, interference with the thalamus generally has more effect on pain than with the cortex. Electrical stimulation of the ventrobasal region may produce sensations of pricking pain, and of the central regions a general sense of intense unpleasantness. Lesions of the thalamus can have widely varying effects ranging from relief from pre-existing chronic pain to the production of unendurable spontaneous pain, while the sensation of pain is usually unaffected, or at most slightly reduced, by cortical damage. Correspondingly, stimulation of cortex has never been reported as producing pain sensations.

The central pathways for pain are in fact rather complex and poorly understood, partly because the sensation of pain is itself very complex. The relation between the type or intensity of a stimulus and the degree of pain that is felt is a highly variable one that depends to a large extent on the emotional state of the subject and on any implications or meaning that the pain may have. We have all had the experience of injuring ourselves inadvertently and of not feeling pain until we actually see what we have done. In states of excitement, as frequently reported by soldiers severely wounded in battle, there may be a general insensitivity to injuries that would certainly be painful under normal circumstances. In one study, more than a third of patients admitted to an emergency clinic said that they felt no pain when they were injured. Conversely, some patients, perhaps when particularly apprehensive, may show exaggerated responses to quite mild stimuli: in the dentist's chair, we may respond violently to almost any unexpected dental stimulus. One might almost go so far as to call pain an *emotion* that is simply triggered off by certain patterns of cutaneous stimulation in certain behavioural circumstances but not others, in much the same way that, for example, the very same pattern of skin stimulation may produce erotic sensations when done by one person but not by another. One of the clearest pieces of evidence that there is a degree of separation between peripheral neural discharges and the objective sense of the existence of a noxious stimulus on the one hand, and actually *feeling* the pain on the other, comes from patients who have undergone frontal leucotomy to relieve intractable pain. As described later in Chapter 13, on questioning they may indicate to the doctor that they sense the pain, yet from their attitude and mood it is evident that they do not, in any normal sense, 'feel' it.

Pain is also influenced to a larger extent than other sensory modalities by other modes of skin stimulation, being reduced, for example, by warmth and by mechanical stimulation such as rubbing or for that matter by acupuncture; self-stimulation with implanted electrodes has been used successfully for many years for the relief of certain kinds of intractable pain. Conversely, in certain circumstances

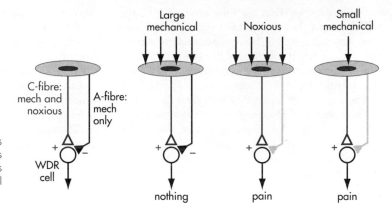

FIG. 4.15 Lateral inhibition in WDR cells between large and nociceptive afferents increases specificity to noxious stimuli, as well as causing pain from mild, small mechanical stimuli.

specific damage to the larger cutaneous afferents may result in an increased sensitivity to painful stimuli. A plausible model of the neural mechanism for this antagonism between the large cutaneous afferents and the small pain fibres has been proposed by Melzack and Wall (1962). Interneurones in the substantia gelatinosa, in layers I and II of the dorsal horn, receive excitatory information relayed from incoming large mechanical fibres, and inhibit the neurones of the ascending anterolateral system; thus the size of central response to a nociceptive stimulus will depend in general on the balance between the degree of stimulation of the large and small fibres. Although the precise details of this gating mechanism are unclear and to some extent controversial, recordings from the anterolateral neurones show that the majority of them, called *wide dynamic range* or WDR cells, do indeed have the kinds of properties that would be expected from such an arrangement. Typically, they have a concentric receptive field arrangement in which the centre responds to light touch as well as noxious stimuli, but the surround is inhibited by mechanical stimulation (Fig. 4.15). One can think of this as a mechanism for making the signals that are sent to the brain more specifically nociceptive than the Aδ fibres themselves that respond to mechanical stimulation as well as noxious stimuli; with purely mechanical stimuli, provided they are large enough, the effects of centre and surround will cancel each other out, and an erroneous pain message will not be transmitted. Here, a kind of lateral inhibition is used not to reduce the effects of spatial overlap but rather to reduce overlap between modalities. In addition, this has the further desirable property that sufficiently *small* mechanical stimuli will also cause pain before they actually cause tissue damage. It is a matter of common experience that such stimuli – a thorn, the point of a drawing pin – do indeed cause pain

without damaging the skin in the slightest; the advantage of responding in this way when walking barefoot is obvious enough.

Direct evidence that the feeling of pain is not linked in any simple, direct way to 'pain' fibres has come from recording from C fibres in conscious human subjects. Heat is applied to the skin until pain is just felt, and the frequency of discharge is noted. Then pressure is applied instead, and increased until the nerve is firing at the same frequency: yet no pain is felt until the pressure is increased much further and the frequency is some four or five times higher than the original threshold.

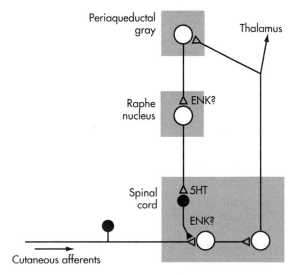

FIG. 4.16 A system associated with the neuropeptide enkephalin (ENK) that may serve to modify the transmission of afferent impulses generating the feeling of pain and associated responses.

Some of the descending control exerted by the brain on the transmission of pain messages seems to be related to the release of the natural opiates, the *endorphins* and *enkephalins*. The functions of these neuropeptides, that are widely distributed as transmitters throughout the nervous system and to some extent as hormones as well, are not yet fully understood. Some of them produce marked analgesia when injected either intravenously or into particular regions of the brain. One such area is the *periaqueductal grey*; it is thought that an excitatory pathway exists from this region to the raphe nucleus of the medullary reticular formation, which in turn sends descending fibres down into the spinal cord which ultimately inhibit the transmission of afferent pain impulses through a spinal interneurone that itself releases enkephalin (Fig. 4.16). It may well be that one of the ways in which this system is activated is by the pain fibres that project to the periaqueductal grey, providing a negative feedback system by which pain might modify its own transmission.

References

Halata, Z. (1975) The mechanoreceptors of mammalian skin. Ultrastructure and morphological classification. *Advances in Anatomy, Embryology and Cell Biology* 50, 1–77.

Kenshalo, D. R. (1976) Correlates of temperature sensitivity in Man and monkey, a first approximation. In *Sensory Functions of the Skin in Primates*, ed. Y. Zotterman. Oxford University Press, Oxford.

Melzack, R. and Wall, P.D. (1962) On the nature of cutaneous sensory mechanisms. *Brain* 85, 331–356.

Penfield, W. and Rasmussen, T. (1950) *The Cerebral Cortex of Man: a Clinical Study of Localisation of Function*. Macmillan, New York.

NOTES

The skin Useful general accounts include Sinclair, D. (1981) *Mechanisms of Cutaneous Sensation* (Oxford University Press, Oxford); Willis, W. D. and Coggeshall, R. E. (1978) *Sensory Mechanisms of the Spinal Cord* (Wiley, New York); Zotterman, Y. (1976) *Sensory Functions of the Skin in Primates* (Oxford University Press, Oxford).

Page 74 Modalities are just names An example may make this clearer. Imagine a simple-minded creature – perhaps some kind of slug – whose cutaneous sensations fall into only three categories: 'wet', 'earth' and 'nice' – the last being the result of contact with a slug of the opposite sex. A slug who studies physiology and investigates the responses of his own somatosensory neurones would find that some fibres – what we call 'light touch' receptors – fire during both 'earth' and 'nice', while others ('cold') fire during 'wet' and sometimes during 'earth', and so on: he would deduce in fact that his fibres were not modality-specific but that 'earth', 'wet' and 'nice' were coded in the form of particular patterns of activity. A human physiologist would completely disagree: what he would report would be highly specific fibres responding to the traditional categories of 'warm', 'cold', 'light touch' and so on: but the argument would clearly be about the naming of sensory categories, not about the observations themselves.

A thoughtful discussion of this whole area (one that many students find difficult) can be found in Melzack, R. and Wall, P. D. (1962) On the nature of cutaneous sensory mechanisms. *Brain* 85, 331–356.

Page 74 Complexity of skin sensation Two accounts that do justice to this area: Katz, D. (1989) *The World of Touch* (Lawrence Erlbaum, Hillsdale, New Jersey); and Sathian, K. (1989) Tactile sensing of surface features. *Trends in Neuroscience* 12, 513–519.

Page 74 Visceral afferents They – and probably small somatic afferents as well – contain an extraordinary range of peptide transmitters, including VIP, somatostatin, angiotensin, substance P, CCK-like peptides, and so on. What are they all for?

Fig. 4.3 Dermatomes The boundaries between dermatomes are nothing like as sharp as the figure implies, and there is a certain amount of disagreement between authors concerning some of the details. An excellent source, with comparisons with the earlier maps of Head, Elze, Richter and others, is Hansen, K, and Schliak, H. (1962) *Segmentale Innervation. Ihre Bedeutung für Klinik und Praxis* (Georg Thieme Verlag, Stuttgart); another is Keegan, J. J. and Garrett, F.D. (1948) The segmental distribution of the cutaneous nerves in the limbs of man. *Anatomical Records* 102, 409–437.

Page 75 Morphology of endings See for instance Iggo, A. and Andres, K. H. (1982) Morphology of cutaneous receptors. *Annual Review of Neuroscience* 5, 1–31; and Halata, Z. (1975) The mechanoreceptors of mammalian skin. Ultrastructure and morphological classification. *Advances in Anatomy, Embryology and Cell Biology* 50, 1–77.

Page 79 Slip and grip See for example Johansson, R. S. and Westling, G. (1987) Signals in tactile afferents from the fingers eliciting adaptive motor responses during precision grip. *Experimental Brain Research* 66, 141–154. Robot hands designed for grasping and lifting objects are sometimes provided with a similar sense, in the form of microphones built into the gripping surfaces whose output is used in a feedback loop to increase the pressure when the object is slipping.

Page 79 Single units of the human hand See for example Johansson, R. S. (1978) Tactile sensibility in the human hand: receptive field characteristics of mechanoreceptive units in the glabrous skin area. *Journal of Physiology* 281, 101–127; Johansson, R. S. and Vallbo, Å. (1979) Tactile sensibility in the human hand: relative and absolute densities of four types of mechanoreceptive units in glabrous skin. *Journal of Physiology* 286, 283–300; Vallbo, Å., Olsson, K. Å., Westberg, K.-G. and Clark, F. J. (1984) Microstimulation of single tactile afferents from the human hand. *Brain* 107, 727–749.

Page 81 Overlap providing redundancy This principle seems to extend right up to higher levels of the sensory pathways. Recordings from sensory cortex in conscious cats have shown that local anaesthesia in the periphery can cause an almost immediate restructuring of cortical receptive fields, with the appearance of new areas that previously had no effective contribution. See Metzler, J. and Marks, P. S. (1979) Functional changes in cat somatosensory and motor cortex during short-term reversible epidural blocks. *Brain Research* 177, 379–383.

Page 84 Lability of cortical maps See for instance Merzenich, M.M. (1989) Representational plasticity in somatosensory and motor cortical fields. *Biomedical Research* 10, 85–86.

Page 84 Pain Intelligent accounts may be found in Holden, A. V. and Winlow, W. (1984) *The Neurobiology of Pain* (Manchester University Press, Manchester); and Melzack, R. and Wall, P. D. (1982) *The Challenge of Pain* (Penguin, Harmondsworth).

Page 85 Injury without pain See Wall, P. D. (1985) Pain and no pain. In *Functions of the Brain*, ed. C. W. Coen. Clarendon, Oxford.

Page 86 Gating theory This theory generated a quite astonishing degree of hostility when it was first proposed, partly, one suspects, because people did not like to have their comfortable, simplistic ideas of 'one fibre, one modality' unsettled. See Melzack, R. and Wall, P. D. (1982) *The Challenge of Pain*. (Penguin, Harmondsworth), p. 233.

Page 86 Human single C fibres See van Hees, J. and Gybels, J. M. (1972) Pain related to single afferent C fibers from human skin. *Brain Research* 48, 397–400.

NEUROLAB

Pacinian corpuscle

Page 75

This exhibit has already been described, in Chapter 3: see p. 70.

Spinal tracts

Page 77

A simple self-testing exhibit covering the ascending and descending tracts of the spinal cord. Click on one of the buttons round the edge of the cross-section (ascending paths on the right, descending on the left). The name of the corresponding tract will appear in the box at top right. Alternatively, click on the button to the right of the box to bring down a list of tracts: click on one, and its corresponding button will display.

Anatomical pathways

Page 77

A database of nuclei and other areas in the CNS, and the tracts and pathways that join them, that you can use for reference or for self-testing. The two upper windows list sources and destinations, the lower one has the names of tracts that join them. If you click on the name of a tract, its origin(s) and destination(s) appear in the upper windows. To restore the full lists, click on Show all. If you click on a source in one of the upper windows, the destination window lists the major areas to which it projects, and the corresponding tracts are listed below. Similarly, clicking on a destination shows the sources and their linking tracts. Double-clicking on a destination takes you one stage further on, by treating it as a source and showing you *its* destinations; similarly, double-clicking on a source takes you one stage further back.

Lateral inhibition

Page 82

This exhibit demonstrates various aspects of lateral inhibition. Some of the items in it are essentially visual, and are described in Chapter 7, p. 168. The section which is more general is on the left, which shows a spatial stimulus (blue) and the spatial pattern of its response (green). The radio buttons choose as stimulus either a single line or point, an edge or a pair of lines. The buttons just to the right generate either blur or lateral inhibition, and can be used repetitively to increase the effect: Restore returns to the original state. At top right, the slider called Completeness determines how much lateral inhibition is applied. Look first at an edge, blur it once, and then apply lateral inhibition once; do this for several settings of completeness. With full completeness, the steady DC component on each side of the edge is completely removed. Using a point stimulus, notice how lateral inhibition counteracts blur, at least up to a point. With a double stimulus, notice that if you add blur to the point where the two stimuli cannot be distinguished, lateral inhibition does not separate them

again: in other words, strictly speaking lateral inhibition does not improve acuity.

Cortical regions

Page 84
A simple map of functional cortical areas, for self-testing. Click on one of the radio buttons designating an area of cortex, and the name and Brodmann number will appear in the box at right. Alternatively, click on the pull-down button at the right of the box to display the whole list, and click on an item: the corresponding radio button will be selected.

5

PROPRIOCEPTION

Muscle proprioceptors 90
Joint receptors 94

Conscious proprioception 94
The vestibular apparatus 95

This chapter is concerned with those mechanoreceptors that provide us with information about ourselves: about the positions and movements of our limbs, the forces generated by our muscles, and our attitude and motion relative to the earth. The main use to which this information is put by the brain is of course in the control of movements; consequently a discussion of the functions of these proprioceptive modalities is left until Chapters 10 and 11, which deal with the control of muscle length and of posture.

MUSCLE PROPRIOCEPTORS

Two distinct kinds of proprioceptors are found in voluntary muscles, specialized for providing information about two quite different quantities: *muscle spindles* that respond to muscle *length* and rate of change of length; and *Golgi tendon organs* that signal muscle *tension* or force. Both of these are in essence stretch receptors: their difference in function comes about because of their different situation in the muscle as a whole (Figure 5.1). Whereas the spindles are in *parallel* with the main contractile elements in the muscle, so that their stretching is simply a measure of the degree of stretch of the muscle itself, the tendon organs are situated in the muscle tendons, in *series* with the contractile elements and the load, so that their stretch is proportional to the tension exerted by the muscle.

Spindles

Muscle spindles are found in practically all the striated muscles of the body, but are greatly outnumbered by the striated muscle fibres themselves: in cat soleus, there is only one spindle for every 500 or so ordinary fibres. Each consists of a fluidfilled capsule some 2–4 mm long and a few

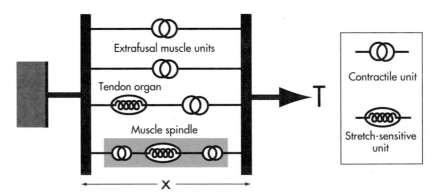

FIG. 5.1 Schematic representation of contractile and stretch-sensitive elements in muscle. The contractile elements within the spindle (intrafusal) are innervated separately from the main (extrafusal) muscle fibres, and make only a negligible contribution to overall muscle tension *T*. Thus, whereas tendon organs respond essentially to muscle tension, spindles respond to length, *x*, but in a manner modified by the activity of their own contractile elements.

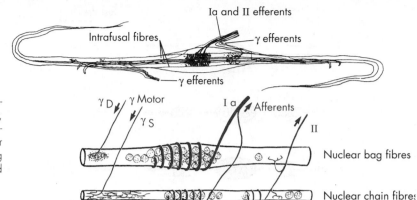

FIG. 5.2 A typical mammalian muscle spindle (simplified from Barker, 1948). Below, schematic representation of the central region of a nuclear bag and nuclear chain fibre, showing the afferent Ia and II innervation, and the two kinds of γ fibre.

hundred micrometres in diameter, whose ends are attached to the exterior sheaths of neighbouring muscle fibres (Figure 5.2). Inside is a small number of modified muscle fibres called *intrafusal* fibres (the 'fus-' root means 'spindle'), each having contractile ends, and a region in the middle that is not contractile but contains the nuclei. Two main types of intrafusal fibre are found, differing in the way in which these nuclei are distributed. *Nuclear chain* fibres are thinner, and their nuclei are lined up in a row along the central portion like peas in a pod; *nuclear bag* fibres have a pronounced bulge in the middle in which the nuclei are bunched together. A typical spindle has some half-dozen intrafusal fibres, the nuclear chain fibres generally being in the majority. Two kinds of afferent or sensory fibres innervate the spindle: the larger, *primary* fibres, belonging to group Ia, send branches to the central portions of both types of fibre and have annulospiral endings; the smaller *secondary* fibres are of group II and terminate partly as annulospiral and partly as flower-spray endings mainly on the nuclear chain fibres, more peripherally than the Ia endings.

These two kinds of nerve fibre respond very differently to muscle stretch. The secondary fibres are in a sense the simpler: their signals are more or less directly proportional to the degree of stretch of the spindle at any moment so that their frequency of firing, whether the muscle is suddenly stretched to a new length, stretched more slowly, made to shorten, or alternately stretched and relaxed in a sinusoidal manner, mirrors quite accurately the instantaneous value of the muscle length (Figure 5.3). These fibres are thus essentially non-adapting or *static*. The Ia fibres, in contrast, are dynamic and show very pronounced adaptation. During a sudden stretch they fire maximally during the period of stretching and only at a reduced rate when the muscle is held at its new length; during a slow stretch they again respond most during the movement, at a frequency nearly proportional to the rate of stretch; and during sinusoidal stretching their maximum firing is not at the moment of maximum stretch but near the point of maximum *rate of change* of stretch. In other words, they respond partly in proportion to muscle length (though rather little at rest) but mostly in proportion to its rate of change or velocity.

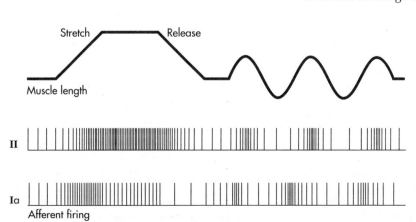

FIG. 5.3 Idealised responses of primary (Ia) and secondary (II) fibres to various patterns of muscular stretch. (After Matthews, 1964)

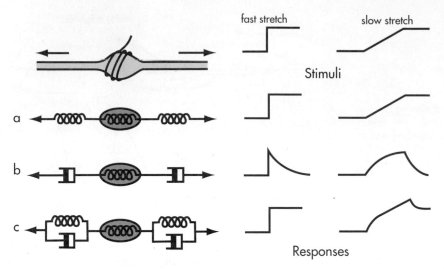

FIG. **5.4** Left, three simple models of the mechanical properties of fibres: **(a)** peripheral region purely elastic; **(b)** purely viscous; (spindle **c**) mixed (viscoelastic). Right, the response of each model, assumed to be proportional to stretch of the central region, to a sudden stretch and to slow stretching. Actual Ia fibres behave most like (c), group II fibres like **(a)**.

Now we saw in Chapter 3 that adaptation in sensory receptors can in general be due to several distinct processes: there may be energy filtering, in which static information is wholly or partly thrown away before it even reaches the transducer element itself, or there may be membrane adaptation, in which even a steady conductance at the ending results in a fall-off in firing frequency. Whereas in the Pacinian corpuscle both of these mechanisms contribute almost equally to the adaptation that is observed, in the case of the muscle spindle it appears that nearly all is of the energy-filtering kind, and not very different from what is produced by the concentric lamellae of the Pacinian corpuscle. The contractile portions of the intrafusal fibres behave as if they were very much more viscous than the central portion (this is particularly true of the nuclear-bag fibres), so that the mechanical properties of the fibres as a whole may be represented by a mechanical model like that of Figure 5.4. In a brief stretch, there is no time for the viscous elements to lengthen, and the stretch is entirely taken up by the central region, where the annulospiral endings are; but if the stretch is maintained, the viscous elements gradually yield, releasing the strain on the middle portion, and thus resulting in a lower frequency of firing. The difference between the non-adapting properties of the secondary fibres and the marked adaptation of the primaries seems partly to be due to the fact that the former go only to chain fibres, which are less viscous, and also to the fact that they innervate more peripheral parts of them.

Besides the two kinds of afferent fibre, spindles also receive a motor innervation from the γ-fibres, (belonging to group Aγ) and around 6 μm in diameter. There are two types of fusimotor fibre, called γ_s and γ_d – static and dynamic – and they innervate respectively the nuclear chain (mostly) and nuclear bag fibres (Figure 5.2), causing contraction of the peripheral regions. For any given muscle length, such a contraction must of course stretch the sensory elements and thus increase the firing of the afferent fibres, and in fact the effect of γ stimulation is in general much the same as if an extra stretch had been applied to the muscle as a whole, though they may also increase the *sensitivity* of the endings to stretch. Figure 5.5 shows some recordings of the firing frequency of stretch receptor afferents in response to different degrees of stretch, when the corresponding γ fibres were also stimulated at different rates: the interaction between external stretch, and the internal stretch produced by the γ activation, can be clearly seen. The static and dynamic γ fibres produce slightly different effects on primary and secondary afferent responses, as would be expected from their differing distribution to the bag and chain fibres. Dynamic γ fibres increase the sensitivity of group Ia fibres but have no effect on group II fibres, whereas the static ones increase the sensitivity of both the secondaries and primaries to static stretch but actually decrease the primary sensitivity to rate of stretch. Thus the central nervous system can, through the γ efferents, control not just the sensitivity of the spindle afferents

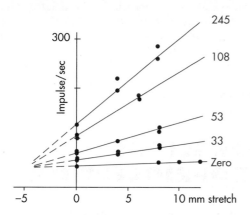

FIG. 5.5 Effect of γ fibre stimulation on afferent response to stretch in an eye muscle from the goat; the rates of stimulation are shown on the right. (Data from Whitteridge, 1959)

but also in a sense their adaptational properties. The way in which this control is actually used by the motor system is left for consideration in Chapter 10.

Golgi tendon organs

The *Golgi tendon organs* have received much less attention from experimenters. In appearance they are very similar to the Ruffini organs in the skin (Chapter 4), and like them appear to respond to tension in the fibres with which they are associated, in the tendon; they are innervated by afferents of group Ib. At one time their importance was underestimated because they seemed to have such high thresholds: large forces had to be applied to the tendon as a whole before they could be induced to fire. But it is now clear that this was because in these circumstances the total tension applied is in effect shared out amongst the tendinous fascicles, so that each tendon organ feels only a small fraction of it: they respond in fact very briskly to the modest tensions generated by the actual muscle fibres to which they are joined. Because they register tension rather than muscle length, during active movements their discharge generally has a reciprocal relationship to that of the muscle spindles: extrafusal activity simultaneously increases the tension in the tendons and decreases muscle length but during passive movements, both kinds of response are normally in step with one another.

Central pathways

The central pathways of both these sensory modalities are quite similar. Fibres enter the dorsal roots in the usual way, and the majority synapse in a spinal nucleus called Clarke's column with fibres that ascend in the homolateral *posterior spinocerebellar tract* to an extremely important region in the control of movement, the *cerebellum* (Figure 5.6). However, Clarke's column fades out above T1 or so, and more rostral afferents turn upwards and ascend to the *accessory cuneate nucleus* of the medulla, from which fibres run in the *cuneocerebellar tract*. Another route by which both cutaneous and proprioceptive information may reach the cerebellum is via the *spino-olivary tract* to the inferior olive, which in turn projects through climbing fibres to the cerebellar cortex (see Chapter 12). Apart from ascending to the cerebellum, branches of fibres from muscle proprioceptors are involved in various reflex mechanisms within the spinal cord, notably the *stretch reflex* (which in its simplest form consists of a monosynaptic excitation of a motor neurone by a Ia afferent) and the *clasp-knife reflex*: these are discussed in Chapter 10. There is also some projection of muscle proprioceptors to the cerebral cortex, via the ventral posterior thalamus.

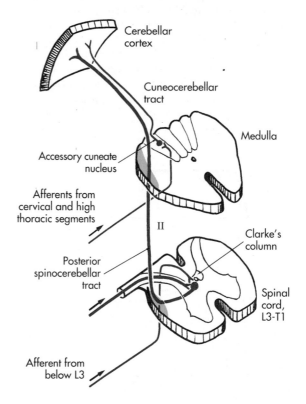

FIG. 5.6 Schematic representation of the principal spinocerebellar pathways. An additional route, not shown, is via the inferior olive and climbing fibres (I, II: first- and second-order fibres).

JOINT RECEPTORS

Another important source of information about limb position and movement comes from the mechanoreceptors that are found in the ligaments and capsules of joints. They are of a variety of morphological types, some very similar or identical to those found in the skin. Thus Pacinian corpuscles and Golgi-like endings are found with large axons (group I), Ruffini endings (II), and also small nerve fibres with unencapsulated endings. Some show complete adaptation and are thus more sensitive to rate of change but most show incomplete adaptation and thus signal limb position as well (Figure 5.7). The patterns of response are complicated to a certain extent by the fact that few receptors are able to respond over the whole range of movement that a joint is capable of: their 'excitatory angle' is typically less than half the entire possible range, thus increasing sensitivity to changes in position within that range. This means that information about the position of a limb is partly coded by frequency of firing but also by *which* neurones are firing. Although in some joints, most of the afferent fibres fire preferentially at extremes of joint position and are presumably intended to give warning that the joint is about to become dislocated, nevertheless there appear to be sufficient fibres responding at midrange positions to provide adequate proprioceptive information; in other joints the majority are midrange anyway. Afferent information from joints follows the same route as that from

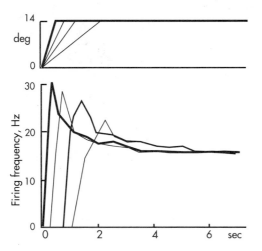

FIG. 5.7 Firing frequency of an afferent from a cat's knee-joint in response to flexion through a fixed angle at the different rates shown at the top, demonstrating incomplete adaptation. (Data from Boyd and Roberts, 1953)

Pacinian and other corpuscles in the skin (see Figure 4.5): fibres ascend in the ipsilateral posterior columns, relay in the cuneate and gracile nuclei, cross and proceed via the medial lemniscus to the ventral posterolateral thalamus and thence to the somatosensory cortex; some also contribute to the spinocerebellar pathways.

CONSCIOUS PROPRIOCEPTION

How are these sources of information actually used by the brain in sensing the position of our limbs? For a long time this question was the subject of bitter controversy between those who believed that such sensations came only from the muscles and those who favoured joint receptors, each side seeking to show that the other mechanism contributed nothing at all. It seems strange in retrospect that the modern view that *both* contribute, and indeed other sources of information such as the skin as well, was not grasped sooner.

The main evidence that mechanoreceptors in joints contribute to proprioception comes by anaesthetizing the receptors either by direct injection into the synovial fluid or by putting an inflatable cuff around the limb in such a way that it stops the blood flow to the joint but not to the muscles that move it. The sense of limb position is then greatly impaired, though the subject will generally still be able to sense movement: static proprioception is more affected than dynamic. It is clear, therefore, that the joints contribute to proprioception but that they are not the *sole* source. Indeed, after operations in which the hip joint is replaced with a prosthesis and the mechanoreceptors are entirely lost, the patient can still sense joint position (though with reduced sensitivity), presumably by using information from muscles and from the skin. Conversely, it is not difficult to demonstrate the muscle contribution directly. Conscious patients have often reported a sense of limb movement when surgeons pull on exposed tendons without moving the joint. A less traumatic way of stimulating the stretch receptors is to apply a vibrator to a muscle or its tendon, which acts preferentially on the Ia endings because of the high rates of stretch it generates. Such a stimulus produces an illusion that the muscle is shortening even though it is in fact held stationary, as can be seen if the subject is asked to match the felt position of the vibrated arm with the other one: this feeling is greatly enhanced if at the same time a cuff has been applied in such a way that the corresponding joint is anaesthetized. Under these conditions it can be shown that the illusion is essentially one of a roughly constant *rate* of movement rather than of static position.

Experiments like these leave little room for doubt: both joints and muscles play a part in providing proprioceptive information, with limb position being sensed more by joint receptors, and velocity by spindles; it also seems highly probable that skin receptors round joints play a part as well, though this is less well established. The other sensation that we seem to get from our muscles is that of the forces we exert with them, and the sense of weight. In this case it is clear from experiments that as well as mechanical information from the skin, an important factor is the sense of *effort*, the size of the commands that we send to them. In circumstances where an extra effort is needed for the same load, because a reflex contribution from sensory receptors has been blocked by local anaesthesia or with muscle fatigue, subjects feel that loads are heavier and that they are generating greater tensions. It may be that Golgi tendon organs also contribute to the sense of load, but this has not been demonstrated unequivocally.

Box 5.1 **Contributions to sense of limb position and muscle loading**	
Muscle	Predominantly change of position
Joints	Predominantly static position
Skin	Predominantly load; may also contribute to position sense
Efference copy	Predominantly load

THE VESTIBULAR APPARATUS

The vestibular apparatus forms part of the *labyrinth* of the inner ear. As its name suggests, it is a complex structure that has partly evolved from the lateral line organ in fishes. This is a system of tubes lined with ciliated sensory cells and in communication with the surrounding water; the cells are stimulated by the flow of water through the tubes as a result either of something moving in the outside world and setting up fluid currents or of the fish's own motion through the water. In the course of time, this system sealed itself off from the outside world, and its two functions – one exteroceptive, one proprioceptive – came to be carried out by two separate organs: the *cochlea*, signalling movement of the surrounding air in the form of sound waves (discussed in Chapter 6), and the *vestibular apparatus*, signalling movement of the head itself.

The vestibular part of the labyrinth is divided functionally into two components: the *semicircular canals*, of which there are three on each side of the head, and the *otolith organs*, of which there are two on each side, the *saccule* and *utricle* (Figure 5.8). The ciliated sensory cells are very similar in all parts of the vestibular apparatus, and will be described first; it is the accessory structures that enclose them that make them specifically responsive to different types of stimuli.

Box 5.2 **Divisions of the vestibular apparatus**	
Vestibular apparatus	**Semicircular canals** (horizontal, anterior, posterior) angular velocity
	Otolith organs (utricle, saccule) linear acceleration, and hence angular position relative to gravity

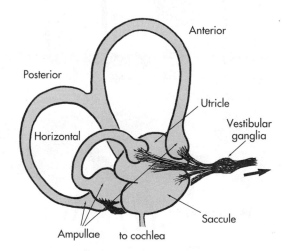

FIG. 5.8 Gross structure of the vestibular part of the labyrinth, viewed laterally (somewhat schematic).

The sensory cells

The sensory epithelium of the vestibular apparatus is made up of a mosaic of sensory cells and supporting cells, the former being divided into two morphological types: a flask-shaped *type I* cell, and a roughly cylindrical *type II* cell. Each sensory cell has a characteristic pattern of cilia projecting from its upper surface, consisting of a single flexible *kinocilium*, whose root is near the edge of the receptor, and between 60 and 100 *stereocilia*, relatively thin and stiff, and arranged in a regular array in the more central area. The latter are graded in size rather like a set of organ pipes, the longest ones being nearest to the kinocilium (Figure 5.9). The kinocilium is a much more elaborate structure than the stereocilia, having the 'nine plus two' arrangement of longitudinal filaments characteristic of motile cilia, and basal bodies. The asymmetrical arrangement of kinocilium and stereocilia defines a direction of polarization for each cell, and it is found that bending in the direction of the kinocilium leads to excitation, while bending in the opposite direction gives inhibition. The deformation caused by bending alters the ionic permeability of the stereocilia through mechanisms that are presumed to be essentially the same as in the hair cells in the cochlea, discussed in more detail in the next chapter, and probably involve direct attachments from mechanically opening channels at the tip of one stereocilium that are linked by filaments to its longer neighbour. This generates currents that alter the membrane potential of the far end of the cell, causing calcium entry and release of transmitter, which is probably glutamate.

The sensory cells are innervated by branches of the *vestibular nerve*: type I cells are almost completely enclosed in a nerve calyx or chalice, and there are often regions of close apposition which, together with the large synaptic area, suggest that the transmission process here may be partly electrical as well as chemical in nature. Type II cells generally receive more than one ending; the terminals are smaller in size, and some of them are efferent rather than afferent. There seems to be much more convergence from type II cells on to their afferent fibres than in the case of the type I cells, and more still in the case of the efferent fibres: there are only some 200 fibres in a cat's vestibular nerve going to the receptors, in contrast with the 12 000 or so afferents. Sensory and efferent fibres travel together in the vestibular division of the VIIIth nerve to the region of the *vestibular nuclei*, of which the lateral nucleus is the origin of the efferents. Most of the afferent fibres terminate within the nuclei, but some carry on through and project ultimately to the cerebellum. Most afferent fibres fire spontaneously, and one finds that a stimulus that

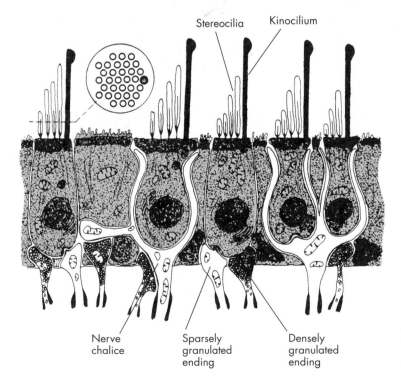

Stereocilia   Kinocilium

Nerve chalice   Sparsely granulated ending   Densely granulated ending

FIG. 5.9 Diagrammatic cross-section of sensory epithelium of vestibular system, showing type I and type II cells with their innervation. Inset, a typical arrangement of the cilia seen in horizontal section.

bends the kinocilium in one direction accelerates the rate of firing, and in the other decreases it: thus each cell has a specific direction of *polarization,* which is generally similar to its neighbours'. Different cells tend to have different spontaneous firing frequencies so that they function over different parts of the total possible range of stimulation, in a manner reminiscent of joint receptor afferents.

Otolith organs (utricle and saccule)

The utricle and saccule are a pair of hollow sacs containing *endolymph,* a fluid whose ionic composition is of the intracellular type (with a high K^+/Na^+ ratio), and continuous throughout the whole of the labyrinth. Surrounding the endolymphatic sac is a second sac containing *perilymph,* whose composition is low in K^+ and more like that of a typical extracellular fluid. The receptor cells of the otolith organs are confined to a special region of the sac called the *macula,* and their projecting cilia are embedded in a jellylike mass, the *otolith,* whose density is increased by the incorporation of large quantities of calcite crystals called otoconia. If the head is tilted, this mass moves relative to the macula, bending the cilia and thus resulting in stimulation of the afferent nerve fibres (Figure 5.10). The cells also respond to linear accelerations of the head, since in this case the otoliths tend to get left behind and hence cause the same sort of bending. Thus the afferent signals from the otolith organs are dependent simply on the vector sum of the acceleration due to gravity and any linear acceleration that may be occurring at the same time: in other words, on the *effective* direction of gravity (Figure 5.10). There is necessarily no way in which the brain can distinguish between head tilt and linear acceleration – since 'gravity' is itself of course simply a kind of linear acceleration – nor is it particularly desirable that it should. From the point of view of controlling posture (as for example in trying to stand upright in a bus that suddenly accelerates) it is the *effective* direction of gravity that matters (see Chapter 11, p.217).

Information about the direction of the acceleration vector is available because the maculae of utricle and saccule lie in different planes – in the utricle roughly horizontal, in the saccule roughly vertical – and also because in each case the direction of polarization of the hair cells varies in a systematic way over the macular surface (Figure 5.11); recordings from individual

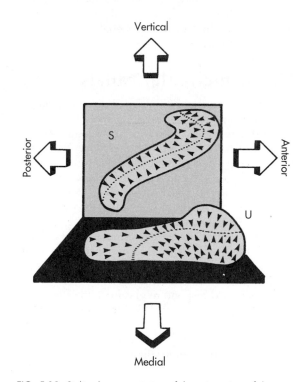

FIG. 5.11 Stylized representation of the orientation of the utricular (U) and saccular (S) maculae in the head. The small arrows indicate the approximate direction of polarization of receptors at different points on the surface.

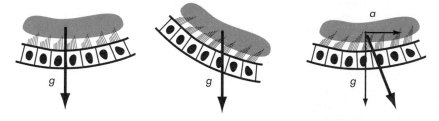

FIG. 5.10 Equivalence of head tilt and linear acceleration. Schematic representation of action of macular receptors (left) at rest, (middle) with head tilt, and (right) under horizontal linear acceleration. The last two conditions are indistinguishable as far as stimulation of the hair cells is concerned.

otolith fibres show that each one fires maximally at a particular orientation of the head, and that there is a fall-off in frequency as the head is tilted away from that position. Thus the pattern of discharge from the whole population of receptors provides information about the direction of acceleration. As might be expected, most units show little adaptation, and for the most part faithfully signal head position without decrement over indefinitely long periods of time. Some do, however, show adaptation, firing most rapidly during changes of head position, but their adaptation is not complete and their tonic discharge still gives a measure of head position: it is the semicircular canals that primarily signal *changes* in the attitude of the head.

The semicircular canals

Each canal consists of a looped tube containing endolymph and having a swelling at one point along its length, the *ampulla*, into which projects a crest, the *crista*, which is covered with sensory hair cells (Figure 5.12). Their cilia are embedded in a jellylike structure called the cupula, forming a kind of flap which can swing backwards and forwards in response to movement of fluid along the canal, thus bending the cilia and causing neural excitation. Unlike the otolith, this jelly does not contain calcareous granules, and is in fact of exactly the same density as the endolymph surrounding it: it is very important that this should be so, as otherwise the hair cells would respond to gravity in the same way as the muscular receptors. What they do respond to, in fact, is *rotation* of the head. When the head is turned, the fluid in the canals tends to get left behind and pushes on the trapdoorlike cupula, thus bending the sensory cilia.

Because the three canals on each side of the head are arranged in more or less mutually perpendicular planes (Figure 5.13) they are able to signal rotations about any axis in space. In most animals, with the head in the normal upright position, the horizontal canals are parallel with the ground, and the superior and posterior canals lie at about 45° to the sagittal plane. The cells in each crista are all oriented in the same direction: thus turning the head to the left stimulates fibres from the left horizontal canal but decreases the frequency of firing of those from the right (Figure 5.13), and similar mutual antagonisms exist between the superior canal of one side and the posterior canal of the other. Corresponding to this arrangement, one finds cells in the vestibular nuclei that are excited by a particular canal but inhibited by its opposite number on the other side, thus effectively

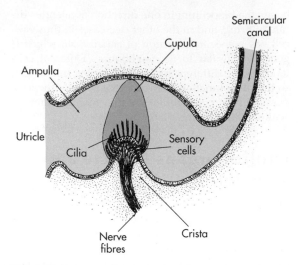

FIG. 5.12 Diagrammatic section through a single canal in the region of the ampulla, showing the cupula, the hair cells of the crista and their innervation.

combining the signals from the two sides in a 'push–pull' manner. For this reason, rotation is not a good stimulus to use if we want to test each of a subject's vestibular organs separately; instead, we need to use a stimulus that only acts on one side at a time. In clinical practice, *caloric* stimulation of the canals is sometimes used; the outer ear is irrigated with warm

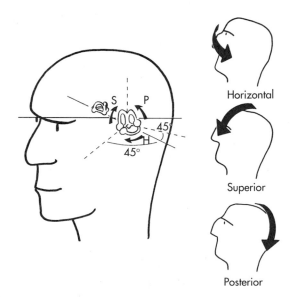

FIG. 5.13 Left, approximate orientation of the semicircular canals in humans (S, superior; H, horizontal; P, posterior); the arrows show the direction of fluid movement that is stimulatory in each case. Right, directions of head movement that stimulate each of the canals on the left side of the head.

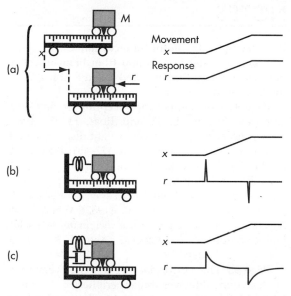

FIG. 5.14 Mechanical model of the action of the cupula in semicircular canals. **(a)** A small truck of mass *M* representing endolymph inertia rests freely on a larger truck representing the head. The reading *r* of the pointer provides a measure of the position *x* of the big truck, since the little one remains stationary. **(b)** If the two trucks are coupled elastically, *r* indicates not position but acceleration, *a*. **(c)** Actual cupular movement is as if the coupling were partly elastic but predominantly viscous: this produces an adapting *velocity* response.

water, which appears to set up convection currents in the endolymph of the canals and thus produces unilateral vestibular stimulation.

The adaptational properties of the canals are very important, and are almost entirely of the 'energy-filtering' type. If the cupula were completely unrestrained, and moved in unison with the fluid of the canal, then the bending of the cilia of the sensory cells would simply signal rotational position of the head; the endolymph would be acting rather like the gyroscope in an inertial guidance system. A mechanical model of such a system is illustrated in Figure 5.14a. A large railway truck, representing the head, has a smaller truck that is free to move on top of it, representing the cupula and the inertial mass *M* of the endolymph. If the big truck moves a distance x, the small truck will remain (in absolute terms) exactly where it was before, resulting in a relative displacement between the two – in effect, what is signalled by the hair cells – of *x*, the new *position* of the big truck.

But consider now what would happen if the little truck, instead of being completely free to move, were coupled to the big one by an elastic element, a spring (b). The system is now no longer a position detector; what we have done is to make it into an *acceleration* detector or accelerometer. For if the truck moves off with acceleration a the spring will experience a force equal to *M.a*, and will therefore stretch by an amount that is simply proportional to the acceleration. Does the cupula in fact behave as a rotational accelerometer? It is perfectly true that it is indeed elastic, and if pushed to one side exerts a restoring force that tends to bring it back to the middle. But it turns out that the cupula and the endolymph are both very *viscous* (Figure 5.14c) and the effect of this viscosity is to slow down the mechanical response. Consider a subject on a swivel chair that is suddenly set into rotation at constant angular velocity. A true accelerometer would give a brief response only at the instant at

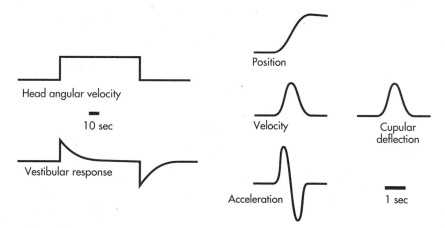

FIG. 5.15 Responses of the semicircular canals. Left, during a head rotation at constant angular velocity, canal response declines exponentially over some 20 seconds; on stopping the movement, there is an opposite response that again declines in the same way. Right, time-course of head angular position, velocity and acceleration during a natural turn of the head (left). Cupular deflection (right) behaves more like the velocity curve than either of the others. (Courtesy Dr T. D. M. Roberts)

which the rotation started, since this is the only time at which acceleration occurs; but recordings of the firing frequency of vestibular units from the canals show that in these circumstances the period of response is very much drawn out by the damping effect of the viscosity, lasting for some 20 seconds or so after the acceleration has stopped. Under *natural* circumstances – continual rotation of the head in one direction is not after all very common in real life! – the frequency of firing mirrors much more closely the instantaneous rotational *velocity* of the head than its acceleration (Figure 5.15).

In fact, the semicircular canals are not really rotational acceleration detectors at all but rather *velocity detectors*. It is only under very peculiar laboratory conditions that their acceleration sensitivity (which can be thought of as an adapting velocity response, just as velocity sensitivity is equivalent to an adapting positional response) manifests itself. A consequence of this adaptation is that a subject who has been set spinning at constant velocity has a gradually decreasing sense that he is actually rotating; even with his eyes open, after 20 seconds or so he has the strong impression that he is actually sitting still, and that the world is spinning round him, as anyone who has had a ride in a fairground 'rotor' will know. Furthermore, if the chair is then suddenly stopped, his cupula, which had previously resumed its resting position, will now be pushed in the opposite direction by the tendency of the endolymph to retain the previous motion of the head; he will then have the very strong impression of rotating in the opposite direction, although he is in fact stationary. Some postural consequences of these adaptational properties are discussed in Chapter 11.

References

Barker, D. (1948) The innervation of the muscle spindle. *Quarterly Journal of Microscopical Science* 89, 143–186.

Boyd, I. A. and Roberts, T. D. M. (1953) Proprioceptive discharges from stretch-receptors in the knee-joint of the cat. *Journal of Physiology* 122, 38–58.

Matthews, P. B. C. (1964) Muscle spindles and their control. *Physiological Review* 44, 219–288.

Whitteridge, D. (1959) The effect of stimulation of intrafusal muscle fibres on sensitivity to stretch of extraocular muscle spindles. *Quarterly Journal of Experimental Physiology* 44, 385–393.

NOTES

Page 92 Spindle motor innervation Chain fibres also receive some innervation from branches of α-fibres, sometimes (unhelpfully) called ß-fibres. Their function is unclear.

Page 94 Conscious proprioception Some useful accounts: Brodie, E. E. and Ross, H. E. (1984) Sensorimotor mechanisms in weight discrimination. *Perception and Psychophysics* 36, 477–481; Burgess, P. R., Wei, J. Y., Clark, F. J. and Simon, J. (1982) Signalling of kinaesthetic information by peripheral sensory receptors. *Annual Review of Neuroscience* 5, 171–187; Matthews, P. C. B. (1982) Where does Sherrington's 'muscular sense' originate? Muscles, joints, corollary discharges? *Annual Review of Neuroscience* 5, 189–218.

Page 95 The vestibular apparatus A very thorough account of the vestibular periphery is Wilson, V. J. and Melvill Jones, G. (1979) *Mammalian Vestibular Physiology*. (Plenum, New York).

Page 99 Caloric nystagmus Not *entirely* through convection currents, for it still occurs under zero-gravity conditions: see Schere, H., Brandt, U., Clarke, A. H., Merbold, U. and Parker, R. (1986) European vestibular experiments on the Spacelab-1 mission. 3. Caloric nystagmus in microgravity. *Experimental Brain Research* 64, 255–263.

NEUROLAB

Adaptation

Page 91
This exhibit, which demonstrates various aspects of adaptation, has already been described in Chapter 3: see p. 70.

Spinal tracts

Page 93
A simple self-testing exhibit covering the ascending and descending tracts of the spinal cord. Click on one of the buttons round the edge of the cross-section (ascending paths on the right, descending on the left). The name of the corresponding tract will appear in the box at top right. Alternatively, click on the button to the right of the box to bring down a list of tracts: click on one, and its corresponding button will display.

6 HEARING

The nature of sound 101
Sound spectra 103
The structure of the ear 106
Fourier analysis by the cochlea 108

Responses from auditory fibres 110
Spatial localization of sound 114
Central pathways and responses 116

THE NATURE OF SOUND

To appreciate the working of the ear it is necessary first to have some acquaintance with the properties of the sound waves to which it responds, a topic that too often seems to get squeezed out of the school physics curriculum.

Sound is generated in a medium such as air whenever there is a sufficiently rapid movement of part of its boundary – perhaps a moving loudspeaker cone or the collapsing skin of a pricked balloon. What happens is that the air next to the moving boundary is rapidly compressed or rarefied, resulting in a local movement of molecules that tends to make the pressure differences propagate away from the original site of disturbance at a rate that depends on the

density and elastic properties of the medium: this velocity is around 340 m/sec in air, and about four times as great in water. If the original sound source is undergoing regular oscillation – as in the case of the prongs of a tuning fork – the sound is propagated in the form of regular waves of pressure. The *wavelength* of these waves – the distance from one point of maximum compression to the next – is equal to their velocity divided by their *frequency*, the number of vibrations made every second by the source. *Pitch* is the sensory perception that corresponds with frequency, just as colour corresponds with the wavelength of a light, but there is not always an absolutely direct relationship between the two.

Strictly speaking, not all vibrations of this kind are sound; to be audible, the waves must have a frequency lying somewhere between about 20 and 20 000 Hz. The simplest of all vibrations are those in which the variations of pressure along the wave are sinusoidal

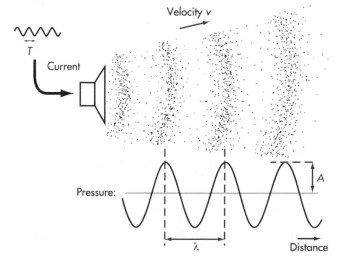

FIG. 6.1 A loudspeaker driven by a sinusoidal current of period T, or frequency $f = 1/T$. The resultant waves of compression and rarefaction of the air travel with a velocity v and are of wavelength λ, where $v = \lambda f$. The amplitude A is the difference between the mean pressure and the peak pressure.

as a function of time, in other words proportional to sin($2\pi ft$), where f is the frequency and t is time. In such a case we may describe the wave completely by means of its frequency and its *amplitude,* the value of the additional pressure at the peak of compression (Fig. 6.1).

Sound waves also of course carry energy: the rate at which energy is delivered per unit area, the *intensity* of the sound, is proportional to the square of its amplitude, and also to the density of the medium and the square of the frequency: it obviously takes more energy to vibrate something backwards and forwards very fast than if it is done more slowly. Because the range of intensities to which the ear can respond without damage is a very large one indeed – a factor of some 10^{14} – it is convenient to use a logarithmic scale to describe sound intensities. For this purpose, a standard reference level is used (its value being near the threshold of hearing under ideal conditions, 10^{-16} W/cm^2), and the log of the ratio of the actual intensity to this standard gives the intensity of the sound in Bels (named after Alexander Graham Bell, an inventor of the telephone). In practice, the unfortunate custom has grown up of dealing in tenths of a Bel, or *decibels* (dB), so that the formula becomes:

$$\text{Intensity in decibels} = 10 \log_{10} \frac{\text{Intensity of unknown}}{\text{Intensity of standard}}$$

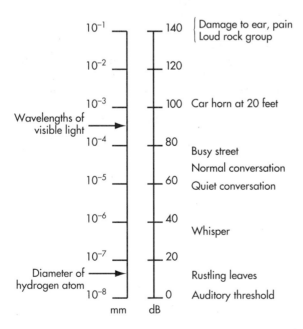

FIG. 6.2 Approximate intensities of various sounds, measured in absolute decibels (dB) and also in terms of the amplitude of the corresponding movement of the molecules in the air (0 dB = 0.0002 dyne/cm^2)

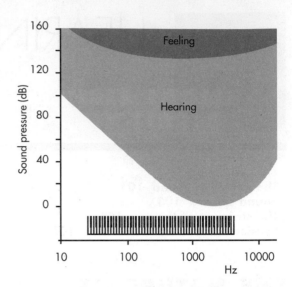

FIG. 6.3 Audiometry curve: the shaded region shows the intensities of sounds that may be heard or felt at different frequencies, averaged over many subjects. (Data from Dadson and King, 1952). The piano keyboard may help relate the frequency scale to ordinary musical pitch.

Figure 6.2 shows the intensity of some common kinds of sound, expressed in decibels. Because intensity is proportional to the square of the amplitude, multiplying the latter by a factor of 10 results in a 20 dB increase in intensity. Finally, although the measure defined above is an absolute scale of intensity, decibels can also be used to express the ratio of two intensities: thus if one sound has one-tenth the intensity of another, it can be described as having a relative intensity of -10 dB or as being *attenuated* by 10 dB.

The smallest intensity that can just be perceived, the auditory threshold, depends very markedly on frequency; a graph of measurements of threshold as a function of frequency is called an *audiometric curve* (Fig. 6.3), and often has clinical diagnostic value. The minimum threshold of around 10^{-16} W/cm^2 corresponds to an amplitude of about 0.0002 dyne/cm , and a movement of the air molecules that is considerably less than the diameter of a hydrogen atom.

One other parameter that is necessary to describe a sinusoidal vibration in certain circumstances is its *phase.* A sinusoidal wave of constant amplitude and frequency that is sampled simultaneously at two fixed points in space – as, for example, by the two ears – will by definition have the same amplitude and frequency at each point, but the compressions and rarefactions at the one point may not occur at the same moment as those at the other. In general, one wave will appear to be displaced in time with respect to the other, and the phase difference between the two is a measure of the fraction of a whole cycle by which one appears to be shifted (Fig. 6.4). It is conveniently expressed as an angle, so that a phase shift of 180° brings the waves into antiphase, the peaks of one then corresponding to the troughs of the other, and a further 180° shift, making 360° (or 0°) in all, brings them back into coincidence.

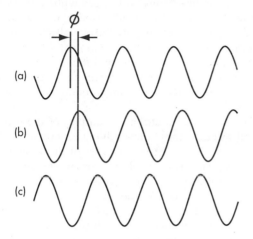

FIG. 6.4 Phase. The sine wave **(b)** has the same frequency and amplitude as (a), but is shifted in phase by an angle φ (in this case a phase advance of 60°). **(c)** A sine wave shifted by 180° relative to *(a)*, or in antiphase to it.

SOUND SPECTRA

Now pure sinusoidal waves are actually rather uncommon in real life: musical instruments, for example, produce waves whose profile, though repetitive, is not sinusoidal (Fig. 6.6). However, there is a theorem due to the French mathematician Fourier that every repetitive waveform is made up of the sum of a series of simple sinusoidal components, whose frequencies are integral multiples of the frequency (*fundamental* frequency) of the original wave. Thus a square wave of frequency f (Fig. 6.5) can be synthesized by adding together sine waves of frequency f, $3f$, $5f$, $7f$ and so on, with amplitudes in proportion to 1, 1/3, 1/5, 1/7, etc. We can represent a recipe for a Fourier synthesis of this kind in the form of a Fourier *spectrum* that shows in graphical form, as a function of frequency, the amplitude and phase of each of the components (*harmonics*) that make it up; in practice, the phase information is often omitted, for reasons that will become apparent later. Figure 6.6 shows the sound spectra of a number of different kinds of musical instrument: in each case, the line of lowest

frequency shows the amplitude of the fundamental, and those of higher frequency show the amplitudes of the harmonics. The Fourier spectrum and the shape of the waveform itself are thus in a sense interchangeable: each contains the same information as the other, for if we know the spectrum, we can add all the components together and recreate the original waveform, and conversely it is possible by a process of Fourier analysis to translate any given waveform into its equivalent spectrum.

Furthermore, it turns out that Fourier analysis can even be applied to waveforms that are not repetitive: unpitched sounds like that of a boiling kettle or transients of the kind produced by dropping a teapot. To see why this is so, consider what happens as we continuously lower the frequency of a repetitive waveform of given shape. Since the individual components of the spectrum are spaced out on the frequency axis by f, the fundamental frequency, it follows that the smaller f is, the closer and closer become the lines of the spectrum. In the limit, when the frequency of the wave becomes zero – in other words when its wavelength is infinite, and it never repeats itself at all – the spectral components are infinitely close together: so the spectrum, instead of being a sequence of discontinuous spikes, is now a smooth curve. Thus repetitive waveforms give rise to

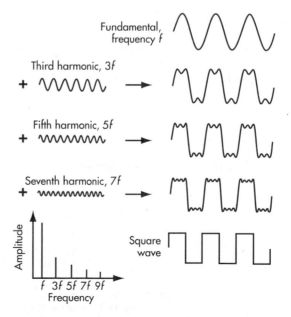

FIG. 6.5 Fourier synthesis: in this case, the gradual approximation to a square wave achieved by adding together successive sine waves of frequency f, $3f$, $5f$ etc.; their amplitudes are proportional to 1, 1/3, 1/5, etc., as shown in the amplitude spectrum at bottom left.

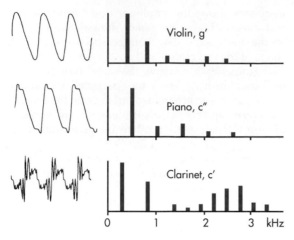

FIG. 6.6 Waveforms (left) and amplitude spectra (right) for different notes played by different musical instruments. (After Wood, 1930)

spectra with discrete harmonics, whereas unrepetitive waveforms produce continuous spectra. In either case, it turns out that the quality of a sound – for example, the timbre of a musical instrument – is much more closely related to the overall shape of its spectrum than to the shape of its waveform. Musical instruments with lots of high harmonics sound bright and strident (trumpets, clarinets, Fig. 6.6); those with most of their energy in the fundamental sound smoother and more rounded. Sharp sounds, hisses, clicks all have continuous spectra with prominent high frequencies (the only difference between a hiss and a click is in fact in the phase relationships of its components), whereas thumps, roars and rumbles have their energy concentrated at the low-frequency end.

To summarize, we have two different and largely independent psychological sensations that arise from a sound that are closely related to two different aspects of the sound's spectrum. On the one hand, *pitch* depends on the fundamental frequency: two instruments may have spectra of entirely different shapes but will be recognized as playing the same note if their fundamental frequencies are identical (and sounds like bangs and hisses with continuous spectra have no pitch at all). *Timbre,* on the other hand, is governed entirely by the overall shape of the spectrum, regardless of the fundamental frequency; an oboe playing a succession of different notes is still recognizably the same instrument, because the general shape of its spectrum remains essentially unchanged.

One of the most striking examples of the use of sound spectra comes from studying the human voice. The larynx, isolated from the rest of the voice-producing apparatus of head and throat, is essentially not very different from the double reed of an instrument like the oboe. As the air passes between the vocal cords, they are alternately forced apart and spring back, producing a repetitive series of compressions and rarefactions whose frequency can be modified by altering the shape and tension of the cords themselves; the resultant spectrum is roughly of the form shown in Figure 6.7. But in real life, the sounds it produces have to pass through a number of hollow cavities – the throat, nose and mouth – before they reach the outside world; these cavities tend to resonate, absorbing certain frequencies and reinforcing others, so that the original sound spectrum becomes distorted (Fig. 6.7). The two or three main resonance peaks in this spectrum simply reflect the fact that the tongue effectively divides the mouth

TABLE 6.1 Information carried by sound waves

Physical quantity	Sensory correlate	Coding
Amplitude	Loudness Interaural differences contribute to localization (higher frequencies)	Total neural activity (including recruitment)
Frequency	Pitch (lower frequencies)	Predominantly temporal periodicity
Spectrum	Timbre (higher frequencies); also contributes to monaural localization	Predominantly spatial pattern
Phase	Interaural differences contribute to localization: (lower frequencies)	Temporal

cavity into separate compartments, and each compartment acts as an independent resonator, at a frequency that depends mainly on the shape of the tongue and the degree of jaw opening. What is striking is that different vowel sounds are associated in a closely reproducible way with particular positions of these resonant peaks (called *formants),* and these characteristics are largely independent of the speaker, the pitch of his or her voice, and whether the vowel is spoken or sung: yet the *waveforms* produced by different speakers pronouncing the same vowel are generally completely different from each other. In other words, it seems that vowels are recognized, independently of the quality of the voice or its pitch,

by the overall shape of the spectrum and not by the shape of the wave itself. It is the frequency of the fundamental that produces the sense of the pitch of the voice, and very often conveys information in its own right (as in the different emphasis in 'I *love* you' and 'I love *you*'), particularly of an emotional nature.

Finally, it seems to be the fine structure of the spectrum, the little bumps and hollows on it that are the results of idiosyncrasies of the way our own particular mouths and throats are constructed, that enable us to differentiate one speaker from another. It turns out, as we shall see, that almost the first thing the ear does to the sound waves it receives is to Fourier-analyse them, and the pattern of activity of the fibres

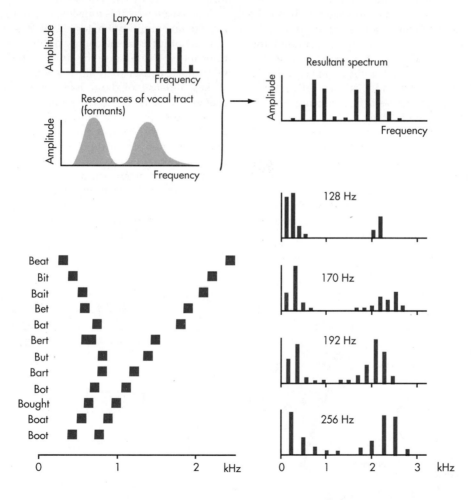

FIG. 6.7 The human voice. Above left, the spectrum of vibrations of the larynx is modified by the resonances of the vocal tract (shaded) to produce the spectrum of the sound finally emitted (right). Below left, the approximate positions of the two principal formants for a number of different English vowel sounds. Right, the vowel sound in 'EAT' sung at the various frequencies indicated. Although the spacing of the spectral lines increases as the frequency rises, the overall shape, defining the vowel quality, remains largely unchanged. (After Wood, 1930)

of the auditory nerve is – at least for medium and high frequencies – in effect a representation of the spectrum of the sound that is heard: only at low frequencies is information about the actual shape of the waveform available to the brain. (See Table 6.1)

THE STRUCTURE OF THE EAR

External and middle ear

The visible external ear, or *pinna,* has little effect on incoming sound except that of colouring it by superimposing little idiosyncratic resonances on it in the high-frequency region, that are dependent on the direction from which the sound is coming and can, as will be described later, provide quite accurate information about the position of a sound source. The auditory canal, the *external meatus,* similarly does little in humans except to add its own rather broad resonance peak around 3000 Hz. In other animals with less vestigial pinnae, they may have a more significant part to play in gathering sound, and if movable, can provide a great deal more information about where a sound is coming from.

At the end of the meatus, the sound impinges on the *tympanic membrane* ('eardrum' in sensible English) that separates the outer ear from the middle ear. On the inner side, the tympanic membrane is attached to the *malleus* ('hammer'), the first of a set of three tiny bones, the *ossicles,* whose function is to transform vibrations of the eardrum into vibrations of the fluids that fill the inner ear (Fig. 6.8). The malleus is joined to the *incus* ('anvil') which in turn bears on the *stapes* ('stirrup'), whose footplate rests on the *oval window,* a membrane separating the middle and inner ears (Fig. 6.8). This chain of ossicles acts as a kind of lever system, converting the movements of the eardrum, which are of comparatively large amplitude but small force, into the smaller but more powerful movements of the oval window; this increase in the pressure of the vibrations is further enhanced by the fact that the tympanic membrane is much larger in area than the oval window. Thus the amplitude is reduced by a factor of nearly 200, and force increased by the same amount.

The reason why this transformation is necessary – it is not an amplification, for like all passive systems it does not increase the energy of the waves that are transmitted – is because the fluid of the inner ear is very much denser than air. If a sound wave in air strikes a dense medium like water, the pressure changes of the air are too small to make more than a slight impression on the fluid, and most of the sound is reflected back. To ensure the most efficient transfer of energy from air to fluid, we need some way of increasing the pressure changes in the sound wave to match the characteristics of the new medium, and this *impedance matching* appears to be the primary function of the middle ear; without it, only some 0.1 percent of the sound energy reaching the eardrum would reach the inner ear.

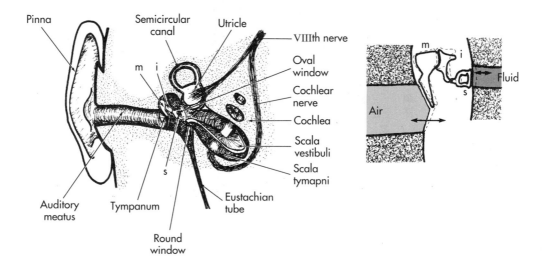

FIG. 6.8 Left, diagrammatic section through the ear. Right, how the ossicles convert low-pressure waves in the air into high-pressure, small-displacement waves in the cochlear perilymph: m, malleus; i, incus; s, stapes.

A second function of the middle ear is that it is capable of acting as a kind of censor: it contains muscles – the *tensor tympani* and *stapedius* – that effectively disable the transmission system when they contract, protecting the inner ear from damagingly powerful sounds. In addition to all this, the middle ear also further shapes the audiometric spectrum, mostly by reducing low-frequency sensitivity.

Inner ear

The inner ear is simply the labyrinth, described in the previous chapter; the part of it that is concerned with sensing sounds is the *cochlea,* in effect an elongated sac of endolymph some 35 mm long, shaped as if it had been pushed sideways into a corresponding tube of perilymph, rather like the sausage in a hot dog (Fig. 6.9). The upper half of the perilymph is called the *scala vestibuli,* the lower is the *scala tympani,* and the endolymphatic sausage is the *scala media.* At the far end of this structure, the two perilymphatic regions join up through an opening called the helicotrema; and finally the whole thing is rolled up into a conical spiral, giving it the shape of a snail shell. In cross-section (Fig. 6.9) one may see that the scala vestibuli and scala media are separated by only a

very thin membrane, *Reissner's membrane,* whilst the boundary between scala media and scala tympani is much more complicated and contains several layers of cells, including the receptors themselves, resting on the *basilar membrane.*

The oval window faces onto the scala vestibuli, while a similar structure, the round window, separates the scala tympani from the air of the middle ear. (This air, incidentally, is in communication with the outside atmosphere through the eustachian tube which joins it to the pharynx. This tube is normally closed, but opens briefly during swallowing and yawning, causing a characteristic modification of one's hearing: one may get relief in this way from the eardrum pain sometimes experienced in air travel as a result of pressure differences between the atmosphere and the middle ear.)

Now endolymph and perilymph are virtually incompressible fluids; so any movements of the oval window must result in corresponding movements of the round window. In other words, sound energy has no option but to pass from the scala vestibuli to the scala tympani, either by crossing through the endolymph or by travelling right to the end of the cochlea and traversing the helicotrema. In the former case, it will cause the basilar membrane, with all its elaborate superstructure, to vibrate as well.

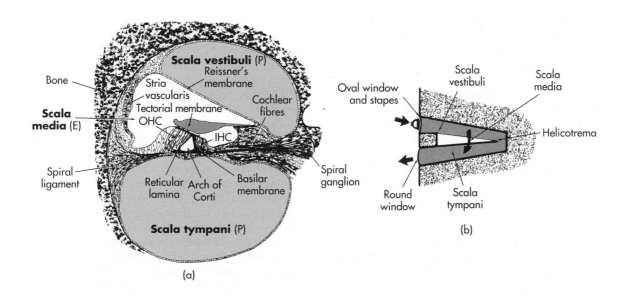

FIG. 6.9 Left, section through the cochlea, showing the organ of Corti. OHC, IHC, outer and inner hair cells; E, endolymph; P, perilymph. Right, a highly stylized representation of the relationship between scala vestibuli, scala media and scala tympani, and the path of sound through them.

Now the cochlear receptors – the hair cells – are peculiarly well adapted to respond to exceedingly small up-and-down movements of the basilar membrane. Their cell bodies are attached at the bottom to the membrane itself, and at the top to a rigid plate called the *reticular lamina*, which is in turn attached to a strong and inflexible support called the *arch of Corti* that also rests on the basilar membrane. Consequently any movement of the basilar membrane results in an exactly similar displacement of the hair cells. These hair cells are very like the vestibular hair cells described in the previous chapter; they possess a number of stereocilia, arranged this time in a characteristic V- or W-formation and graded in size, but the auditory hair cells of adults do not appear to have kinocilia. The cilia project through holes in the reticular lamina, and in the case of the outer hair cells the tips of the cilia are lightly embedded in the lower surface of the *tectorial membrane*, a flap of extracellular material analogous to the cupula or otolith, that extends from the inner boundary of the scala media and lies along the top of the inner and outer hair cells. The cilia of the inner hair cells do not appear to make contact with the tectorial membrane, but lie just short of it.

A consequence of the geometry of this arrangement is that any up-and-down movement of the basilar membrane will result in horizontal sliding, or shear, between the reticular membrane and the tectorial membrane. This in turn will bend the cilia of the hair cells through an angle which will be enormously greater than the original deflection of the basilar membrane (Fig. 6.10). There is then a further stage of mechanical amplification, since the actual mechanism by which bending gives rise to permeability changes seems to be that protein filaments run from the tip of one filament to the tip of its shorter neighbour, where they appear to be linked directly to the opening of membrane channels. Once again, a small angle of ciliary bending will generate a disproportionate mechanical effect. This permeability change gives rise to generator currents that eventually lead to depolarization of the terminal, calcium entry, release of transmitter and stimulation of the auditory fibres. An electrode in the vicinity of the cochlea can be used to pick up the summed receptor potentials of the hair cells, giving a recording that is closely related to the form of the original sound waves called the *cochlear microphonic potential*. If amplified and used to drive a loudspeaker, the result is quite a faithful reproduction of the sound entering the animal's ear. But although it is fairly clear how the cochlea may act as a transducer of sounds into nervous energy, nothing has yet been said about whether it also carries out

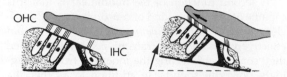

FIG. 6.10 Shear amplification. Vertical deflection of the basilar membrane causes shear between the reticular lamina and the tectorial membrane, thus bending the cilia of the hair cells. (For clarity the movement of the basilar membrane is of course vastly exaggerated.)

any analysis of the sound at the same time, in the way that, for instance, the cones of the retina begin the analysis of colour by responding preferentially to light of different wavelengths. In fact it turns out that different regions along the length of the cochlea are especially responsive to different sound frequencies, providing a rough kind of Fourier analysis of the type described earlier in this chapter. Before going on to discuss the electrophysiological responses of auditory nerve fibres, it is useful first to consider the mechanical properties of the cochlea that enable it to do this.

FOURIER ANALYSIS BY THE COCHLEA

The physicist and physiologist Hermann von Helmholtz (1821–94) was the first to appreciate the general way in which sound quality was related to its frequency spectrum. Observing that the basilar membrane gets wider as one approaches the helicotrema, he suggested that it might be the cochlea itself that carried out this Fourier analysis. His notion was that individual transverse fibres of the basilar membrane might act rather like the strings of a piano, tuned to different frequencies and resonating in sympathy whenever their own particular frequency was present in a sound. (If you open the lid of a piano and sing loudly into it with the sustaining pedal depressed so that the strings are undamped, you will hear it sing back to you as particular strings are set into sympathetic vibration: and if there were some device that signalled which strings were vibrating and which weren't, you would have a kind of Fourier analyser.) However, direct measurements of the mechanical properties of the basilar membrane show that it cannot in fact behave in this simple mechanical way. There is too much longitudinal coupling of the membrane, much as if neighbouring strings in the piano were glued together; and in any case it is easy to show, simply by cutting it and observing that it does not twang back, that there is hardly any tension in the basilar membrane at all, and certainly not enough to make it resonate in the way Helmholtz suggested.

Nevertheless, it is clear from a number of pieces of evidence – for instance, that lesions of the basal end of the cochlea are associated with the specific loss of high-frequency auditory sensitivity – that different regions of the cochlea really are sensitive to different frequencies, in a systematic way. The foundations for our knowledge of the mechanism by which this comes about were laid when Georg von Békésy, some 40 years ago, applied his superlative experimental skill to an investigation of the way the basilar membrane actually responded during stimulation by sounds of different frequencies. What he found was that at any particular frequency, as one explored from the base towards the apex, the amplitude of the vibration of the membrane increased relatively slowly up to a maximum and then fell off again more sharply. The position of this maximum along the cochlea was dependent on the frequency, and the lower the frequency the nearer it was to the helicotrema: by 50 Hz or so the maximum had more or less reached the end of the cochlea. There were also phase differences at different points along the membrane: the greater the distance from the basal end, the greater the phase lag between the movement of the membrane and that of the oval window. Consequently when one looked at the basilar membrane as a whole, the appearance was of a travelling wave progressing towards the apex, growing larger as it went until the point of maximum response was reached, and then abruptly decaying to zero (Fig. 6.11). More recent work using preparations in a more physiological condition than von Békésy's cadavers has shown that the peak of amplitude is actually much sharper than shown in the figure, for reasons that will become apparent. But this remains a good description of the passive contribution of the basilar membrane, considered in isolation.

The mechanical properties that give rise to this behaviour are rather complex, and an elementary account must necessarily be oversimplified. In essence, what happens is something like this: the sound waves, entering the scala vestibuli at the oval window, can only get out again through the round window, but there is a choice of routes by which they can get there. They might, for example, cross straight through the basilar membrane at the basal end: the membrane is stiffer here but on the other hand this would be a short route involving less movement of

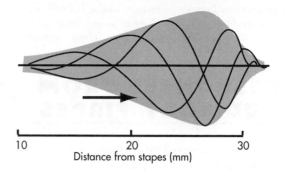

Distance from stapes (mm)

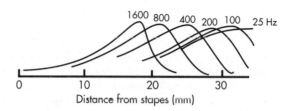

1600 800 400 200 100 25 Hz

Distance from stapes (mm)

FIG. 6.11 Above, three consecutive 'snapshots' of the displacement of the basilar membrane in response to a sine wave (vastly exaggerated in amplitude, as usual). The whole waves moves from stapes to helicotrema, with an envelope (shaded) that depends on the frequency. Below, peaks of the envelopes associated with waves of the frequencies indicated. (After von Békésy, 1960. Had the displacements been measured using modern techniques, the peaks would be seen to be much sharper.)

perilymph. Alternatively, the sound waves might prefer to travel further along the cochlear duct before crossing into the scala tympani, involving a longer mass of fluid to have to move but an easier crossing because of the decrease in stiffness of the basilar membrane at increasing distances from the base. Now the relative hindrance offered by the stiffness of the membrane and the inertia of the perilymph depends very much on what the frequency of the sound is; the energy required to move a mass backwards and forwards increases enormously with increasing frequency, so that at high frequencies the path of least resistance is for the sound to cross from scala vestibuli to scala tympani near the base. At very low frequencies, the opposite is true: it is not much trouble to move the entire mass of perilymph backwards and forwards, and by doing so the sound can make the easier crossing at the apical end, where the stiffness is least. In other words, the preferred route will represent a compromise between the relative disadvantages of membrane stiffness and perilymph inertia, and the structure as a whole will act as a kind of auditory prism, sorting out vibrations of different frequencies into different positions along the membrane: behaving, in fact, like a Fourier analyser. One can find out how well it carries out this task by looking at the responses of the auditory fibres themselves.

RESPONSES FROM AUDITORY FIBRES

The synaptic connections between primary auditory fibres and the hair cells are broadly similar to those found in the vestibular system; corresponding to the distinction there between type I and type II cells, there are clear differences in innervation between the *inner* and *outer hair cells* (IHC, OHC) of the cochlea; both probably release glutamate. Each inner hair cell has afferent connections from some 20 or so radial fibres (Fig. 6.12), each of which appears to terminate on a single receptor. By contrast, the spiral afferents that innervate the outer cells run along the cochlea for a millimetre or so, and send afferent terminals to large numbers of receptors; about 10 percent of the auditory nerve fibres come from outer hair cells and 90 percent from inner. Thus there is a great deal of convergence from outer hair cells on to the afferent fibres but little or none from the inner hair cells. There is a rough analogy here with the rods and cones of the retina: the outer hair cells have (like rods) a low threshold for stimulation – partly because their cilia actually stick into the tectorial membrane – and are grouped together in large receptive fields; whereas the inner hair cells, like cones, have reduced sensitivity but a more discrete connection with the brain, suggesting that here too the inner hair cells

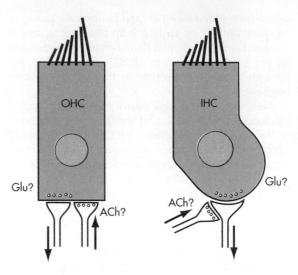

FIG. 6.13 Differences in the innervation of individual outer and inner hair cells. Outer hair cells (OHC) receive afferent and direct efferent innervation; inner hair cells (IHC) receive direct afferents only, but the terminals themselves are presynaptically influenced by the efferent innervation.

may have better 'acuity', in this case to small differences of frequency; there are some 400 IHC per octave or more than 30 per semitone. The hair cells also receive an *efferent* innervation, originating from a nucleus in the brainstem called the superior olive; these fibres, which are probably cholinergic, terminate directly on outer hair cells but presynaptically on afferents to inner hair cells (Fig 6.13).

There are two different sorts of electrical response that can be measured in the cochlea; with microelectrodes one can record action potentials from the auditory nerve fibres, and with larger electrodes in various areas within and around the cochlea one may in addition record several kinds of slower potential. The hair cells have resting potentials that are some 40 mV negative to the scala tympani, while an electrode in the scala media records a standing potential of some 80–90 mV positive with respect to perilymph: this endocochlear potential appears to come about through an electrogenic Na^+/K^+ pump in the stria vascularis, and has the desirable consequence that the voltage difference across the top end of the hair cells is half as big again as that which is usually found across neural membranes, implying that any given conductance change will give 50% more than the usual generator current, thus presumably increasing sensitivity. One may also record *cochlear microphonic* potentials with large electrodes almost anywhere in the vicinity of the cochlea. These are thought simply to be the summed generator potentials

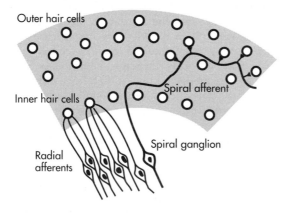

FIG. 6.12 Afferent innervation of outer hair cells (right) and inner hair cells (left), showing convergence in the former case and divergence in the latter.

of large numbers of hair cells, and appear to be more or less proportional to the local displacement of the basilar membrane; they thus follow the shape of the sound wave itself quite accurately, though with different degrees of frequency filtering at different distances from the oval window.

The auditory nerve fibres show similar properties to primary vestibular fibres, most having a spontaneous resting discharge whose frequency is increased when the basilar membrane moves towards the scala vestibuli and decreased when it moves in the opposite direction. Outer hair cells seem to respond to the actual deflection of the basilar membrane at any moment, whereas inner hair cells seem to respond to its velocity, probably because their cilia are only viscously coupled to the membrane rather than being directly linked. Different fibres have response curves lying on different positions along the displacement axis, and the effect of stimulation of the efferent fibres seems to be to reduce their sensitivity. This effect is rather small under experimental conditions, being some 15 dB, and it is difficult to believe that this is all they are for. We shall see later that there is good reason to think they have a much more fundamental part in receptor tuning.

Because of the frequency analysis performed by the mechanical properties of the basilar membrane, individual auditory fibres show a marked frequency selectivity (Fig. 6.14). A feature of this selectivity, most noticeable when the preparation is in good condition, is that the cells are much more sharply tuned – the range of frequencies is much narrower – than one would expect from von Békésy's measurements of the response of the membrane itself to pure tones. It seems as though there must be some extra mechanism – a *second filter* – that makes the responses more selective than they would otherwise be. It has been shown in some species that individual hair cells respond in a frequency-selective manner even to electrical stimulation at auditory frequencies (which of course bypasses the mechanical filter provided by the basilar membrane), suggesting that the second filter is an intrinsic property of the receptors themselves. It also appears to be an active, energy-requiring process rather than the kind of passive filtering provided by the basilar membrane's mechanics, for, under the influence of anoxia or cyanides, the tuning curves revert to something more like what von Békésy originally observed for the basilar membrane (Fig. 6.15).

The mechanism is likely to be some kind of resonant circuit generated in the outer hair cells by mutual interactions between mechanical displacement and electrical depolarization. It is not hard to imagine a process in which not only does ciliar

displacement cause a change in potential but changes in potential, with consequent calcium entry, in turn generate mechanical forces on the cilia (in most ciliated cells the cilia are, after all, motile). If this were so, one would expect the second filter to be observable not only in the electrical responses of the cells but also (since their cilia are coupled to the basilar membrane) in the sharpness of the membrane's tuning. Recent observations of the pattern of movement of the basilar membrane appear to support this idea.

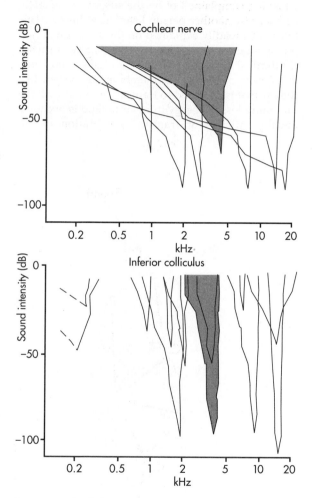

FIG. 6.14 Threshold response curves for individual units in cochlear nerve (left) and inferior colliculus, as a function of frequency. (After Katsuki, 1961)

If great care is taken to maintain the animal in reasonable condition, and to cause minimal interference with the membrane itself, the envelope of the travelling wave appears to be much more sharply tuned than was originally observed, and corresponds more closely to the tuning curves of the hair cells themselves (Fig. 6.15).

Many other observations point in the same direction. One of the distressing symptoms of the high-frequency hearing loss associated with progressive disorder of the cochlea is *tinnitus*, imaginary sounds taking the form of continuous high-pitched whistling (as in the well-known case of Ludwig van Beethoven) or hissing noises. Occasionally, there have been reports of 'objective' tinnitus in which the whistling complained of by the subject can actually be heard by another person listening at his ear. This too can be readily explained on the assumption that the spontaneous oscillation of the hair cells causes rhythmical movements of their cilia and thus movement of the basilar membrane. A system like the ear that is designed to transfer vibration with the minimum loss of energy from air to fluid is of course equally efficient at transerring vibration in the opposite direction. Similarly, with a sensitive microphone in the auditory meatus one may record cochlear echoes to very brief sound pulses, resulting from a shortlived ringing of the resonant mechanism: the phenomenon can be used to estimate the integrity of the auditory periphery in very young babies. In manmade systems, instability of this kind is a very common problem with highly resonant feedback systems: if the feedback is too great it can easily turn into spontaneous oscillation. It may well be that the function of the efferent fibres to OHCs in particular is to provide some general kind of central control of the feedback, incidentally detuning their selectivity.

A further mechanism that helps to sharpen up the spatial patterns of neural activity in response to auditory stimulation is the existence, as in all sensory systems, of lateral inhibition. If one determines the tuning curve for a single auditory unit using a single tone, and then adds to this a second tone of different

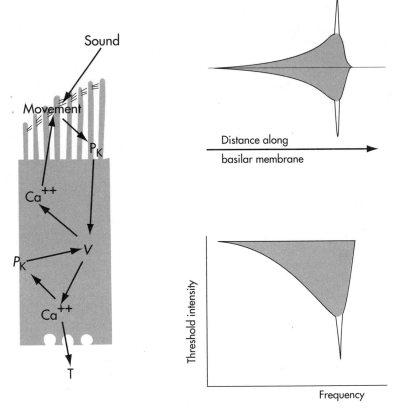

FIG. 6.15 The second filter: sharpening of hair cell tuning by a mechanism within the OHCs. Left, two ways in which such intrinsic tuning might arise. Changes in potential cause calcium entry, which in turn increases P_K: if the delay round this feedback loop were large enough it could cause resonance. In addition, the calcium can cause the cilia to move, creating another feedback loop through the transducer mechanism itself. Right, the effect of the second filter on cochlear function. A typical basilar membrane envelope for one frequency is shown above, a typical tuning curve for a cochlear afferent below, both in highly schematic form. The shaded area shows what the form would be in the absence of the second filter, for example after poisoning (or with poor experimental techniques).

frequency, one finds that in the regions immediately neighbouring on the original tuning curve the response of the cell is actually reduced by the extra sound. In other words, each fibre has – in terms of frequency – a central excitatory area and an inhibitory fringe, which serves further to sharpen its selectivity. For various reasons, however, it is clear that lateral inhibition is not, as elsewhere, due to inhibitory synaptic connections but rather to some intrinsic property of the interaction between basilar membrane and hair cells that is not fully understood.

The mechanisms of frequency analysis described so far provide a means whereby the spectrum of a sound can be coded into a spatial neural pattern, giving rise to the sense of timbre or tone quality. They operate essentially at medium and high frequencies, and indeed at frequencies above a kilohertz or so there is no other way that information about frequency could be transmitted to the brain except by peripheral analysis and recoding, since individual nerve fibres are incapable of firing more frequently than about 1000 times a second at the very best, and hence cannot reproduce the pattern of the sound waves reaching the ear. But this is not the case at low frequencies, and in any case we saw in Figure 6.11 that the frequency analysis produced by the basilar membrane begins to become ineffective at low frequencies because the maximum of activity has nearly reached the helicotrema. Recordings from single auditory units show that as the frequency of a stimulating tone is decreased, there is an increasing tendency for firing to be *phase locked* to the stimulating frequency; even if the frequency is too high for any one fibre to be able to fire once in every cycle, it may do so every two cycles or every three or more (Fig. 6.16). So although no single fibre will be firing at the frequency of the stimulus, the average activity over the whole set may nevertheless be modulated at this frequency.

In practice, phase locking is not quite as rigid as this: even at low frequencies where the fibres would be perfectly capable of following the imposed frequency, unless the stimulus intensity is very great what one observes is simply that there is an increased *probability* of firing during one part of the cycle rather than another. At all events, phase locking provides a method of conveying auditory information to the brain without peripheral frequency analysis, and has the advantage that it retains information about the phase of incoming sound, information which is thrown away at high frequencies, above some 5 kHz. (Though phase information contributes very little to sound quality, we shall see later that it is extremely important in localisation.) This mechanism of phase-

locking, working at low frequencies, is of course much better suited to transmitting information about the fundamental frequency of a sound than its harmonics, and a number of kinds of observations suggest very strongly that it is the frequency at which the activity in the auditory nerve repeats itself that generally determines the pitch of a sound. Frequencies higher than those that can be coded by phase-locking are not heard as pitches at all, which is why the piano keyboard stops where it does rather than at our high-frequency hearing limit: the top notes on a piano (above 3 kHz) sound more like clicks than tuned notes, just as the top notes on a violin have a hissing rather than a truly musical quality. Sounds which are modulated in amplitude at an auditory frequency generally appear to have the corresponding pitch, even though there is no energy at that frequency and no corresponding peak of neural

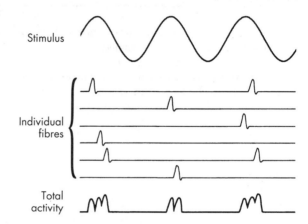

FIG. 6.16 The principle of phase locking. Although no one fibre out of the whole ensemble fires in every cycle of the sound wave, nevertheless the modulation of the total activity reflects the frequency of the original stimulus. With a larger amplitude wave, the probability of firing per cycle would increase.

activity along the cochlea. Finally, human subjects who have been provided with auditory prostheses in the form of an implanted electrode that stimulates the cochlea or auditory nerve report that although they cannot perceive speech very well (a task that requires analysis of the shape of the spectrum, which their prosthesis cannot provide since it can generate only temporal patterns), they can still perceive pitch, though not very accurately. It is clear that much of the sense of pitch must be due to central analysis by the brain rather than something that is done by the cochlea, since in this case it has been bypassed altogether.

To summarize, it seems that the perceived *pitch* of a sound depends essentially on the periodicity of the afferent neural activity – i.e. on its *temporal* pattern – whereas the sensation of *timbre* or quality, which requires the detailed perception of the high-frequency power spectrum of the sound, is coded by the relative activity of fibres from different parts of the cochlea, i.e. by their *spatial* pattern of activity. *Loudness* is presumably simply a matter of the total amount of auditory activity; as auditory intensity is increased, there is both an increase in the firing of any one fibre, and also an increase in the total number of fibres that are firing at all, through recruitment.

SPATIAL LOCALIZATION OF SOUND

There are two components to localization – distance and direction – and these are carried out in very different ways by the auditory system. Since the energy of a sound wave decreases with the square of the distance it has travelled, one could in principle judge distance if one knew in advance the power of the

sound source and the degree of absorption of the intervening structures but in practice intensity can give only very approximate information. Rather more useful is the fact that not all frequencies suffer equal attenuation with distance: in an ordinary sort of environment, shorter wavelengths tend to be reflected or absorbed by physical objects, whereas long wavelengths simply ignore them. For this reason, the further one is from a sound source, the more of its high frequencies are lost: as a marching band approaches, it is the bass drum and then the tubas and euphoniums one hears first. Or again, when listening to a radio play one has a clear sense of how far the actors are from the microphone from the ratio of high to low frequencies in their speech sounds. Close to, the consonants – particularly sibilants like 'S' – are predominant, whereas with increasing distance it is the lower frequency components – mostly vowels – that are heard most prominently.

Locating the *direction* of a sound source is a much more precise business, and is carried out by at least three separate mechanisms. Contrary to popular belief, one can localize sounds quite accurately using one ear alone. As was mentioned earlier, the peculiar pattern of bumps and whorls that decorate our pinnae add a coloration to all the sounds one hears, a pattern of small peaks and troughs in one's frequency

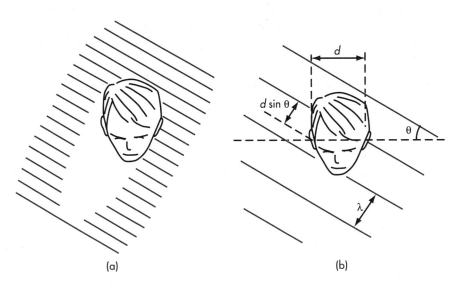

(a)   (b)

FIG. 6.17 Two binaural methods of localising sounds. **(a)** Sounds of sufficiently high frequency cast a sound shadow on the far side of the head: the wavelength λ must be less than the order of magnitude of the head diameter, *d*. **(b)** A sound coming from a direction at a bearing θ is associated with a phase difference between the ears of 360 $(d \sin \theta/\lambda)$ degrees, equivalent to a time difference of $(d \sin \theta)/v$ milliseconds, where *v* is the velocity of sound in km/sec and *d* is expressed in metres.

sensitivity curve that is dependent on the angle at which the sound waves impinge on the ear. In the course of growing up one presumably learns that particular kinds of coloration are associated with particular directions, and in the adult this mechanism has been shown to provide localization of sound accurate to a few degrees. Using both ears produces only a slight improvement, to perhaps 1–2°.

The extra information provided by binaural listening is of two distinct kinds: differences in interaural intensity and in interaural phase. Intensity differences come about because the head casts a 'sound shadow' that screens the ear to a certain extent from sounds coming from the opposite side (Fig. 6.17a). For the head to cast a shadow of this kind, it needs to be at least of the order of magnitude of the wavelength of the sound itself; thus screening of this type can only cause significant effects at frequencies higher than some 2–3 kHz. You can explore this effect for yourself by using a transistor radio as a source of sounds of different frequencies, covering one ear and listening to the changes in the intensities of low- and high-frequency components as you move the radio around your head. Intensity differences alone, even at high frequencies, do not permit sounds to be localized very accurately unless one is also allowed to move one's head to find the direction for which the intensity is most nearly equal in the two ears.

Phase differences arise because a sound coming from one side takes slightly longer to reach one ear than the other (Fig. 6.17b). Since by using phase information alone a subject may detect movement of a sound source of only 1–2°, one can calculate that the

Box 6.1 Contributions to auditory localization		
Distance		
Spectral pattern		
Horizontal direction		
Monaural	Spectral pattern	
Binaural	Phase difference (low frequencies)	
	Intensity difference (high frequencies)	
Vertical direction:		
Monaural	Spectral pattern	
Head movement	Resolves ambiguity	

brain must be sensitive to interaural time differences of the order of 10 microsec or about one hundredth part of the duration of an action potential! However, although phase differences can give accurate information about the direction of sounds, pure tones cannot be localised in this way if their frequencies are higher than some 1–2 kHz. The reason for this is that once the wavelength of the sound is less than the distance between the ears, ambiguities can occur, in the sense that a given phase relationship could be the result of more than one possible source direction (Fig. 6.18). In any case, we have already seen that information about phase is simply not transmitted by auditory nerve fibres at high frequencies.

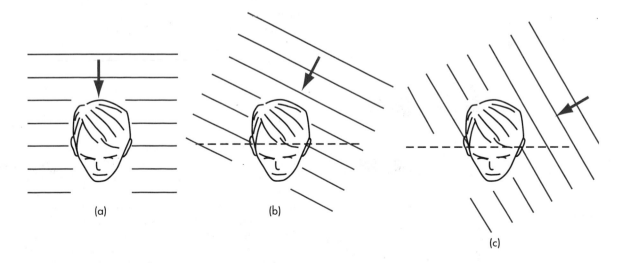

(a)   (b)   (c)

FIG. 6.18 At high frequencies, a given phase difference (in this case, zero) could be due to more than one sound direction.

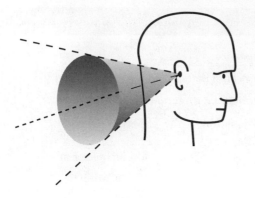

FIG. 6.19 The cone of confusion. A sound producing a given phase delay, even at low frequencies, may lie anywhere on the cone which is the locus of all points lying at a given angle from the axis formed by the two ears. (This is not strictly the case if the source is close to the head.)

Thus the two fundamental binaural mechanisms of location are – rather conveniently – exactly complementary to one another. At low frequencies, only phase can be used, and at high frequencies, only intensity: the crossover point is a function of the size of the head. With such a system one might expect to

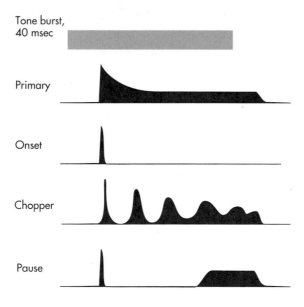

FIG. 6.20 Responses from cochlear nucleus. Typical, simplified profiles of summed responses from some categories of neurone found in the cochlear nucleus are shown, in response to a 40 msec tone burst, shown in grey. The heights of the curves effectively represent the instantaneous probability of a spike occurring.

be able to cancel out a time delay on one side by increasing the corresponding intensity; this kind of time–intensity *trade* can in fact be demonstrated quite easily in the laboratory by arranging for a subject to hear a click delayed in one ear, and asking him to adjust the relative loudness in each ear until they sound as if coming from straight ahead – a sort of titration.

Neither of these binaural mechanisms can do more than tell you the angle between the direction of a sound source and an imaginary line joining the two ears (Fig. 6.19); in particular, they cannot distinguish between a sound lying immediately behind the head, immediately in front or somewhere overhead in the sagittal plane. For a complex sound of known frequency composition, this extra information can be provided by the monaural mechanism of directionally selective coloration described earlier. When this is impossible, then moving the head can provide an extra 'fix' on the sound that will enable its exact three-dimensional direction to be established, as when a dog cocks his head on one side when trying to locate the source of a sound.

CENTRAL PATHWAYS AND RESPONSES

After leaving the cochlear ganglion, the primary auditory fibres synapse first in the *cochlear nuclear complex*, a group of three nuclei, each of which has a systematic tonotopic representation of the basilar membrane, so that neighbouring areas correspond to neighbouring frequencies. Functionally, the cells of the dorsal and anteroventral parts have very different properties and project to different areas, with the intermediate posteroventral nucleus showing a mixture of the two types. The *anteroventral* cells behave very like auditory nerve fibres, showing relatively simple responses to particular frequency bands and an incompletely adapting response to tone bursts; at low frequencies they show phase locked responses. In the *dorsal* region one finds cells with entirely novel and complex specializations. Some show only a brief burst of activity at the start of a sustained tone, while others respond with a slow increase in activity or with repetitive bursts of spikes (Fig. 6.20). Many show tuning curves in which the main excitatory peak is flanked by prominent areas of inhibition that narrows the range of frequencies to which they respond.

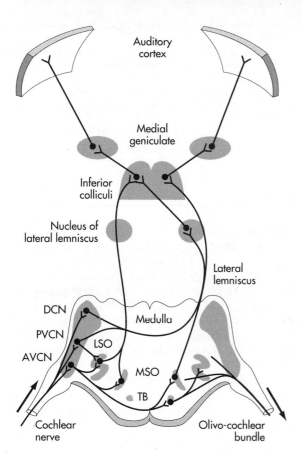

Auditory cortex

Medial geniculate

Inferior colliculi

Nucleus of lateral lemniscus

Lateral lemniscus

DCN

PVCN

AVCN

Medulla

LSO

MSO

TB

Cochlear nerve

Olivo-cochlear bundle

FIG. 6.21 Schematic diagram of ascending auditory pathways: first- and second-order fibres are shown thicker than the others.

The central auditory pathways are complex (Fig. 6.21) and not fully understood. Cells in this dorsal region project straight up to the next highest level in the ascending pathway, the (contralateral) *inferior colliculus*, whereas those in the simpler, ventral region, first have to undergo an additional stage of processing in the *superior olive* of the brainstem. This may well correspond with the fact that while some spectral information has already been analysed in the cochlea, at medium and high frequencies, and is available as a spatial code, low frequencies are still coded in temporal form and require further processing in the brainstem. In addition, information from the two ears needs to be compared to compute spatial information. The superior olive is the lowest level at which information from one ear meets information from the other, and seems to be concerned with auditory localization rather than recognition. Cells in the lateral part of the superior olive are typically excited by the ipsilateral ear and inhibited by the contralateral one (through a relay in the nucleus of the trapezoid body), and are concerned mostly with high frequencies: it seems very likely, therefore, that they form the neural basis for the use of interaural intensity differences in judging the direction of a sound. In the medial part of the superior olive the cells are

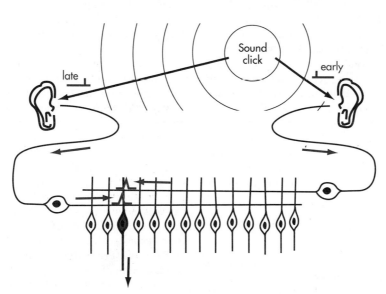

FIG. 6.22 A possible neural mechanism for binaural sound localization. Two neurones with axons pointing in opposite directions are driven each by one ear. When a sound arrives sooner at one ear than the other, the resultant neural response will have travelled further than its opposite number when they meet. An array of cells responding only when excited simultaneously by both axons would then code spatially for different interaural time differences.

predominantly low-frequency and appear to be interested in *time differences*: many of the cells respond best when there is a particular time-interval between the arrival of sound at each ear, so that sounds from different directions preferentially stimulate different neurones. (Fig. 6.22).

At the inferior colliculus the two pathways recombine, bringing together information about the kind of sound and about where it is. Cells here may show the same types of complexity in their response as can be seen in the dorsal cochlear nucleus, as well as coding for localization; in some species a systematic topological mapping of the directional responses has been described, with some somatosensory responses as well. Crossed and uncrossed projections ascend to the next highest level of the auditory system, the medial geniculate nucleus, which in turn relays to auditory cortex. Cells in the ventral part of the medial geniculate show much the same properties as those in the inferior colliculus, and relay to the primary *auditory cortex* (AI). But in the medial part, and in the secondary cortex (AII) to which it projects, some neurones seem to respond specifically to more complex sounds. Whereas AI is essentially tonotopically arranged, this is much less obvious in the adjoining areas of auditory cortex. Many units can be found that are not simply tuned to one particular frequency: some respond best to two different frequencies (the kind of response needed to recognize speech sounds), to changing frequencies, or react preferentially to such specialized, 'real' stimuli as clicks, whistles, hisses and voices. When, in the next chapter, we look at the way the visual cortex processes information from the eye, we shall see that there are cortical cells that respond very specifically to fragments of the retinal image such as lines and edges and thus provide detailed information from which one's recognition of visual objects could easily be derived. It would be nice to demonstrate a similar process unequivocally in the case of the auditory cortex, but it has been a less fashionable area of study and we simply do not have enough data, from enough species, to be able to make the same kinds of generalizations.

References

Carpenter, M. B. and Sutin, J. (1983) *Human Neuroanatomy.* Williams and Wilkins, Baltimore.

Dadson, R. S. and King, J. H. (1952) A determination of the normal threshold of hearing and its relation to the standardisation of audiometers. *Journal of Laryngology and Otolaryngology* 66, 366–378.

Katsuki, Y. (1961) Neural mechanisms of auditory sensation in cats. In *Sensory Communication*, ed. W. A. Rosenblith. MIT, Boston.

Spoendlin, H. (1968) Ultrastructure and peripheral innervation pattern of the receptor coding of the acoustic message. In *Hearing Mechanisms in Vertebrates*, ed. A. V. S. de Renck and J. Knight. Churchill, London.

von Békésy, G. (1960) *Experiments in Hearing*. McGraw-Hill, New York.

Wood, A. (1930) *Sound Waves and their Uses*. Blackie, Glasgow.

NOTES

Hearing Excellent general accounts of the physiology and psychophysics of hearing include: Gelfand, S. A. (1981) *Hearing: an Introduction to Psychological and Physiological Acoustics* (Marcel Dekker, New York); Moore, B. C. J. (1989) *Introduction to the Psychology of Hearing* (Cambridge University Press, Cambridge); Pickles, J. O. (1988) *An Introduction to the Physiology of Hearing* (Academic, London); Stebbins, W. C. (1983) *The Acoustic Sense of Animals* (Harvard University Press, Massachusetts).

Page 102 Auditory sensitivity To see what this astonishing sensitivity means in practical terms, in theory a 10 watt loudspeaker of moderate efficiency situated in London and sending out a 1 kHz tone ought to be audible in Cambridge, 50 miles away! In fact, of course, not only would much of the sound be absorbed by intervening structures but prevailing background noise will tend to drown the incoming signal: maximum sensitivity can only be obtained when all other sound sources are silenced. Nevertheless, there are well-authenticated reports from World War I of heavy shelling at a particular location being heard over wide areas in Europe.

Page 103 Fourier analysis The best general book on Fourier analysis and synthesis is probably still Bracewell, R. (1965) *The Fourier Transform and its Applications* (McGraw-Hill, New York).

Page 104 Musical instruments There are many good accounts of specifically musical aspects of hearing: see for instance Pierce, J. R. (1983) *The Science of Musical Sound* (Scientific American Books, New York); and Roederer, J. G. (1973) *Introduction to the Psychophysics of Music* (Springer, New York).

Page 107 Protective function of middle ear The reaction time of such a response to intense sounds is such that it cannot in fact provide much protection against things like loud bangs, since by the time the muscles contract the damage has been done. But in discos and other hostile environments they may help by acting as automatic earplugs.

Page 109 von Békésy His *Experiments in Hearing* (1960) (McGraw-Hill, New York) still makes stunning reading.

Page 110 IHCs per octave This happens to be of the same order of magnitude as what a musician can discriminate; but since pitch discrimination is more likely to be a central phenomenon, based on periodicity, this appears to be simply a coincidence.

Page 112 Hair cell mechanisms See for instance Ashmore, J. F. (1991) The electrophysiology of hair cells. *Annual Review of Physiology* 53, 465-476; and Dallos, P. and Corey, M. E. (1991) The role of the hair cells in cochlear tuning. *Current Opinion in Neurobiology* 1, 215-220.

Page 116 Binaural localization These mechanisms are obviously of very great importance in the design of stereo audio systems. Ordinary stereo heard through a pair of loudspeakers is not very realistic for a number of reasons. First of all, it can provide an impression only of right – left localizsation and not of vertical localization; but more important, it messes up the normal time delays between the ears that are vital in low-frequency localization. Each ear hears the sound from both speakers, so that a single recorded click reaches the brain as four separate clicks, two to each ear. This problem can obviously be got round by listening through headphones; but although this can certainly give a greatly improved sense of localization, one is then up against a different problem. In order to achieve good balance between different instruments in an orchestra or band, sound engineers like to use a vast array of microphones scattered about in different locations, and then mix them all together to form the two stereo channels. As a result, the phase relations between the same sound on the two channels are more confused than ever, and a single click is likely to end up as many dozens of clicks by the time it reaches the listener. Since most people listen through loudspeakers which muddle up the phase relationships anyway, this is not thought to matter much, but it means that recordings of this type do not work very well even through headphones.

A very great improvement is the use of dummy head microphones. Here each channel is recorded through its own single microphone, which is placed in a dummy head, carefully designed, sometimes with detailed modelling of the external ears, in such a way that it produces the same kind of directional coloration that a real head would. If one now listens to the recording through headphones, the effect is extraordinarily realistic, partly because both amplitude and phase information is preserved, and also because for the first time it is possible to perceive the vertical localization of a sound. The one snag, which is true of all headphone systems, is that moving the head moves the sound image with it, reducing the illusion.

Page 118 Binaural coincidence One might speculate on whether a similar mechanism, with signals from the same ear sent in from *both* directions, might not serve to convert the periodicity of lower frequency auditory signals into a spatial pattern suitable for processing by higher levels.

NEUROLAB

♫ Sound and Fourier analysis

Page 103

This exhibit lets you explore the relationship between the waveform of a sound and its spectrum. If you have a Soundblaster card or equivalent, you can listen to the waves that you create, by clicking on the Listen panel. On the right is a list of radio buttons which select various preset waveforms, ranging from a simple sine wave to an extremely complex sound with many spectral components. Examine each of them in turn, and compare the waveform with the spectrum displayed in the window at bottom left, and listen to them as well if your equipment allows you to. You can edit the spectrum by choosing a harmonic with the horizontal scroll-bar at the bottom, and altering its amplitude with the vertical one on the right; there is also a row of radio buttons to the right which select different phases. When the spectrum is ready, press Make new wave, and the corresponding waveform will appear in the waveform window.

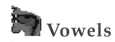 Vowels

Page 104

This exhibit allows you to select various vowel sounds, with the radio buttons on the right, to examine either their waveform or spectrum, and – if you have a Soundblaster card or equivalent – to listen to the result. Selecting Larynx alone shows the unfiltered sound from the vocal cords, with a comb spectrum in which all the harmonics are of the same amplitude. Choosing High, Medium or Low frequency selects the pitch generated by the larynx, and you can see that at high frequencies the harmonics are spaced further apart. The effect of changing the configuration of the vocal tract to generate different vowels is to add an envelope to the spectrum, which in this simple model has two peaks or formants (in real life there are three or four). The positions of the formants change for different vowels, but they do not vary with pitch. Note that although the spectra associated with different vowels are relatively simple, the resultant waveforms are extremely complex.

 ## The basilar membrane

Page 109

This exhibit shows, very schematically, how a travelling wave passes along the basilar membrane at different frequencies. Choose a frequency with the radio buttons on the right. The corresponding envelope will then appear in the window (note that it does not incorporate the action of the second filter, which in real life makes the peak of the envelope much sharper). Click on Start, and you will see a sequence of snapshots of the deflection of the basilar membrane (highly exaggerated in amplitude, of course) at equal intervals of time, giving the appearance of the travelling wave as it passes along the membrane.

 ## Phase locking

Page 113

This exhibit illustrates the principle of phasing locking or circus firing in auditory fibres. Click on Sweep, and you will see a sinusoidal sound wave (red, at top), and below it the pattern of action potentials in eight individual fibres, together with their total activity at the bottom (light blue). Although there is a degree of randomness about the behaviour of any one fibre, and – particularly at high frequencies – fibres may fire on average only every other cycle or

less often, nevertheless because the probability of firing is determined by the sound pressure the activity of the nerve bundle as a whole reflects the frequency of the stimulus, even when this is so high that no one fibre can follow it. You can alter the amplitude and frequency of the sound with the two sliders.

 ## Interaural delay

Page 117

This exhibit show how a pair of delay lines conducting in opposite directions, with a row of neurones that detect coincidence, can convert interaural delays into a spatial pattern for sound localization. Click at some point in the main window: this represents a brief pulse of sound, and you will see a wave front spread out from it. The two bottom corners of the box represent the two ears. When the wave reaches them, they are transformed into neural activity that moves at a steady rate along the corresponding horizontal delay lines. Where activity in the two lines meets, the corresponding neurone lights up red to signify detection of coincidence. If you click in the middle, a middle neurone eventually lights up; if to one side, a contralateral neurone is activated. In general, interaural delay is converted into spatial position.

Cortical regions

Page 118

A simple map of functional cortical areas, for self-testing. Click on one of the radio buttons designating an area of cortex, and the name and Brodmann number will appear in the box at right. Alternatively, click on the pull-down button at the right of the box to display the whole list, and click on an item: the corresponding radio button will be selected.

7 VISION

Light and dark 122
Image-forming by the eye 124
The retina 129
Retinal interneurones 135
Mechanisms of adaptation 137

Visual acuity 141
Visual form recognition 149
Colour vision 155
Visual localization 160
Visual proprioception 164

Light is a form of energy propagated by electromagnetic waves travelling at an immense velocity – some 300 metres per microsecond – and carried in discrete packets called quanta or photons. Only a very small range of all the wavelengths of electromagnetic radiation known to physicists are *visible* (Fig. 7.1). The longest waves that we can just see, forming the red end of the spectrum, are some 0.7 µm in length, slightly less than twice as long as the shortest waves at the blue end.

In nature, most electromagnetic radiation is generated by hot objects: the hotter they are, the more of this energy is radiated at shorter wavelengths. The peak of the spectrum of light from the sun – an exceedingly hot object – corresponds roughly with the range of wavelengths seen by the eye. Of man-made sources of light many, like the ordinary incandescent electric lamp, radiate as hot bodies and have a smooth and broad emission spectrum: others are quite different, and emit light only at a few

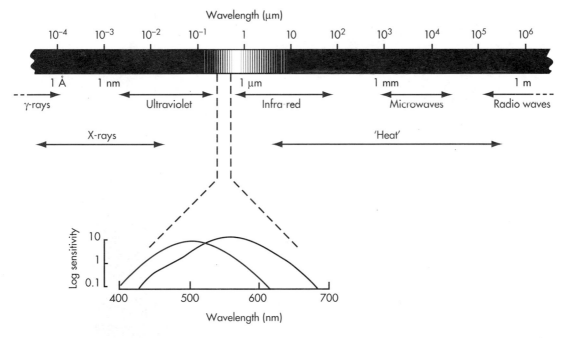

FIG. 7.1 The electromagnetic spectrum: vertical shading indicates the approximate energy distribution of radiation from the sun. Below, the visible portion of the spectrum expanded, showing the relative sensitivity of the human eye to different wavelengths in the dark-adapted (red curve) and light-adapted (black) state.

discrete wavelengths. The sodium lights used for street lighting, for example, are effectively monochromatic, their energy being concentrated in a very narrow band in the yellow region. Domestic fluorescent lamps have a spectrum consisting of a number of emission lines superimposed on a continuous background. *Colour* is a function of the relative energy in different parts of the spectrum.

LIGHT AND DARK

Colour is in a sense a measure of the quality of a light. Determining its quantity is called photometry, and is complicated by the fact that there are two kinds of photometric measurements: firstly, how much light is *emitted* by a source of radiation, and secondly, how much light is *received* by an illuminated object. The *candela* is a measure of the rate of emission of light by an object: an ordinary 60 watt bulb is equivalent to about 100 candela. The amount of light received by an object per unit area is its *illuminance*, and is measured in *lux*. This unit is defined as the degree of illumination of a surface one metre from a source of

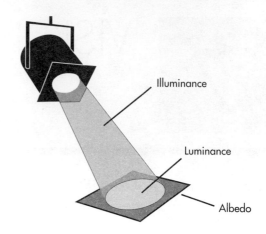

FIG. 7.2 Illuminance measures how much light falls on a surface; luminance measures how much it emits. Albedo is a measure of the extent to which a surface scatters back the light that falls on it: a perfect diffuser has an albedo of one.

one candela radiating in all directions. Full sunlight may provide about 100 000 lux.

Now objects in the real world scatter back some of the light that falls on them, so that in general an illuminated surface is also a luminous one, emitting a

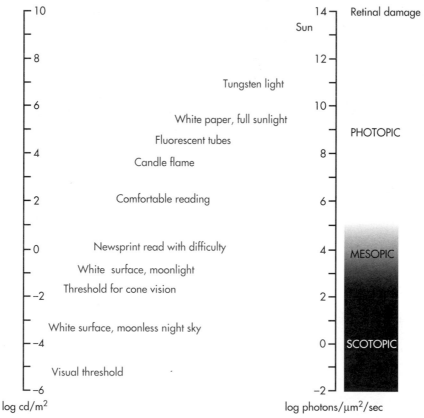

FIG. 7.3 The range of luminances (left) and retinal illumination (right, approximate) found in the natural world.

certain amount of light per unit area: this is described by its *luminance,* measured in candelas per square metre (cd/m²). Finally, the ratio of luminance to illuminance in these conditions is a measure of the surface's whiteness or *albedo* (Fig. 7.2). If we shine one lux on a perfectly white object that is also a perfect diffuser, it will have a luminance of about 0.32 cd/m², and such a surface is said to have an albedo of unity. Ordinary white paper has an albedo of about 0.95; paper printed with black ink, about 0.05. The photometry of coloured objects, which scatter back light of a different spectral composition from that which illuminates them (so that their albedo is a function of wavelength), is more complex and requires special definitions and methods of measurement.

Figure 7.3 gives some idea of the range of luminances found in nature. It can be seen that the brightest lights tolerated by the eye without damage are some 10^{15} times more intense than the dimmest that can just be perceived. This is an extraordinary performance that few man-made imaging devices can emulate: one need only think of the absurd level of lighting that is apparently necessary in television studios.

Adaptation: a sliding scale

In practice, however, at any one moment the actual range of luminances to which the eye is exposed is very much smaller than this. Because the albedos of natural objects vary only from about 0.05 to 0.95, the range of luminances that you see, for instance as you look round a uniformly illuminated room, is only about 20:1, and this ratio is of course unaffected by changes in the overall level of illumination. Black objects seen in daylight look black because they lie at the bottom end of the range of luminances in the environment, even though absolutely they may radiate very much *more* light than white objects seen under dimmer artificial light at night. Although not very bright in absolute terms, the latter look white because they are at the top end of the range of luminances in the vicinity (Fig. 7.4).

Black and white are thus relative terms: the eye operates on a sliding scale of brightness that can be moved up and down the whole 15 log unit range in such a way as to match the prevailing level of luminance; this property is the result of various mechanisms of *adaptation.* It follows that the eye responds not so much to the luminance of natural objects as to their albedo, a much more useful sensory quality since albedo is an intrinsic property of objects, whereas their luminance depends on how much they happen to be illuminated.

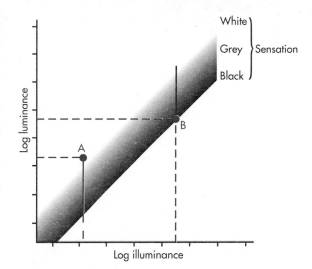

FIG. 7.4 The eye's sliding scale of brightness. A piece of white paper that is dimly lit (A) looks white because its luminance lies at the top of its local scale, even though this luminance may be *less* than that of a piece of black paper that is brightly lit (B). The latter looks black because it is at the bottom of its local scale.

There are several distinct mechanisms that contribute to this ability of the eye to adapt to the prevailing level of illumination, and they are discussed in more detail on p. 137 below. Some respond quickly to a sudden change in the ambient level, others more slowly. If we go from daylight to a dark room we find that it takes nearly 40 minutes for the eye to adjust its sensitivity fully to the reduced level of illumination. The simplest way to demonstrate this process of dark adaptation is to measure a subject's absolute threshold – the luminance of the dimmest light he can just perceive – at regular intervals during this adapting period. Such curves normally show two distinct components (Fig. 7.5): an initial one that levels off after some 8 minutes, and a further, slower increase in sensitivity that takes another 30 minutes or so to reach completion.

This dual response is due to the presence in the retina of two different types of receptor: *cones,* that function at high light levels (the *photopic* region of Fig. 7.3) but cannot respond to luminances lower than some 0.1 cd/m², and *rods,* which are much more sensitive and respond throughout the *scotopic* range but are overloaded by bright lights and cannot contribute much in the photopic region. Between scotopic and photopic is a *mesopic* region where both types of receptor contribute to vision. The cones adapt relatively quickly and are responsible for the first branch of the adaptation curve; the rods adapt more slowly, and provide the final and more gradual

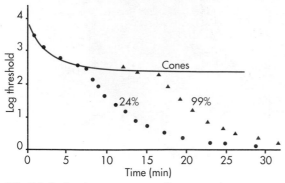

FIG. 7.5 Dark adaptation curves. The points show measurements of absolute threshold at different times after a strong light that bleached 99 percent (triangles) or 24 percent (circles) of the pigment in the rods. The red line indicates the approximate timecourse of recovery of sensitivity of the cones alone. It is clear that recovery occurs in two stages: the first is due to cones, and the second, delayed, stage to rods. (Data from Rushton and Powell, 1972)

component of dark adaptation. Animals that are specialized for night vision have only rods in their retina, which means that they are unable to respond effectively to the enormous range of luminances that can be appreciated by an eye of mixed type such as our own. We shall see later that cones have further properties that are useful in vision. In particular, they respond preferentially to different narrow bands of the spectrum, providing a mechanism by which the visual system can respond to the *quality* (i.e. the colour) of a source of light, as well as its quantity.

Some of the differences between photopic and scotopic vision are summarized below. Further explanation of some of the terms used is given in the sections that follow.

IMAGE-FORMING BY THE EYE

But the eye is not just a device for sensing light and dark: it forms an image of the outside world, and encodes it as neural messages for the brain. When parallel rays of light pass into a denser medium with a convex surface or a less dense medium with a concave surface, they are brought to a focus at a distance that is a function of the radius of curvature and of the ratios of the refractive indices of the two media. In the eye, there are three surfaces of this sort that act together to bring the images of distant objects to a focus on the retina: they are the *cornea*, and the front and back surfaces of the *lens* (Fig. 7.6). The refractive index of the aqueous humour that separates the cornea and lens is much the same as that of the vitreous humour that fills the rest of the eye, and is about 1.34; that of the crystalline lens is only slightly greater than this, being about 1.42, so that most of the refractive power of the eye is due to the cornea rather than the lens. Ophthalmologists describe the power of refractive surfaces by the reciprocal of their focal length in metres, and these units are called *dioptres*

Box 7.1 Vision under photopic and scotopic conditions		
	Photopic	**Scotopic**
Sensitivity	Low; best vision in fovea	High; best vision outside fovea
	Light entering periphery of pupil less effective than centre (Stiles–Crawford effect)	No Stiles–Crawford effect
Spatial properties	High acuity; contrast sensitivity reduced at low spatial frequencies (lateral inhibition)	Low acuity; less lateral inhibition
Temporal properties	High flicker fusion frequency; reduced sensitivity at low frequencies (fast adaptation)	Low flicker fusion frequency; less fast adaptation. Increased latency
Wavelength	Most sensitive at around 550 nm	Most sensitive at around 500 nm (Purkinje shift)
	Trichromatic colour discrimination	Monochromatic

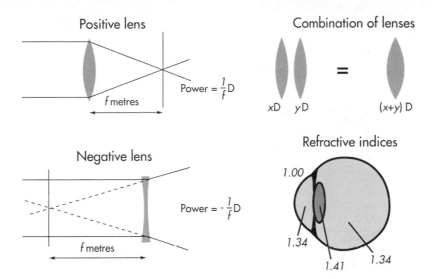

FIG. 7.6 Left, a positive (convex) lens with focal length *f* metres has a power of (1/*f*) dioptres; for a concave lens, the power is negative. Above right,,for thin lenses, close together, dioptres simply add linearly. Below right, images are formed in the eye by refraction at several interfaces between media of different refractive indices; the lens itself contributes less than might be expected, because its refractive index is not very different from what surrounds it.

(D). The effective total refracting power of the human lens and cornea when the eye is focussed on a distant object is some 60 D. Of this, only a little more than a quarter is due to the lens rather than the cornea.

Accommodation and the lens

The lens does not contribute much to the total refractive power; but its main use lies in the fact that it can alter its shape and hence change the eye's effective focal length: this function is called *accommodation*. The lens presents something of a design problem for nature, since it obviously cannot have a blood supply. It obtains its nutrients and oxygen from the *aqueous humour* that bathes it both sides, a fluid similar to plasma but with only some 1% of its protein concentration and a peculiarly high concentration of ascorbic acid. It is continuously secreted by the ciliary body (Fig. 7.7), and passes through the iris into the anterior chamber where it eventually filters its way out into the *canal of Schlemm*, where it contributes to tears and from there to veins. The resistance to its outflow generates an intraocular pressure of some 10–20 mmHg. Blockage may raise this pressure to the point where the flow of blood into the eye is hindered, a serious condition called glaucoma which is a common cause of blindness. The aqueous humour is able to penetrate the lens because it is fibrous, made of remarkably long (10 mm)

threadlike cells, rectangular in cross section and – for transparency – lacking nuclei, knitted together in a series of concentric layers like zip-fasteners by ball-and-socket joints that provide flexibility. There are also large numbers of gap junctions between them.

The lens is encircled at a distance by a ring of fibres called the ciliary zonule, to which it is joined by the radial *suspensory ligaments*; his ring can be made smaller by contraction of the radially arranged fibres of the *ciliary muscle* (Fig. 7.7). When the ciliary muscle is relaxed, the suspensory ligaments exert a radial pull on the edge of the lens that tends to flatten it; in accommodation, the ciliary muscle contracts under the influence of its parasympathetic innervation (Fig. 7.8) and thus allows the lens to revert to its natural, more biconvex and optically more powerful shape.

The range of accommodation can easily be measured by finding the positions of the *near and far points* of the eye, the nearest and furthest distances at which objects can just be brought into focus. For a normal or *emmetropic* eye with accommodation fully relaxed the far point will be at infinity, and the range of accommodation will be given by the reciprocal of the distance of the near point in metres: for a young subject, the near point will generally lie at around 80 mm, corresponding to 12 D of accommodation. As one gets older, however, the elasticity of the lens declines, and by the age of 60 the possible amplitude of accommodation may have fallen to 1 D or so, a condition known as *presbyopia* (Fig. 7.9). The near point will then be typically further than a metre, so

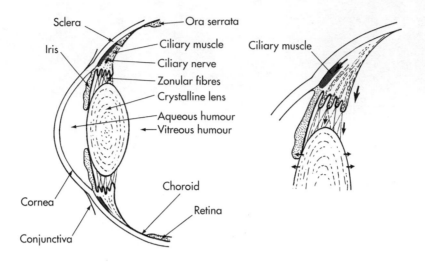

FIG. 7.7 The anterior part of the human eye, shown in parasagittal section.

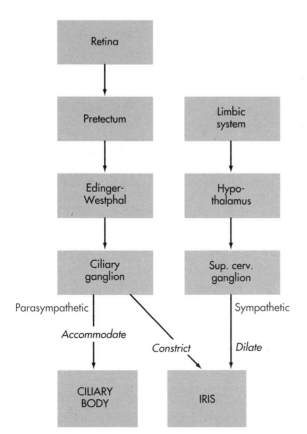

FIG. 7.8 Origins of signals controlling accommodation and pupil size.

that convex spectacles have to be worn if reading matter is to be brought within a comfortable holding distance.

Errors of refraction

But few people are exactly emmetropic, and what is normally found is that when the accommodation is fully relaxed the total refractive power is either too great or too small in relation to the distance from the cornea to the retina. If it is too great, images of distant objects are brought to a focus in front of the retina, and the eye is said to be *myopic* or short-sighted: under these circumstances the far point will not be at infinity but nearer to the eye. Such a condition may be corrected by the use of concave or negative spectacle lenses. *Hypermetropic* or far-sighted subjects are precisely the opposite, and require convex or positive lenses in order to focus at infinity with relaxed accommodation (Fig. 7.10). In either case, the degree of disability may be indicated by the power and sign of the lens needed to bring the eye back to emmetropia: thus a mildly short-sighted patient might require a correction of -1.75 D. This is called the *spherical* correction, and in general is not the same in both eyes.

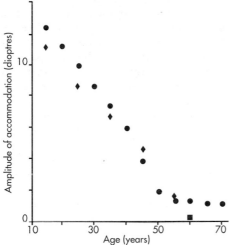

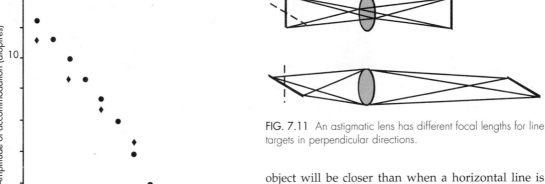

FIG. 7.11 An astigmatic lens has different focal lengths for line targets in perpendicular directions.

FIG. 7.9 Presbyopia: decline in the amplitude of accommodation as a function of age in three large groups of subjects. (Data from Fisher, 1973)

Another common defect is *astigmatism:* here the refractive power of the eye is found to be different in different meridians (Fig. 7.11), generally because of non-uniformities of the radius of curvature of the cornea. If, for example, it has a smaller radius of curvature in the horizontal plane than in the vertical, the far point when measured with a vertical line as test object will be closer than when a horizontal line is used. Opticians test for astigmatism by means of a target like that of Figure 7.12, called an *astigmatic fan;* an astigmatic subject will see some of the lines more sharply than others, and this will tell the optician the angle at which a cylindrical lens should be placed in front of the eye to make the refractive power as nearly as possible equal in all meridians. The power of the cylindrical lens that is needed to do this, together with its meridional angle, make up the cylindrical correction that is the second part of a prescription for spectacles. (A cylindrical lens is in effect a section cut from a cylinder, just as a spherical lens is cut from a sphere: it focuses only in one meridian (Fig. 7.13).

Astigmatism and incorrect refractive power are not the only faults that may be found in the eye's optics, and as in many man-made optical systems,

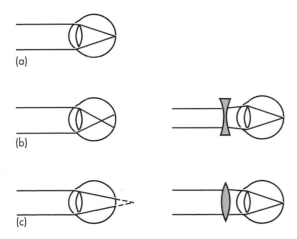

FIG. 7.10 Errors of focusing. **(a)** shows an emmetropic eye with relaxed accommodation that focuses parallel rays exactly on the retina. A myopic eye **(b)** brings parallel rays to a focus that is too close to the lens: the defect may be corrected with a negative (concave) lens (right). A hypermetropic eye **(c)** cannot bring parallel rays to a focus at all: a positive lens is needed for correction.

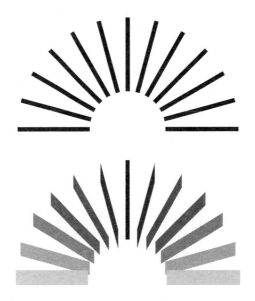

FIG. 7.12 Above, an astigmatic fan, a target used for testing for astigmatism, and its appearance (below) to a subject with marked astigmatism in the horizontal/vertical directions.

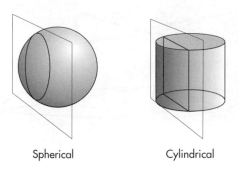

Spherical   Cylindrical

FIG. 7.13 The origin of spherical and cylindrical lenses.

the cornea and lens together produce a number of different types of optical *aberration*. The first of these is due to the fact that the refractive indices of the various optical media of the eye depend on the wavelength of the incident light. In general, the refractive index increases with decreasing wavelength, so that blue light is refracted more than red. This phenomenon is called dispersion and gives rise to defects in the resultant image, in the form of coloured fringes, called *chromatic aberration* (Fig. 7.14). This means that if one looks at a blue object and a red object lying side by side at the same distance from the eye, they cannot both be in focus simultaneously, and a subject who is emmetropic when his far point is measured in red light will be shortsighted if it is measured in blue: his far point will then be only a metre or so away. This forms the basis of a simple clinical test for errors of refraction, consisting of an

illuminated screen divided into three portions that are red, green and white: identical test figures are superimposed on each field, and the subject is simply asked which figure he sees most clearly. The emmetrope will see the one on the white background best, while the hypermetrope and myope will see most clearly those lying respectively on the green and red backgrounds.

The second major type of aberration is one that is common to all systems formed of spherical refracting surfaces, and is called *spherical aberration*. This arises because the shape of refracting surface needed to bring parallel rays to a point is not strictly speaking a spherical one at all, but an ellipsoid. For surfaces that are small in comparison with their radii of curvature the difference is slight, and spherical aberrations are often negligible. But in the case of the eye, the aperture is of the same order of magnitude as the radius of curvature of the cornea, and the result is that rays entering near the periphery of the cornea are bent too much, and form a closer focus than those entering near the centre (Fig. 7.14). To some extent nature has compensated for spherical aberration, first of all by making a cornea that is not exactly spherical but tends towards the desired ellipsoid, and secondly in that the refractive index of the lens is not constant throughout but graded from a maximum of some 1.42 at its centre to about 1.39 at the edge, thus cancelling out, to some extent, the extra bending of peripheral light rays. The degrading effects of both spherical and chromatic aberration, and of other defects due to irregularities of the refracting surfaces, get worse as the *pupil* or aperture of the eye increases, and this in turn is under the control of the *iris*.

The control of the pupil

Unlike the lens, the size of the pupil is under the control of two different muscles: one, the sphincter pupillae, lies circumferentially round the iris, and the other, the dilator, lies radially. The two muscles thus have opposed effects, the first causing contraction of the pupil and the second dilatation, and they are respectively under the control of the parasympathetic and sympathetic systems (Fig. 7.8). It is not entirely clear which of the two branches of the autonomic nervous system is responsible for normal tonic control of pupil size, and one may cause mydriasis (enlargement of the pupil) by drugs that either block the action of acetylcholine on the sphincter (e.g. atropine) or simulate the effect of noradrenaline on the dilator (e.g. phenylephrine). The advantages of a large pupil size are first that the eye receives more

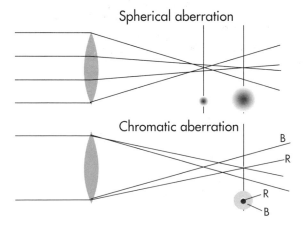

Spherical aberration

Chromatic aberration

B
R

R
B

FIG. 7.14 Aberrations. Spherical aberration (above) arises because the focal lengths of different regions of the lens are not the same. Below, chromatic aberration is the result of focal length depending on wavelength (B = blue; R = red).

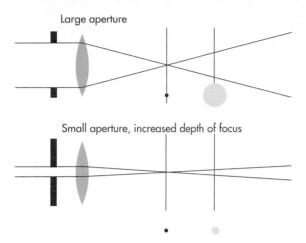

Large aperture

Small aperture, increased depth of focus

FIG. 7.15 A small pupil minimizes the effects of bad focus on the size of the image, so it increases the depth of focus as well as reducing the effects of the aberrations.

light (over the normal range of pupil diameters, about 2–8 mm, the amount of light caught by the eye varies by a factor of 16), and secondly that the diffraction effects that always occur when light passes through a small aperture are minimized. The advantages of a small pupil, on the other hand, are an increased depth of field (a greater tolerance of errors of focus) and a reduction in the magnitude of the optical aberrations (Fig. 7.15): the extent of this effect can be seen for oneself by looking through a pinhole, which acts as a very small artificial pupil. The effects of pupil size on visual acuity are discussed in more detail later in this chapter, on p. 144.

Thus the ideal size for the pupil is something of a compromise, and depends on the ambient light level. Under bright photopic conditions the eye can take advantage of the excess light by reducing the pupil and improving the quality of the retinal image. In scotopic conditions, however, the eye needs all the light it can get and the quality of the retinal image is of secondary importance: in any case, we shall see later that the rods are not capable of passing on accurate information about the detailed structure of the retinal image. It is important to emphasize that pupil dilatation contributes very little to the enormous changes in sensitivity that accompany dark adaptation, since it can only vary the incoming light by a factor of 16 at most or 1.2 log units. The control of the pupil is also closely linked to accommodation: when the ciliary muscle contracts in order to focus on a near object, there is normally an associated constriction of the pupil (the *near reflex*). As these responses are usually also combined with binocular convergence movements of the two eyes, the whole pattern

of response (constriction, accommodation, convergence) is also known as the *triple response*. Under certain clinical conditions, notably in neurosyphilis, one may find that the pupillary response to near objects remains despite loss of the response to bright lights: this condition is known as the Argyll Robertson pupil, and is an important diagnostic neurological sign. The fact that pupil dilatation is also a measure of general sympathetic activity and of emotional or sexual excitement also has its uses.

THE RETINA

One might hope to be able to see another person's retina directly by eyeball-to-eyeball confrontation: if both eyes are emmetropic and relaxed, each retina should be clearly in focus on the other (Fig. 7.16). The reason why this doesn't in fact work is that the presence of the observer's eye also prevents light falling on the other's retina, so that nothing can be seen: under normal conditions the pupil of the eye is always dark. The *ophthalmoscope* is a device that gets round this problem by projecting a small beam of light into the subject's pupil at the same time. It also has an arrangement whereby one of a set of negative and positive lenses can be introduced into the optical pathway: the power of the lens that exactly brings the subject's retina into sharp focus is equal and opposite to the combined refractive errors of observer and subject. Thus so long as an oculist knows his own

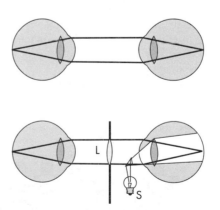

FIG. 7.16 The principle of the ophthalmoscope. If an observer looks into a subject's eye and both are emmetropic, the retina of one will be focused on that of the other. But the observer's eye prevents light from reaching the subject's retina, so that nothing can be seen (above). But the ophthalmoscope (below) introduces an extra source of light, S, to illuminate the subject's retina, and is fitted with a set of lenses (L) that correct for errors of refraction.

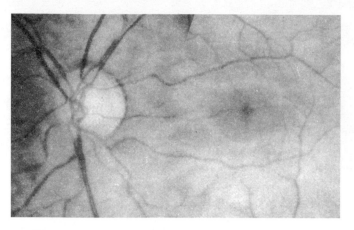

FIG. 7.17 Photograph of a living human retina, showing blood vessels, optic disc and blind spot (left) and macula lutea, with fovea at its centre (right). (Courtesy of J. Keast-Butler, FRCS)

correction, the ophthalmoscope provides an objective method for determining what spectacles the subject requires, as well as permitting the examination of the retina for signs of disease.

Two features of the retina are immediately obvious when seen through the ophthalmoscope (Fig. 7.17), both of them the consequence of a massive error of judgement on the part of nature, namely the decision to have the retina inside out with the neurones between the receptors and the incoming light. As a consequence, the nerve fibres from the retina find themselves inside the eye when they want to be outside; what they do is come together to form the optic nerve, and crash their way out, together with the central retinal artery and vein, through a region called the *optic disc* at about 15° to the nasal side of the optical axis. Since this area is incapable of responding to light, subjectively it forms the *blind spot*. Although some 5° across, one is usually unaware of its existence because the brain tends to fill it in with whatever background colour or pattern immediately surrounds it (Fig. 7.18).

The other gross feature of the retina visible with the ophthalmoscope is an area about 5° across very close to the centre of the retina that is free of large blood vessels – they arch around on each side to sup-ply it from the edge – and is also distinctly yellower than the rest of the field. This is the *macula lutea* (yellow spot), and at its centre is a very small dot – actually a depression or pit – called the *fovea centralis*. When we look at a small object in the outside world, it is the fovea that is directed to the corresponding part of the retinal image: its angular size is about that of one's finger nail with the hand fully extended. The fovea is specialized for high quality, photopic vision: it is quite without rods, and the cones themselves are tightly packed to give the maximum information about image detail (Fig. 7.19). Cones in this region are about 2.3 μm across, corresponding to a visual angle of some half minute of arc. The depression arises because the retinal structures that elsewhere in the retina lie between the receptors and the lens – remembering again that the retina is inside-out in its layered structure – are here displaced to one side so as to cause the minimum scattering of incoming light. The supply of oxygen and nutrients for this region must derive almost entirely from the blood vessels that richly supply the *choroid,* the layer immediately superficial to the receptors and separated from them by the thin *pigment epithelium.*

The retina is quite different from any of the sense organs we have met so far in that a good deal of the

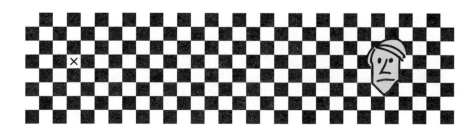

FIG. 7.18 Demonstration of the blind spot. Close the left eye, and fixate the cross with the page at about 35 cm from the eye. The face will disappear, and no discontinuity on the background will be apparent.

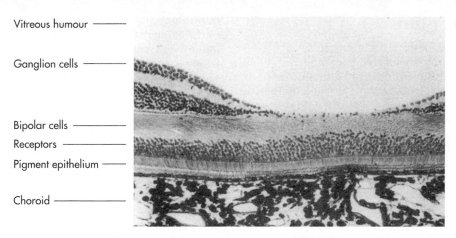

Vitreous humour ————

Ganglion cells ————

Bipolar cells ————

Receptors ————

Pigment epithelium ————

Choroid ————

FIG. 7.19 Section through a monkey fovea. The direction of incident light is from above downwards, passing through the layers of neural elements (which in the central fovea are pushed to one side) before reaching the receptors.

neural processing of the afferent information has already occurred before it reaches the fibres of the optic nerve. No doubt the reason for this is that the eye is a highly mobile organ, and if each of the 130 million or so receptors sent its own individual fibre

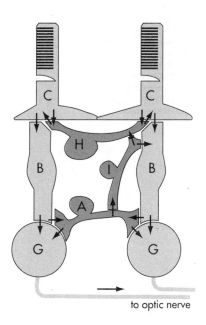

to optic nerve

FIG. 7.20 Retinal neurones and their connections. Schematic representation, showing primate cones (C) forming synapses between the r pedicles and bipolar cells (B) and horizontal cells (H). The bipolars connect with amacrine cells (A) and ganglion cells (G) whose axons form the optic nerve. Interplexiform cells (I) have also been described, feeding back from amacrines to bipolars and horizontal cells.

into the optic nerve, the latter would have to be some 11 times thicker than at present, and would be a considerable hindrance to rapid movement of the eye; and of course the blind spot would be correspondingly larger as well. The fibres of the optic nerve are in fact at two synapses' remove from the retinal receptors, and particularly as far as the rods in the periphery are concerned, there is considerable convergence of information from large groups of receptors. What happens is that receptors synapse with *bipolar cells*, and these in turn synapse with the million or so *ganglion cells* whose axons form the optic nerve. These two types of neurone form consecutive layers on top of the receptor layer – except in the fovea, where we have seen that they are pushed to one side – and are mingled with two other types of interneurone that make predominantly sideways connections. These are the *horizontal cells* at the bipolar/receptor level, and the *amacrine cells* at the ganglion cell/bipolar level. Finally, there is a type of interneurone whose existence remained undetected until very recently, because it does not take up the Golgi stain: the *interplexiform cell*. This actually appears to conduct information backwards, from the amacrines back to the horizontals and bipolars. The arrangement of the connections of all these types of interneurone is shown schematically in Figure 7.20; the general arrangement is quite constant across species, though details vary. We shall see that there are marked differences in the electrical behaviour of all these neurones: although ganglion cells and amacrines show spike discharges in response to retinal stimulation, the bipolars, horizontal cells and the receptors themselves do not: they are small enough to be able to interact electrotonically without the need for active propagation.

The receptors

Rods and cones both consist of two distinct parts: an outer segment, apparently a grossly modified cilium, and an inner segment containing the nucleus. The outer segment possesses a high concentration of photopigment associated with a richly folded set of invaginations of the outer surface, which are formed at the bottom and gradually move up to the tip over the course of a month or so, then breaking off and being destroyed. In the case of rods they seal themselves off near the bottom, to form a stack of flattened saccules or discs (Fig. 7.21); in the cones they remain partially open. At the base of the outer segment the remains of the ciliary filaments and centrioles can be seen. The inner segment has mitochondria as well as the nucleus, and its inner end forms the synaptic junction with bipolar and horizontal cells. There is no doubt that the *photopigment* straddling the membranes of the outer segment discs plays a key role in

transforming incident light into electrical changes, for if the pigment is isolated from the receptor it is found that its absorption of light of different wavelengths corresponds closely with the spectral sensitivity of the receptors themselves. In the frog, each rod has some 1700 discs, and a disc contains some 1.5 million pigment molecules.

Retinal photopigment consists of two portions: a chromophore called *retinal* or retinene (a derivative of retinol, better known as vitamin A), in association with a protein/oligosaccharide complex with a molecular weight of around 40 000, which may be called *opsin*. It is slight differences in the composition of the opsin part that give rise to the different spectral sensitivities of rods and cones. The first effect of light on the visual pigment found in rods *(rhodopsin)* is to cause an isomerism of the retinal from the normal 11-cis form to the all-trans configuration (Fig. 7.22). This in turn leads to a series of changes in the configuration of the rhodopsin, producing a number of more

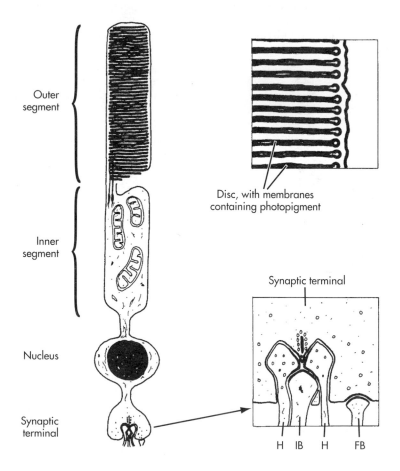

FIG. 7.21 Schematic section of a monkey rod showing inner and outer segments. H, horizontal cell; FB, IB, flat and invaginating bipolars

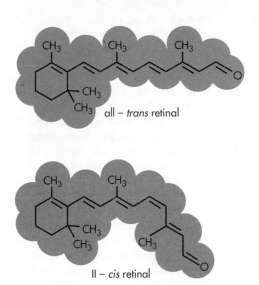

FIG. 7.22 All-trans retinal and 11-cis retinal.

or less shortlived intermediates, that culminates in the complete dissociation of the opsin from the retinal. In vitro, this is the end of the matter, and the pigment is said to be bleached. But in the rods, the bleached pigment can be regenerated by enzymes present in the receptors and in the pigment epithelium that lies behind them. The first stage of this process consists of the reconversion of the free all-trans retinal back to the 11-cis form, a relatively slow

process (Fig. 7.23). The significance of these wanderings of pigment back and forth between receptor and pigment epithelium is unclear.

We shall see later that it is this slow regeneration of pigment that determines the long time-course of recovery of rod sensitivity during dark adaptation that has already been mentioned (Fig. 7.5). In bright light, most of the rhodopsin is in the bleached form: an equilibrium is reached in which the rate of bleaching equals the rate of regeneration. Estimates of the amount of pigment in the receptors of a living eye during particular stimulus conditions may be made by the technique of *retinal reflection densitometry*, in which one measures the amount and spectral composition of the light scattered back from the retina when a light is shone into the eye. In this way it is possible to track continuously the amount of rod or cone pigment in bleached form under relatively natural visual conditions. Alternatively, in microdensitometry, the spectral absorptions of individual receptors may be measured in a preparation on a microscope slide. As far as we know, the reactions that occur in rods and cones are fundamentally similar, though the regeneration of cone pigment is substantially quicker than in rods, and under photopic conditions a smaller fraction of the cone pigment is in the bleached state than is the case for rods. This is one of the reasons why the cones are able to function at much higher light levels.

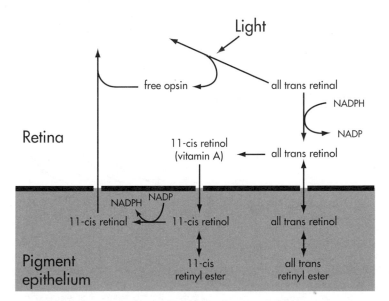

FIG. 7.23 The cyclical sequence of events by which light leads to isomerization of retinal and its dissociation from opsin, followed by the relatively slow processes that lead to the final regeneration of rhodopsin.

Electrical responses to light

The nature of the basic transduction process was outlined in Chapter 3 (p. 45). The bleaching of rhodopsin is coupled by a G-protein – it is not known at what stage – to the activation of phosphodiesterase (PDE) that converts the cyclic nucleotide cGMP to GMP. Since cGMP tonically promotes the opening of sodium channels in the plasma membrane, the effect of light on the outer segment is to reduce sodium permeability by reducing the level of cGMP (Fig. 7.24), and hence hyperpolarize the receptor from a resting

value of some –30 mV to a maximum of –60 mV. As in many such cascades, there is a huge amplification of effects along the way: in rods, each quantum absorbed appears to cause the breakdown of about a million cGMP molecules, although the next stage is a bit of an anticlimax since it takes three cGMPs to open a channel. Measurements of the absolute threshold for seeing dim flashes of light when the eye is fully dark-adapted show that a single rod is capable of responding to a single absorbed photon. Individually, cones are an order of magnitude less sensitive (photopic vision is *several* orders of magnitude less sensitive, because it enjoys less convergence and pooling of neural signals).

The time-course of the hyperpolarization generated by a brief flash of light is very prolonged – a characteristic of indirect transduction with a lengthy cascade – and shows a pronounced plateau with very large stimuli, corresponding to closure of all the sodium channels. If one plots the size of this receptor potential as a function of the intensity of the flash (Fig. 7.25) one finds a characteristic S-shaped or saturating relationship. The effect of different levels of light adaptation is to shift this curve along the intensity axis, providing one of the mechanisms by which the sensitivity of the retina is adjusted to suit the prevailing luminance. Bright backgrounds shorten the response as well as reducing its size; the significance and mechanism of this are discussed later, on p. 137.

Students are sometimes upset to discover that photoreceptors respond to a positive stimulus (light) by what might be regarded as a negative response (hyperpolarization and consequent reduction in the rate of transmitter release at the synaptic ending). It

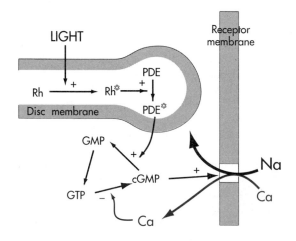

FIG. 7.24 The cascade linking bleaching of rhodopsin (RH → RH*) to sodium entry, as believed to occur in vertebrates. PDE = phosphodiesterase. The entry of calcium at the same time as sodium is believed to be a mechanism contributing to receptor adaptation, in part by slowing the regeneration of cyclic AMP.

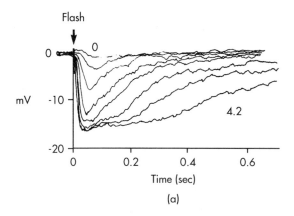

(a)

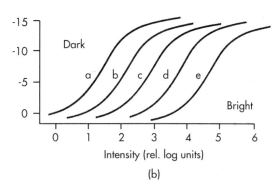

(b)

FIG. 7.25 Electrical responses from turtle cones. **(a)** Hyperpolarizations generated by a very brief flash of various intensities ranging from 0 to 4.2 relative log units in steps of 0.6 log unit. **(b)** Showing the effect of preadaptation to different backgrounds in such an experiment. Each curve is the result of an experiment like the one on the left, where peak electrical response is plotted as a function of the flash intensity. Curve *a* was measured in the dark, *b–e* under different increasing background adaptation levels over a range of some 3.5 log units. (After Baylor and Fuortes, 1970, and Normann and Perelman, 1979)

is understandable enough that a physicist should regard turning on a light as a positive signal; but in the natural world, the kinds of visual objects that are of importance to an animal are much more commonly dark than light. One need only think of a frog's view of an insect flying against the background of the sky or of the sudden and ominous darkening of the field of view that portends the arrival of an unpleasant predator or a descending foot.

RETINAL INTERNEURONES

Horizontal cells and bipolars

The *bipolar* cells represent the next stage in the transmission of visual information from receptors to brain. Photoreceptors tonically release their transmitter, glutamate, from their feet or *pedicles*, and in the light they release less of it. Rods synapse with a particular kind called the *rod bipolar*, with convergence from many rods (Fig. 7.26); rod bipolars depolarize in response to light. Cones make contact with two kinds of bipolars. With one class, the *flat bipolar*, the synapse is at the base of the receptor and is relatively conventional in appearance; the bipolar hyperpolarizes to light. The other kind is of an unusual type in which invaginations of the foot of the receptors receive processes from both *invaginating bipolars* (depolarizing to light – very unusually, the glutamate is inhibitory, indirectly via cGMP-mediated channels) and also *horizontal cells* (hyperpolarizing) in a kind of three-way junction. Here, the receptor affects both horizontal cells and bipolars, and in addition transmission to the bipolar is modulated by the horizontal cells acting on the receptors (they also make conventional GABinergic inhibitory synapses with both types of bipolars).

Since the horizontal cell receives information from receptors over a wide area, this means that the horizontal cells provide a mechanism of lateral inhibition (Fig. 7.27). This can be demonstrated directly by electrical recording from bipolars. Although their electrical responses are generally similar in size and time scale to the slow potentials that can be recorded from the receptors themselves, they show receptive field properties that are quite different from those of rods and cones. Whereas the receptive field of a receptor is very simple (a small area over which light causes hyperpolarization), in the case of a bipolar the field is much larger, and is non-uniform: light falling in its centre has the opposite effect to light falling in the periphery. Thus a cell that depolarizes when a bright spot shines on the centre of its receptive field will hyperpolarize if it is focused on the surround,

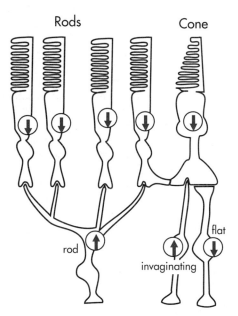

FIG. 7.26 Diagrammatic representation of the functional relationship between primate rods and cones and various types of bipolar cell. Rod bipolars receive information from many rods, and depolarize in response to light. Invaginating and flat bipolars connect with cones, and show opposite electrical responses; through rod–cone electrical connections they may also respond indirectly to rods. (Modified, after Kolb and Nelson, 1984).

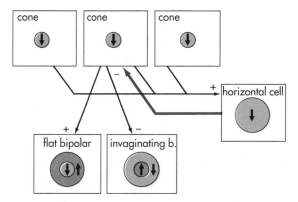

FIG. 7.27 Lateral inhibition in bipolar cells. Left, a set of cones influencing a horizontal cell; bipolar cells may receive a hyperpolarizing input from a receptor and a depolarizing one from the horizontal cell, or vice versa, resulting in a receptive field with opposed centre and surround. Right, responses of bipolar cell to disc (above) and annulus of light, showing antagonism between centre and surround.

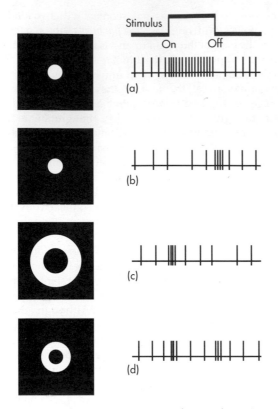

FIG. 7.28 Schematic representation of types of ganglion cell response: **(a)** sustained; **(b)** off-centre; **(c)** on-surround; **(d)** intermediate on–off.

that enables the number of optic nerve fibres to be so much smaller than the number of rods and cones. In the fovea this convergence is much less evident, and most of the bipolars contact only a single cone: acuity is thus preserved at the expense of sensitivity.

Ganglion cells and amacrines

As noted earlier, ganglion cells differ from all the other types of cell except the amacrines in that they respond to light with repetitive spike discharges. Like bipolars, ganglion cells often have receptive fields consisting of a centre region with an antagonistic surround, many of them having in addition the property that they respond only transiently when retinal illumination is suddenly changed from one level to another. Sometimes a transient burst of firing is found in response to an increase of illumination (an 'on response'), and sometimes to a decrease ('off response') and occasionally one may find a burst response both at the beginning and end of a period of steady illumination (an 'on–off response'). A cell with an on response at its centre will normally show an off response in its surround, and vice versa (Fig. 7.28), and show on–off responses in intermediate regions. Thus as far as their field properties are concerned, ganglion cells are similar to bipolars: the new feature of transient sensitivity is probably the result of feedback inhibition from the amacrines, whose responses are very similar to those of ganglion cells and have the right sort of connections for mediating lateral and self-inhibition of the type that would explain the time-course of the ganglion cell responses.

Amacrine cells come in a large number of distinct types, each with a characteristic morphology and often with its own particular synaptic transmitter, including some fancy peptides, and it is likely that each type has a different specialized function but as yet we have little idea as to what precisely these different functions are (Fig. 7.29). Mammalian rod bipolars do not synapse with ganglion cells directly but *only* through amacrines.

Of the ganglion cells, the simplest are W or wide-field cells that show sustained responses to steady light level over a large field, with very slow conduction velocities: clearly some such source of information must be projected into the optic nerve to explain such tonic responses to constant illumination as the tonic pupil light reflex or the various hormonal responses to day length and time of day. But most show more complex responses, and fall into more or less distinct functional classes, often related to their size or the general shape of their dendritic tree. One

and vice versa (Fig. 7.27). The effect of this antagonism between centre and surround is to make the bipolar respond more vigorously to small stimuli in the centre of its field than to large areas that cover both centre and surround; the existence of the two populations of bipolar cell, depolarizing and hyperpolarizing, no doubt corresponds to the need to be able to detect objects that are lighter than their backgrounds as well as those that are darker.

In addition to pooling of information through horizontal cells, direct electrical synapses between the receptors themselves, and also linking horizontal cells, can sometimes also be seen. Pooling of this kind is extremely desirable under scotopic conditions, when it is helpful to average responses over large areas of the retina in order to distinguish feeble stimuli from background noise (but it doesn't, of course, do much for one's visual acuity). In the periphery of the retina, pooling of this kind is also mediated by the bipolars, some of which receive synapses from large numbers of receptors and hence provide the first stage of convergence, the funnelling of information

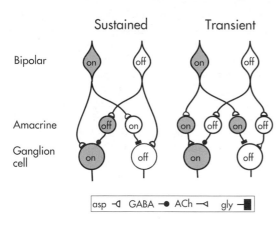

Sustained **Transient**

Bipolar

Amacrine

Ganglion cell

asp ◁ GABA ● ACh ◁ gly ■

FIG. 7.29 Schematic wiring diagram showing how amacrine cells may mediate the transient and field properties of ganglion cells. (Data from Ikeda and Sheardown, 1983)

broad classification is between Y cells (large, with high conduction velocities, responding briskly to movement or changes of light intensity) and the much more numerous X cells (smaller and slower, showing sustained responses with simple linear summation when different parts of the receptive field are simultaneously illuminated). Some of these differences seem to be related to whether their input comes primarily from bipolars (sustained) or from amacrines (transient); in mammals, it appears that no rod bipolars contact ganglion cells directly, so that all signals in the dark-adapted state must be transmitted via the amacrines. Other cells code specifically for colour, for movement in particular directions, and a host of other things; 23 different classes of ganglion cell have been described in the cat retina but not all these kinds of response are found in all species. The complete adaptation shown by the Y cells may correspond with the fact that images that are stabilized on the retina, for example by projection through a device attached to the cornea, disappear from view in a matter of seconds; the function of this kind of fast adaptation were discussed earlier, (p. 52). At all events, it is clear that the pattern of neural activity that is sent from the retina to the brain is not just a simple map of retinal illumination but that various kinds of information have already been computed and extracted from the retinal image, in preparation for the still more specific analysis that is performed by the brain itself.

MECHANISMS OF ADAPTATION

Having completed our tour of the retina, we are now in a position to consider the more difficult and perhaps more interesting problems that arise when we try to correlate what we feel about what we see (the psychophysics of vision) with how we know the brain actually works (the neurophysiology). It is convenient to start with one of the most basic psychophysical phenomena, our extraordinary indifference to very large fluctuations in the illumination of our surroundings.

The fundamental importance of adaptation in the visual system has already been emphasized. It enables the eye to cope over an enormous range of light intensities, a range that defeats all man-made devices. And it allows us to recognize objects through registering their *albedos*, ignoring the accident of how much they happen to be illuminated. It turns out that there are several different mechanisms in the eye that contribute to adaptation. One of them, the *pupillary light reflex*, has already been considered: we saw that in fact it is relatively puny in comparison with the huge dynamic range in which vision has to operate, and contributes rather little to adaptation. The other mechanisms are of two distinct kinds. When we change the overall illumination of the visual scene, part of the resultant change in sensitivity occurs almost immediately, and is simply a function of how intensely the visual field is illuminated at any moment: this kind of adaptation is called *field adaptation*. But in addition, we find that having adapted to bright visual surroundings, when the brightness is subsequently reduced it takes an appreciable time for sensitivity to return to its final value; the time-course of this slower component of adaptation, that persists after the adapting stimulus has been removed, turns out to be closely related to how much of the retinal pigment is in the bleached form: it is called *bleaching adaptation*.

Field adaptation

The simplest way to demonstrate the changes in sensitivity that accompany field adaptation is by means of an *increment threshold* experiment. Here the subject is presented with a background field of steady luminance I, and a test flash of luminance ΔI is suddenly superimposed on it: we adjust ΔI until it can only just be perceived against the background, and the sensitivity is then the reciprocal of this threshold value or

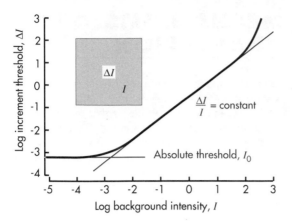

FIG. 7.30 The increment threshold curve. The smallest increment Δ*I* that can just be seen against a background *I* is plotted; for very small values of *I* the curve levels out at the absolute threshold, ΔI_0, while in the midrange Δ*I* is proportional to *I*. At very large values of *I*, saturation occurs, and Δ*I* begins to rise more steeply. (Data from Aguilar and Stiles, 1954)

$1/\Delta I$. It turns out that over a moderate range of background intensities the ratio Δ*I*/*I* is constant: in other words, the sensitivity is inversely proportional to the light level to which one is adapted. This is known as the Weber–Fechner relationship, and the quantity Δ*I*/*I* as the Weber fraction, *k*. This proportionality breaks down both at very high and very low luminances (Fig. 7.30). At the high end, the size of flash needed increases out of proportion to the background: this can be explained very well in terms of the kind of saturation of receptor response shown in Figure 7.24. At low luminances, the value of Δ*I* levels off to a fixed quantity, ΔI_0, which is the *absolute threshold* (i.e. the 'increment' threshold for a flash when there is no background present at all).

But it turns out that a simple modification of the Weber–Fechner formula enables us to fit this part of the curve as well: instead of writing Δ*I*/*I* = *k*,we have

$$\frac{\Delta I}{I + I_0} = k$$

where I_0 ($= \Delta I_0/k$) is another constant. What does this new formula mean?

Clearly, we would not really have expected Δ*I* to get smaller and smaller indefinitely as we turn the background intensity down to zero, for that would imply infinite sensitivity. In fact, the reason why there are some lights so dim that we cannot perceive them is to do with *receptor noise* (see Fig. 7.34). Even when no light falls on them, there is always a certain probability that the rhodopsin molecules will isomerize spontaneously through thermal activation, initiating the same train of events that would nor-

mally be triggered by the arrival of a photon. Consequently, even if no background *I* is present, the receptors will still generate a neural signal against which the test flash must be detected. As far as the rest of the visual system is concerned, this signal will look exactly like a 'real' background; what I_0 represents in the new formula is simply the apparent intensity of this virtual background, often called the *dark light*. When fully dark adapted in a pitch-black room, we can see this dark light for ourselves: the world is not black but rather a kind of shimmering grey. The reason that there is an absolute threshold at all is that visual targets have to be detected against this virtual background.

Now we have already seen that the sensitivity is not constant but gets smaller as the background intensity gets bigger. How might this be done? One possibility is to arrange that the sensitivity be turned down automatically by the prevailing level of the input ($I + I_0$). Such a device is called an *automatic gain control* or AGC, and is used in radio receivers, for example, to maintain a roughly constant average level of output to the loudspeaker despite fluctuations in the strength of the received signal: the analogy with visual adaptation is obvious. In particular, if we arrange for the gain to be equal to $1/(I + I_0)$, then the output in response to an increment Δ*I* will be $\Delta I/(I + I_0)$, and on the assumption that there is some constant threshold at which this is just detectable, the Weber–Fechner law is explained.

Where in the retina is this automatic gain control operating? There are almost too many places where it *might* occur, and at different times various proposals have been made. Any kind of negative feedback could do the trick (see p. 62), and suitable feedback circuits are evident at the ganglion/amacrine cell level and at the horizontal/bipolar level, but on the whole

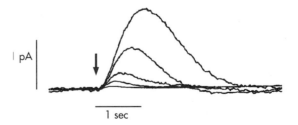

FIG. 7.31 Effect of adaptation on time-course of toad rod response. Stimuli of constant intensity were delivered in the presence of backgrounds of increasing intensity, starting from zero (top trace). It is evident that brighter backgrounds make the response shorter as well as smaller. (After Lamb, 1984, with permission)

they are probably more concerned with adaptation of a slightly different kind, that generates the transient properties obvious in many ganglion cell responses. An attractive candidate is a feedback mechanism that can be demonstrated within the receptors themselves, involving calcium. When light falls on receptors, as we have seen, sodium channels in the outer segment close; but these channels are also permeable to Ca^{++}, so that a consequence of a raised level of illumination is that calcium concentration within the receptor starts to fall. Calcium has several intracellular effects, including one that is relevant to the gain of the transduction process: it inhibits the recycling of GTP to form cGMP, that opens the sodium channels (see Fig. 7.24). So in the light, when calcium levels are low, cGMP is quickly replaced and the responses to light are relatively small and brief (Fig. 7.31).

Bleaching adaptation

Bleaching adaptation is quite different in its properties. It can be demonstrated by means of the same apparatus as for measuring increment thresholds, exposing the subject to an adapting field I which is then turned off before the eye's sensitivity is tested with the test flash ΔI. The results are very different from the previous case. Whereas in field adaptation ΔI depends directly on I, now it is found that ΔI is a function not of I on its own but rather of *how much pigment was bleached* during the adapting period: for fairly short adapting periods this is proportional to the product of I and the time of exposure. The second difference is that the adaptation lasts a considerable period after the adapting field has been switched off, a time that in fact corresponds closely to the time required for the pigment to regenerate (see Fig. 7.5). From our knowledge of the photochemistry of the pigment we might well have expected some such effect: obviously sensitivity must depend in part on the amount of active pigment present, and if, say, 20 percent of it is in the bleached state, then we would expect the eye to be 20 percent less sensitive. But it turns out that the changes in sensitivity that result from pigment bleaching are vastly greater than the simple proportionality that would be expected by this argument. By means of the technique of retinal densitometry (p. 133) it is possible to measure ΔI in this experiment at the same time as monitoring the proportion of pigment that is bleached. In the case of rods, it turns out (Fig. 7.32) that it is not ΔI but $\log(\Delta I)$ that is proportional to B, the fraction of pigment bleached, and that very small bleaches produce very large changes in sensitivity: a 20 percent bleach pro-

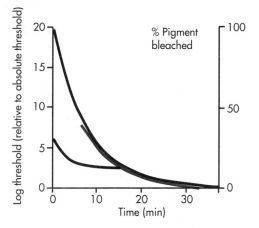

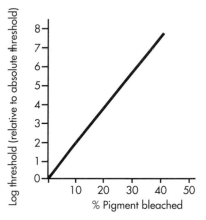

FIG. 7.32 The relation between rhodopsin concentration and sensitivity during dark adaptation. Above, continuous line shows the percentage of rhodopsin in the bleached state at various times during recovery after a full bleach: the curve is closely similar in a normal subject and in a rod monochromat. Also shown are simultaneous measurements of absolute threshold by a rod monochromat (red line) and normal subject (dotted), plotted on a logarithmic scale as shown on the left. Below, the relation between percent pigment bleached and log threshold obtained from this experiment in the case of the rod monochromat: it is evident that the relationship is a linear one, and threshold is proportional to 10^{aB}, where B is the percentage of pigment bleached, and a is a constant. (Data from Rushton, 1965)

duces not a 20 percent reduction in sensitivity but a reduction by a factor of 10 000!

Another feature of bleaching adaptation that shows that it is not just the consequence of a simple lack of pigment is that if we bleach a patch of retina with a pattern that affects some receptors and not others, we find that not only is the sensitivity of the bleached receptors reduced, that of their neighbours is as well. It is difficult to avoid the conclusion that bleached

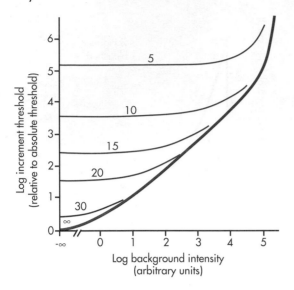

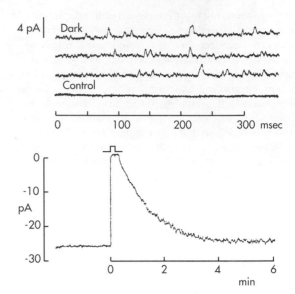

FIG. 7.33 Effect of bleaching on increment thresholds. Increment threshold curves are plotted as in Fig. 7.38, at various times (shown in minutes by the number above each curve) after a very intense bleach of the rods. (Data from Blakemore and Rushton, 1965)

FIG. 7.34 Noise in photoreceptors (toad rods). Above, three electrical records in the dark, with a control record below showing the level of instrumental noise. Below, effect of bleaching a receptor (0.7%) followed by recovery in the dark. The fluctuations in the recovery phase show the same statistical properties as the random responses that would occur during actual illumination. (Baylor *et al*, 1980; Lamb, 1980, with permission)

receptors are sending some kind of message into a pool – perhaps to horizontal cells – that turns down the gain over a relatively wide area.

We can get a clearer idea of how this comes about by measuring the increment threshold curve after bleaches of different sizes: what one then finds is that though the values of ΔI are unchanged at high background luminances, as I is reduced the curve flattens off sooner to a higher value of ΔI_0 the more pigment is in the bleached state (Fig. 7.33). It is as if the presence of free opsin as a result of bleaching caused an increase in the level of retinal noise or dark light, and indeed such curves can be very well explained by supposing that the dark light, I_0, is increased by a factor of 10^{aB}, where a has a value of about 20. In other words, bleaching an area of retina has much the same effect on sensitivity as shining a light of luminance $I_0 10^{aB}$ on it; this imaginary light is called the *equivalent background*. What seems to be happening is simply that bleaching the pigment greatly increases the rate of spontaneous isomerization and hence the background of retinal noise (Fig. 7.34).

But why do we not see this light? The answer is that sometimes we do: after viewing a light that is bright enough to bleach a significant amount of pigment – an ordinary light bulb does very well – we see initially a bright after-image (*positive after-image*) which is in effect $I_0 10^{aB}$; but being stabilized on the retina, it undergoes complete adaptation as already described,

and after some seconds it fades from view. If we now look at an illuminated surface, the after-image may reappear but in its negative form: the areas that have been bleached are less sensitive than the rest of the retina, because of the steady dark light that turns down the AGC, and so the bleached areas look darker than their surroundings. When we go from a brightly lit room into a dark one, the reason we cannot see clearly at first is that everything we look at is superimposed on an invisible background consisting of all the after-images that we have accumulated over the past 20 minutes or so. Although short-term adaptation prevents us from seeing the dark light that is generated by bleaching, the pathways that control the size of the pupil do not show this complete adaptation, and during the course of dark adaptation the pupil responds to the dark light in exactly the same way that it would to real lights. Incidentally, the lack of visual sensitivity in the dark that is caused by vitamin A deficiency can be explained very easily in these terms, since it will result in a pile-up of opsin that cannot be reconverted to rhodopsin, which will increase B and turn the sensitivity down.

What is not clear in this system is how the function 10^{aB} comes about, and whether the dark light signal is conveyed in the same neural pathways as

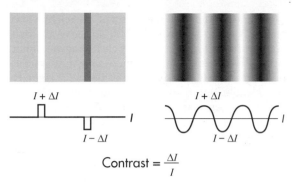

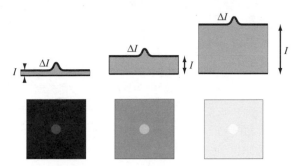

FIG. 7.35 Contrast is defined as $\Delta I/I$ both for light or dark lines on a grey background (left) or for a sinusoidal grating (right).

FIG. 7.37 On not seeing stars. As the sun rises, the contrast of the image of a star will fall as the background intensity I against which it is seen gradually rises, even though ΔI is constant.

those from real lights. It is difficult to think of plausible mechanisms by which a receptor's output would be the sum of a signal corresponding to the amount of light falling on it, i.e. proportional to the rate of bleaching, and a signal so non-linearly dependent on the amount of bleach. The answer almost certainly lies in the complex interactions that occur between the many intermediate products produced by the action of light on the retinal pigments.

Contrast

The existence of adaptation, and particularly of the automatic gain control, has the most profound effects on what we are able to see and how we see it. It is easy to show that in a very wide variety of situations our perceptions are determined entirely by the Weber fraction $\Delta I/I$ and for this reason the ratio has a special name: *contrast*. Contrast can be defined equally well for positive or negative increments on a steady background or for repetitive stimuli called gratings in which the luminance varies – often sinusoidally –

around a mean level I (Fig. 7. 35). In general, we detect an object if its contrast exceeds a certain threshold value, and not otherwise. This explains, for instance, why a very thin white line on a black background may be visible while a black line of identical width on a white background is not (Fig. 7.36). Though ΔI is the same in each case (though of opposite sign), I is not, so the contrast is bigger for the dark background. Or consider stars, which have a fixed ΔI: as the sun rises, I increases and their contrast drops and they disappear one by one (Fig. 7.37).

VISUAL ACUITY

Measurement

Visual acuity is a measure of the fidelity with which the visual system can transmit fine details of the visual world: it is the equivalent of the ability of a camera to produce sharp pictures. In a camera there are essentially two stages at which sharpness may be lost: either through optical defects that blur the patterns of light in the image on the film or by defects in the film itself, such as graininess, that limit the density of detail. These correspond in the eye to the quality of the *optics*, and to the density of the *retinal receptors*. But in the case of the eye there is a third factor: the possible degradation of the image that may occur in the course of the neural processing that takes place in the retina.

In an ideal system, a point source of light such as a star would produce a point of excitation in the neural output pattern; but the effect of the various types of image degradation mentioned above is to blur this final image so that its excitation is spread out over a finite area. The distribution of excitation in the image of a point source is described by the *pointspread function* (Fig. 7.38).

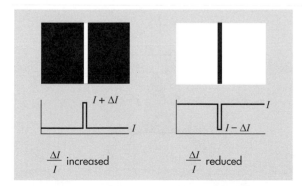

FIG. 7.36 Even though the width of the lines and the intensities of the black and white parts of the targets are matched, the visibility of the white line will always be greater than that of the black because its contrast, $\Delta I/I$, is higher.

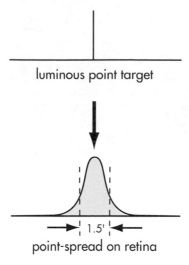

luminous point target

1.5'

point-spread on retina

FIG. 7.38 The pointspread function. An infinitely small point of light generates an image of finite width on the retina, the pointspread function. Its size determines the spatial quality of retinal images.

There are two distinct consequences of spreading of this kind. The first is that since the incident energy from the point source is spread out over a larger area, the maximum intensity at the central peak is necessarily reduced, leading to a decrease in the contrast, $\Delta I/I$, that determines whether it will be seen against its background. For objects of intrinsically high contrast, such as stars seen against the void of space, this will not matter much, and subjects with poor visual acuity as measured conventionally (see below) are not as bad at seeing stars as one might expect, bearing in mind the fact that such objects subtend an almost infinitely small angle. In the dark, whether one sees a star or not is almost entirely a matter of whether a sufficient number of photons from it fall upon a rod summation pool; under other conditions its visibility depends on whether $\Delta I/I$ exceeds the threshold contrast.

The second effect of the spreading of the images of points is a spatial one: it means that images of adjacent points on an object will overlap and lead to obliteration of spatial detail. Consider, for example, a pair of point sources that are close to one another – as, for example, a double star (Fig. 7.39). As the pointspread function is increased in width, there will come a point at which the distribution of excitation in the image will no longer exhibit a dip in the middle, so that an observer will be unable to see that there are two stars present and not just one. For normal observers the angle of separation for which this kind of resolution can just be performed is an order of

magnitude greater than the width of a black line that can just be seen, and is around 30–45 sec of arc. In a case like that of Figure 7.39c, it is clear that we cannot improve resolution simply by increasing the contrast, and such a stimulus may be described as absolutely unresolvable. But in an intermediate case like Figure 7.39b, whether resolution is possible or not will depend on the contrast of the original object as well as on the width of the pointspread function.

This interaction between resolution and contrast can best be investigated by using *grating* patterns as test targets. A grating is simply a regular pattern of stripes. If the stripes are simply bars of black and white, it is called a square-wave grating: if one were to plot intensity as a function of distance in a direction perpendicular to the stripes, it would have a square-wave profile. In the same way, sinusoidal gratings have an intensity profile that is sinusoidal (Fig. 7.35). In each case, one can describe the grating in terms of its *spatial frequency* (i.e. the number of cycles per degree) and its *contrast* (defined as the difference in intensity between the peaks and the troughs, divided by twice the mean intensity). Thus a pattern of alternate pure black and pure white strips, each 1° across, could be described as a square-wave grating of 100 percent contrast and spatial

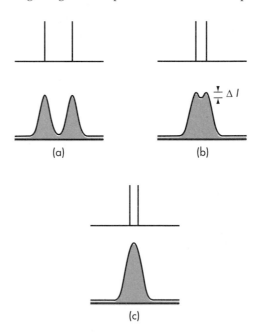

(a)   (b)

$\frac{1}{1}\Delta I$

(c)

FIG. 7.39 Resolution and contrast. As a pair of point sources are gradually brought together (above), their retinal images (below) begin to overlap. **(a)** is easily resolved, so long as the points can be seen at all; **(b)** will be resolved only if the contrast is sufficiently high; while **(c)** can never be resolved, whatever the contrast.

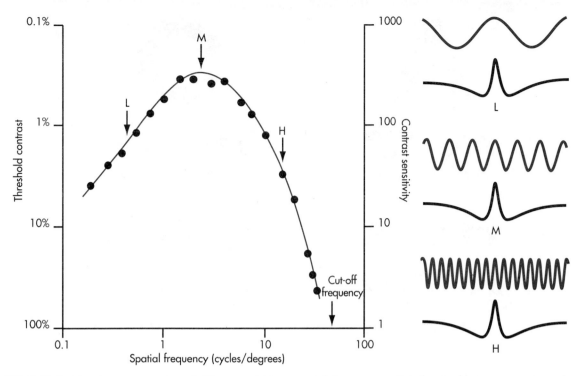

FIG. 7.40 Visibility of sine-wave gratings of different spatial frequency. Left, frequency-sensitivity function for sine-wave gratings, showing a peak (M) around 2–3 cycles per degree and a fall-off in sensitivity both at higher (H) and lower (L) frequencies. Right, schematic representation of a sinusoidally modulated image falling on a receptive field having excitatory centre and inhibitory surround. When the centre is roughly matched in size to the peak of the sine-wave (M), the response is maximum. With lower or higher frequencies (L,H) there is a relative increase in the degree of stimulation of the inhibitory surround. (Data from Campbell and Robson, 1968)

frequency 0.5 cycles per degree. A simple experiment is to ask a subject to view a sinusoidal grating of a particular spatial frequency, and then reduce its contrast until he reports that he can no longer see it. If we plot this threshold contrast as a function of spatial frequency, we typically obtain a curve such as Figure 7.40. Because a blurred pointspread function affects high spatial frequencies much more than low, the contrast required to see the grating increases sharply as its frequency is increased, until at about 40–50 cycles per degree (the cut-off frequency) the subject cannot even see a grating of 100 percent contrast. Because of the steepness of this cut-off, a small amount of extra blur causes a large increase in the contrast needed, and so the method provides a sensitive measure of acuity.

However, it is not an easy one to use in ordinary ophthalmological testing, and simpler tests of resolution are preferred. One such test is the Snellen chart (Fig. 7.41), in which rows of letters of diminishing size are to be read: by discovering the row at which the subject finally stops, and knowing the size of letters and the subject's viewing distance, one can estimate his minimum resolvable angle. In practice, each row is

marked with the distance at which a standard observer should just be able to read it, i.e. the distance at which the details of the letters subtend a minute of arc (Fig. 7.42); a subject who could only read the 8-metre row at 6 metres would be described as having an acuity of 6/8. The difficulty of the Snellen chart for scientific work is that the test is only partly one of resolution, some letters being recognized more easily than others because of their overall shape; and for some purposes the Landolt C chart (Fig. 7.41), used in the same way, is preferable because it provides no extraneous clues to the subject. A novel kind of chart in which all the letters are the same size but are graded in contrast has recently been introduced: it has the advantage of testing for certain kinds of defects in the visual system in which sensitivity to contrast is specifically impaired.

The tests described so far are all genuine tests of acuity in that they require that detail of some kind be resolved. Other tests, that at first sight might also appear to be acuity tests, are really tests of detection or localization, and give apparent acuities far better than 30–45 sec of arc. A well-known example is *vernier acuity*, where a subject is required to move two

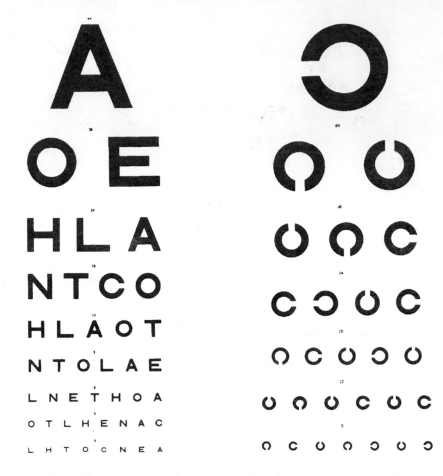

FIG. 7.41 Charts commonly used for routine testing of visual acuity. Left, Snellen chart; right, a similar chart using Landolt Cs: the subject must name the position of the gap in the circle.

lines into alignment, as for instance in the scale of vernier callipers: this can typically be done to a few seconds of arc, because information can be integrated by combining information along the length of the line. Another pseudoacuity task is the detection of stars, which may subtend extremely small angles at the eye (Betelgeuse subtends 0.05 sec of arc, for example). Such figures are irrelevant, however, since their retinal images cannot be narrower than the pointspread function; as explained earlier, whether they are seen depends only on their contrast, and hence on how much light they emit.

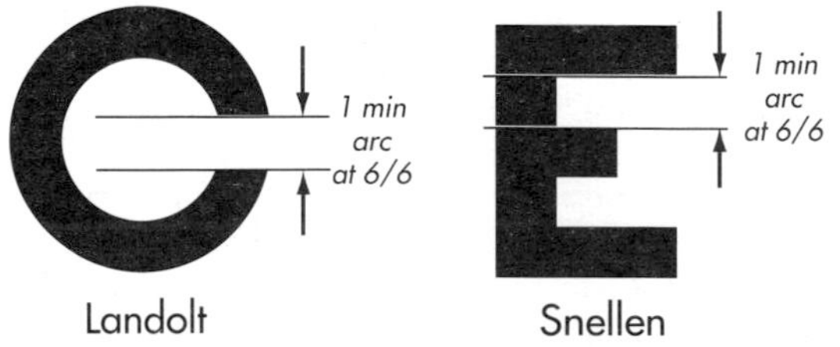

Factors affecting visual acuity

What contributions do the various parts of the visual system make to visual acuity? Clearly, the quality of the image on the retina is an important factor, and this in turn depends on the quality of the optics of the eye. But even if the eye is fully corrected for errors of refraction and astigmatism, the cornea and lens will still introduce a certain amount of blur. There are three sources of this degradation. The first is the existence of the various *aberrations*, already discussed. Chromatic aberration can be reduced by limiting the range of wavelengths in the image: in monochromatic yellow light, visual acuity may be improved by some 25 percent. The only practical way to reduce

FIG. 7.42 Criteria for the Landolt/Snellen charts. At the standard viewing distance, critical parts of the letters subtend 1 minute of arc.

spherical aberration is to limit the area of lens and cornea that contributes to refraction of the incoming rays: other things being equal, the smaller the pupil, the more nearly the optical surfaces will approximate to their ideal forms, and the less noticeable the aberrations will be.

But reducing pupil size cannot improve acuity indefinitely (quite apart from its undesirable effect of reducing the light-catching power of the eye) because of the second of the optical factors to be considered, namely *diffraction.* When light is imaged by a lens or other optical device of finite diameter, the edges of the aperture cause a diffraction blur of the resultant image. The width of the resultant pointspread function is of the order of λ/d radians, where λ is the wavelength and d the aperture of the system. For a pupil of diameter 2.5 mm, and with green light, this amounts to a little less than one minute of arc. In other words, under these conditions acuity is effectively limited by diffraction at the pupil. In the dark, with a pupil of some 8 mm diameter, the corresponding figure is about 17 sec of arc, but the actual pointspread is very much wider than this because of the increased contribution of the aberrations when the lens is widely exposed: in fact, the pointspread function actually gets wider with increasing pupil diameter beyond 3 mm or so. Thus if acuity were the sole consideration, the optimum pupil size would be around 3 mm, and we would expect it to remain fixed at that value. But as we shall see, under conditions of dark adaptation the intrinsic acuity of the neural processing of the retinal image is so low that the poor optics contribute little to the overall blur, and the advantage of being able to increase retinal sensitivity by catching more light with a dilated pupil outweighs the disadvantage of slightly decreased acuity.

The third source of optical blur is *glare,* caused by the diffuse scatter of light from the optical surfaces and media of the eye. Glare is scattered rather uniformly over the retina, so its effect on acuity is due not so much to spatial effects as to the reduction in the contrast of the retinal image that it produces, by superimposing on the image a more or less uniform background whose illuminance is of the order of 10 percent of the mean illuminance of the retina. The effect of this scatter is to reduce the contrast of the retinal image, particularly in dark areas.

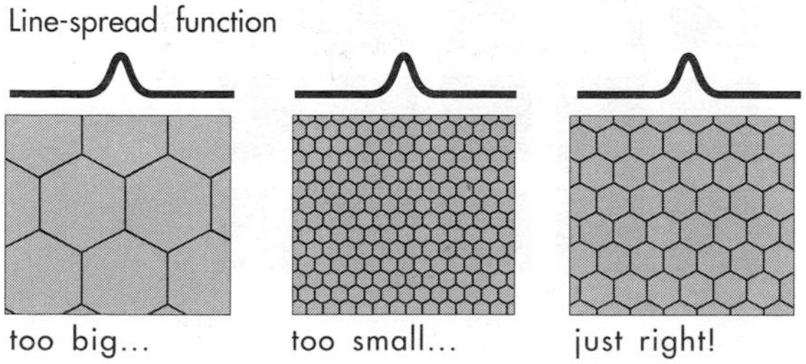

The relative importance of optical as opposed to retinal and neural factors in determining acuity can be determined directly by arranging to project a grating on the retina in such a way that its contrast is unaffected by the quality of the optics. One way of doing this is to generate interference fringes on the retina by means of two point sources of coherent light from a laser: the resulting interference pattern is in effect a sinusoidal grating, whose frequency depends on the separation of the two sources, and whose contrast is substantially unaffected by the quality of the optics. One can then measure the subject's threshold contrast as a function of frequency in the manner already described, and compare the result with what is found when viewing a 'real' sinusoidal grating. Although there is some improvement when the optics are bypassed in this way, even when the eye is fully corrected (as would be expected from our calculation of the limiting effect of diffraction when the pupil is small), it is not very great. This suggests that the retina is in a sense *matched* to the eye's optical properties. Clearly it would make little sense to have a retina with tiny receptors capable of resolving detail that could never be found in the retinal image in practice, because of optical blur. Nor for that matter would it be very sensible to have optics producing beautifully precise images if the receptors were so gross that they were incapable of appreciating them (Fig 7.43).

Under photopic conditions, acuity is thus essentially limited by both optics and receptor size together. It will be recalled that under these conditions it is the central fovea that is used to examine fine detail, and the cones here are spaced some 30 sec of arc apart (i.e. about the same size as the pointspread function) and connected in a one-to-one manner with the optic nerve, so that no further blur is introduced by sideways diffusion of information through neural collaterals. But if the contrast threshold as a function of spatial frequency is measured with a fixed pupil during progressive stages of dark adaptation, one finds a steady decrease in the cut-off frequency (Fig. 7.44), the result of changes in the neural organization of the retina. One of the adaptational responses to reduced light levels, as we shall see, is an increase in the effective size of the ganglion cells' summation pools, so that they can catch more light. But this obviously has the effect of increasing the degree of neural blur, and hence of reducing the overall acuity.

Line-spread function

too big... too small... just right!

FIG. 7.43

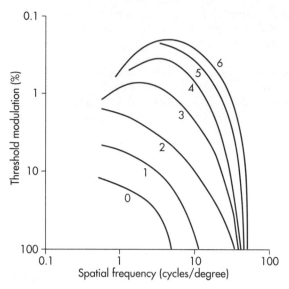

FIG. 7.44 Effect of adaptation level on the visibility of sinusoidal gratings. Each curve is a contrast sensitivity function of the kind shown in Fig. 7.47, measured at a different background intensity level ranging over 6 log units (the number by each curve indicates background intensity in relative log units). (After Van Ness and Bouman, 1967)

To summarize the factors that contribute to visual acuity, we have, first, factors that are properties of the *target*: its contrast, its colour (shorter wavelengths reduce diffraction, and monochromatic targets reduce chromatic aberration) and its luminance (bright targets allow smaller retinal fields and a smaller pupil, very dim targets near the absolute threshold show a further reduction in acuity because of quantum fluctuations). Secondly, there are *optical*

factors: errors of refraction, aberrations, and the effect of pupil size on both of these and on diffraction, and glare from scatter. And finally there are factors related to the *retina* itself: the spacing of the receptors (closer in the fovea, closer for cones than for rods and for red and green cones than for blue, resulting in poor acuity in blue light despite better diffraction), and the size of the receptive fields, being larger in the dark-adapted state and in the periphery of the visual field. In a good light, acuity is limited by diffraction, and thus about as good as could be expected from an eye of the size that we actually have.

Lateral inhibition

The general properties of lateral inhibition, and its desirability in sensory systems, have already been discussed in Chapter 6. It is a very important feature of visual processing, and is indeed one of the first things that the retina does – at the horizontal cell level – to the signals that come from the receptors. It is strikingly demonstrated in the Hermann grid (Fig. 7.45b), and certainly accounts for some of the phenomena of simultaneous contrast (Fig. 7.45a) which, like adaptation, helps to ensure that the subjective sensation of brightness is on a sliding scale and thus more closely related to albedo than to luminance. It can be estimated quantitatively by using sinusoidal gratings to measure contrast threshold as a function of spatial frequency, as already described on p. 142.

We have already seen how the presence of large excitatory receptive fields has the effect of reducing the effective contrast of high-frequency gratings. Lateral inhibition has in a sense the opposite effect: it

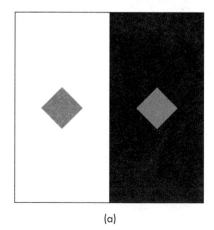

(a)

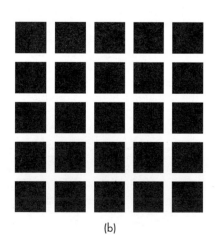

(b)

FIG. 7.45 Two illusions caused by lateral inhibition. (a) Simultaneous contrast: the two grey squares are of equal luminance but appear different in brightness because of the backgrounds they are seen against. (b) The Hermann grid: illusory dark spots are seen at the intersections of the white bars. The effect is much less striking near the fovea than in the periphery.

FIG. 7.46 Demonstration of the low-frequency cut, and thus of lateral inhibition. This sine-wave grating, of low spatial frequency and contrast, is more easily visible at distances of a metre or so than close to, when its spatial frequency is too small.

reduces the contrast of low-frequency gratings. To see why this is so, consider the response of a unit with a receptive field consisting of an excitatory centre and inhibitory surround, as it views sinusoidal gratings of various spatial frequencies (see Fig. 7.40). If the frequency is in effect matched to the dimensions of the field, in the sense that if a peak in the grating corresponds to the peak of the excitatory centre, then the troughs on each side correspond to the inhibitory troughs of the field, and the response of the unit will be a maximum. Increasing the spatial frequency will reduce the response, because of the smudging effect of the central area, already mentioned. But reducing the frequency will also decrease the response, because the bright part of the stimulus will begin to invade the inhibitory surround and lead to inhibition. In the extreme case, at zero spatial frequency when the unit is viewing a field of uniform luminance, the excitatory and inhibitory areas will both be maximally stimulated, and thus exhibit their maximal antagonism. Consequently the shape of the contrast-threshold curve as a function of frequency for such a unit will be shown in Figure 7.40. Just as

the high-frequency cut-off tells us about the size and shape of the excitatory centre, so the low-frequency part of the curve tells us about the inhibitory surround. You can demonstrate the low-frequency cut quite easily for yourself by means of Figure 7.46, which is a sine-wave grating of low contrast and low spatial frequency. Seen at a distance of a metre or so, the grating is easily perceived, but paradoxically the more closely it is examined the more difficult it is to see: eventually it disappears altogether because its spatial frequency is reduced to below the cut-off for the contrast concerned. Lateral inhibition means *sensitivity to change*, and at low spatial frequencies the rate of change is too small to be perceived.

By measuring a number of contrast-threshold curves at different levels of light adaptation, one can follow the changes in effective field configuration as a result of changes in the retina: under bright conditions, the excitatory centre is small and the surround prominent, so that there is a marked low-frequency cut but a good high-frequency response. As the illumination is reduced, the increase in size of the excitatory area brings the high-frequency cut down to lower frequencies, as already described on p. 146, and the simultaneous reduction in lateral inhibition gradually flattens the low-frequency response. At the lowest light levels the low-frequency cut cannot be seen at all, corresponding to the fact that under dark adaptation, inhibitory surrounds of the ganglion cells in experimental animals become progressively less and less prominent, and finally disappear altogether. The fundamental process at work here is one we have met several times: that of a basic dichotomy between sensitivity and resolution. If we try to maximize sensitivity by pooling information over wide areas, this can only be at the expense of acuity.

Temporal properties

Just as the spatial characteristics of vision can be determined with a sinusoidal grating, an area whose luminance is modulated sinusoidally as a function of distance but is constant in time, so its temporal properties can be determined with a stimulus that is spatially uniform but whose luminance is altered sinusoidally as a function of time. With a sinusoidally flickering stimulus of this kind, we can perform an experiment that is analogous to determining the threshold contrast of a sinusoidal grating as a function of its frequency, previously described. But now we ask the subject to reduce the contrast of the flicker until he can only just see it, and determine how this threshold contrast varies with the temporal frequency of the flicker. The resultant curve shows many points of similarity with the spatial one. At the high-frequency end, there is a cut-off frequency (the flicker fusion frequency) at which the flicker cannot quite be seen even with 100 percent contrast; and at the low-frequency end, one again finds that sensitivity begins to fall off as the rate of change of luminance declines, reflecting the inability of the eye to perceive slow changes because of its adaptational mechanisms. A further striking parallel between the two experiments is that if the flicker sensitivity curve is measured at progressively lower light levels, it undergoes very similar changes to those observed with sinusoidal gratings. The increasing sluggishness of the system when luminance is low (see, for instance, Fig. 7.31) is reflected in a progressive lowering of the flicker fusion frequency, while the gradual loss of the fast adaptational component causes a flattening of the low-frequency end. The close parallelism of the two effects, spatial and temporal, tempts one to speculate that the same fundamental mechanism might be responsible for both. Once again, sensitivity is achieved only at the expense of resolution: in time, rather than in space.

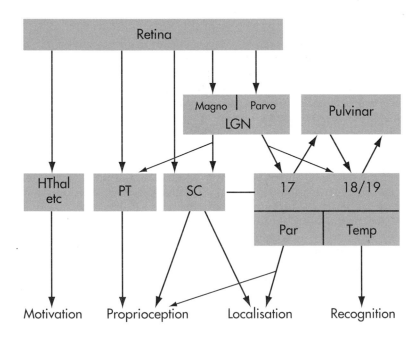

FIG. 7.47 The functional destinations of fibres in the optic nerve. LGN, lateral geniculate nucleus; HThal, hypothalamus; PT, pretectum and other visual proprioceptive areas; SC, superior colliculus; Par, Temp, parietal and temporal cortex.

VISUAL FORM RECOGNITION

We have seen something of the wide variety of signals being sent down the optic nerve from ganglion cells, reflecting the fact that vision is used for a variety of different tasks. Boundary or edge detectors for recognition; movement detectors for proprioception; whole-field tonic units for working out the time of day or controlling the pupil; and so on. Much of this information is packed off to different destinations within the brain that correspond with the three main uses to which visual information is put (Fig. 7.47). We use our eyes first to *recognize* objects in the outside world (primarily a cortical function), secondly to *locate* them (superior colliculus), and thirdly as a source of information about our position and movement relative to the outside world: visual *proprioception*, largely mediated by the pretectum and associated structures in the brainstem. (Small numbers of fibres also project, through pathways that are largely unknown, to the areas of the brain concerned with the control of accommodation and pupil size,

and hormonal responses to light.) Each of these kinds of analysis requires the incoming visual information to be processed in quite distinct ways, and we shall see that this is reflected in the behaviour of the neurones of which they are composed. We shall deal first with the areas that are concerned with the recognition of visual form.

Although both our eyes point forwards and have much the same view of the world, the brain is lateralized in the sense that the left brain is primarily concerned with things on the right side of the body and vice versa, so it is not surprising that the first thing that happens to the optic nerve fibres after leaving the two eyes is that they are sorted out according to which side of the retina they come from, and brought into association with the corresponding fibres from the other eye. This occurs in the *optic chiasm* (Fig. 7.48). A consequence of their rearrangement is that whereas lesions of the optic nerve naturally enough cause blindness in one eye (*unilateral anopia*), a unilateral lesion of the optic tract (the continuation of the fibres after the chiasm) results in blindness of the same half field of each eye (*homonymous hemianopia*); damage to the chiasm itself may give a bitemporal *heteronymous hemianopia*. Not all the fibres

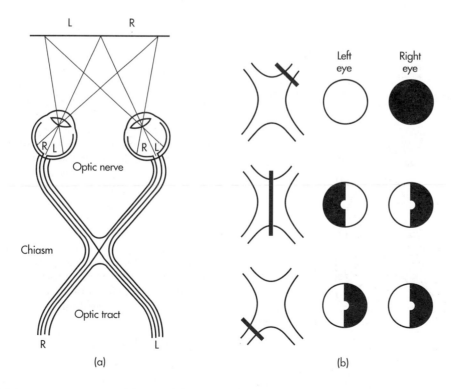

FIG. 7.48 (a) Schematic representation of the partial decussation of the optic nerve fibres in the chiasm. **(b)** The effect on the visual fields of each eye of lesions at three different points on the peripheral visual pathway.

Box 7.2 The three types of visual information

Recognition
Geniculate, cortex: cells respond to specialized features of a stimulus but are relatively uninterested in where it is

Localization
Superior colliculus: cells respond to the existence of a stimulus at a certain place, regardless of what it is

Proprioception
Pretectum, pons: cells respond to movement of the visual field as a whole in a particular direction

decussate completely, however, and the fovea of each eye is to some extent represented in both cerebral hemispheres. This gives rise to the phenomenon of *macular sparing*: lesions that would be expected to produce an exact homonymous hemianopia often show no loss of vision on the affected side near the point of fixation.

Lateral geniculate

In primates, the LGN has six distinct layers of cells, three of which (2,3 and 5) are entirely associated with the ipsilateral eye and the other three with the contralateral one: the functional significance of this arrangement is not understood. Layers 1 and 2 on each side have larger cell bodies *(magnocellular)* and

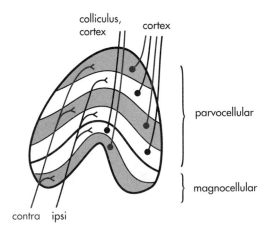

FIG. 7.49 Lateral geniculate nucleus: schematic diagram of the layers, showing the termination of optic nerve fibres from each eye (left) and the cells of origin of the optic tract, to different destination (right).

project more to the superior colliculus and other sub-cortical regions, though some go to the cerebral cortex. The other layers – *parvocellular* – have smaller bodies and project to the cortex, their smaller conduction velocities perhaps reflecting the fact that recognition is a relatively leisurely process whereas information about localization and movement is often urgently required by the motor system.

The receptive fields and responses of geniculate neurones are not markedly different from those of retinal ganglion cells, show the same concentric organization of on and off responses, and may be classified into X and Y types corresponding quite closely to parvocellular (P) and magnocellular (M) cells respectively. Many LGN cells also show centre–surround antagonisms that are wavelength-dependent. A cell of this type might, for example, show an on response to red light in the centre and an off response to green light in the surround or for that matter, vice versa. Yellow-versus-blue cells may be found as well as red-versus-green ones, and some cells show spectral antagonism of this type without having a centre–surround organization. The significance of these spectrally opponent cells in the perception of colour is discussed later, on p. 158. Another general feature of geniculate neurones is that to a far greater extent than ganglion cells their response to light may be modified by nervous activity in other parts of the brain: in sleep, for example, their responses to flashes of light are considerably reduced. This 'gating' of the geniculate cells, allowing some control of what information reaches the cerebral cortex, seems to be a general feature of thalamic relays, and it is important to remember that the thalamus receives many descending fibres from other parts of the brain in addition to its primary sensory projections.

The various layers of the LGN are all strictly in register in the sense that cells driven by the same area of retina form a single radial column, although there is a certain amount of distortion in the sense that central regions have a relatively greater representation than more peripheral ones: this is partly a consequence of the greater degree of retinal convergence found in the periphery. The general features of this map are preserved in the projection of neurones of the lateral geniculate through the *optic radiation* to the occipital lobe of the cerebral hemisphere.

Cerebral cortex

Their destination is Brodmann's area 17, the primary visual cortex, also known as the striate cortex on account of a prominent stripe, the stripe of Gennari, that runs through it that is a consequence of the

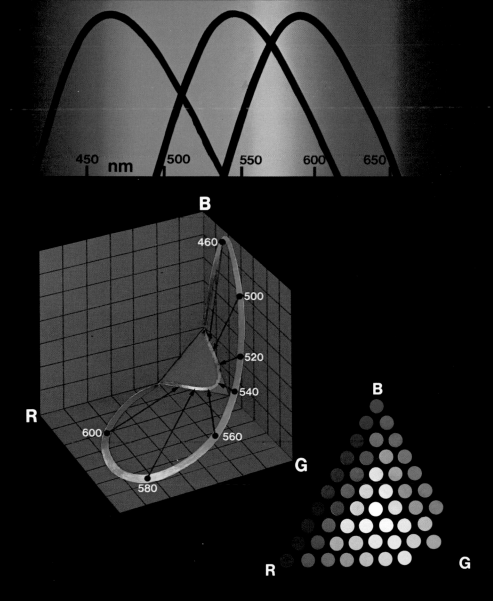

450 nm · 500 · 550 · 600 · 650

B

460
500
520
540
600 · 560
580

R

G

B

R · G

PLATE I Top, visible spectrum, showing the approximate average spectral sensitivities (on log scale) of primate 'blue', 'green' and 'red' cones. (Data from Marks et al., 1964) Middle, the three-dimensional locus traced out by a light of fixed intensity and varying wavlength; at any particular wavelength, the R-, G- and B-co-ordinates correspond to the degree of activation of red, green and blue receptors, as above. The locus may be projected onto the colour triangle, as shown. Bottom, an approximate representation of the colour triangle; the 'real' triangle is of course continuous rather than discrete. (The colours on this plate are not exact, because of the unavoidable problems associated with colour printing – discussed in the text.)

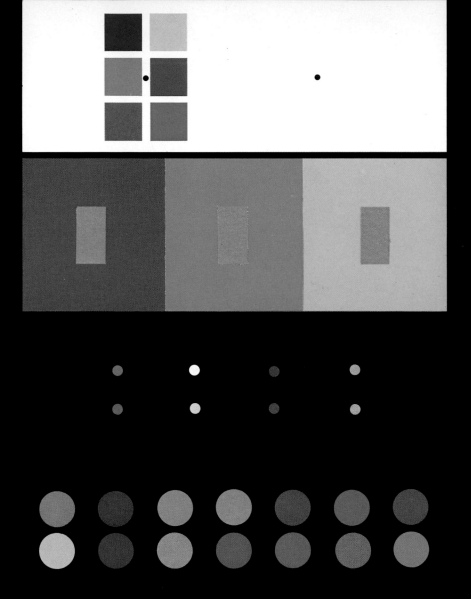

PLATE II Peculiarities of colour vision. From the top: (a) After-images and colours. If the black spot on the left is fixated for half a minute and the gaze shifted to the spot on the right, coloured after-images of the six squares will be seen. The colours in each of the three pairs have been chosen to be approximately complementary to one another so that in the after-image each pair appears to swap over. (b) Simultaneous colour contrast. The central rectangle is in fact the same colour in each case, though it tends to take on the complementary colour to its surround. (c) Tritanopia with small targets. In each of the four pairs, the colours differ only in the degree to which they stimulate the blue channel. When viwed from a distance (at least 5 metres) they appear indistinguishable because of the failure of the blue mechanism (tritanopia) with small targets. (d) Matching by colour-blind subjects. Each pair of colours in the row was accepted as a good match by a fully red–green blind subject; some but not others were acceptable by a subject with partial red–green deficiency.

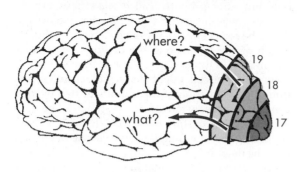

FIG. 7.50 Cerebral cortex, showing the general location of visual areas 17, 18 and 19. Subsequent processing can be divided roughly into two separate strands: of localization and movement, to parietal areas ('where'), and of recognition, including colour and shape, to temporal regions ('what').

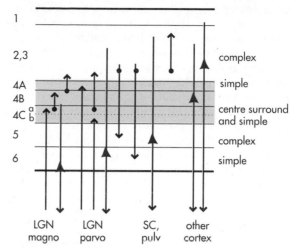

FIG. 7.51 Schematic representation of the segregation of input and output in visual cortex. (After Hubel, 1988

massive inflow of afferent fibres to this region (Figs 7.50 and Fig. 7.51). Area 17 is surrounded by other areas (18, prestriate, and 19, medial temporal or MT) that are wholly visual; further out are associational areas which show many visual features. An alternative system of nomenclature denotes 17 as V1, divides 18 into areas V2–V4 and calls 19 V5. The interconnections between these various areas are partly direct and partly through another thalamic nucleus, the *pulvinar*.

It is a relatively simple matter to record from cells in the visual cortex, and this has been a happy hunting ground for neurophysiologists over the last 40 years or so. As in the retina, there is an enormous range of morphological types of cell within the cortex. Two of the six layers of the visual cortex (Fig. 7.51) contain pyramidal cells whose axons form the output to other parts of the brain, including other cortical areas: in between are interneurones of different kinds, including stellate cells. Although some cells, particularly in layer 4 close to the layer of afferent

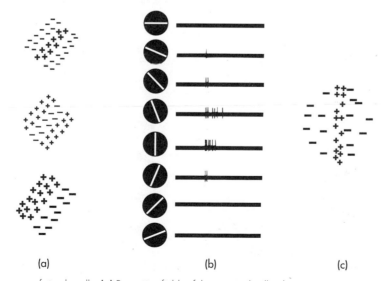

(a) (b) (c)

FIG. 7.52 Visual responses of simple cells. **(a)** Receptive fields of three typical cells, showing regions responding to a localized spot of light being turned on (+) or off (-). **(b)** Responses of a single unit to a bar of light presented at the various orientations shown: it is preferentially stimulated by a vertical bar. **(c)** The receptive field of the unit whose responses are shown in **(b)**. (After Hubel and Wiesel, 1962)

fibres from the geniculate, show receptive field properties that are very similar to the roughly circular and concentric fields seen in retinal ganglion cells and in the LGN, most (and all of them outside area 17) show receptive field properties that are quite novel. Many other cells have fields that are not circular but when mapped with single spots of light, consist of a central strip with antagonistic strips flanking it (Fig. 7.52): the centre may be excitatory or inhibitory, and the orientation of the entire field is different for different cells. As would be expected, what these *simple cells* respond to best is a line of a particular position and orientation: they can be called *line detectors*. Moving or flashed stimuli are in general more effective as stimuli than steady ones, and diffuse illumination is generally completely ineffective: this is of course only what would be expected in a system designed for recognition.

Another type of cortical unit is the *complex cell*; like simple cells, they respond best to a bar or edge of a specific orientation but in this case they will respond to such a target placed anywhere within their field of view. It is not possible to map out excitatory and inhibitory areas of their fields as it is with simple cells because they do not respond to single spots of light. Moving stimuli are again more effective, and the neurones often show responses of opposite sign to movement in the opposite direction. One can think of a complex cell as extracting information about what kind of object is present while throwing away information about exactly where it is: recognition without localization. Some cells, originally called *hypercomplex*

cells but now properly called *end-stopped complex cells*, are even more fussy: not only has the orientation to be correct in order to obtain a response but the length of the stimulating bar or line must also lie within certain limits (Fig. 7.53). It is easy to imagine how a simple cell might derive its receptive field from the summation of the outputs of two or more geniculate cells arranged in a straight line; and although it is tempting to extrapolate this notion by supposing that the complex cell response might similarly be the result of the summation of the outputs of simple cells, it appears that in fact this is not so, and that both types of response are actually the result of appropriate connections from geniculate afferents. Responses to colour are less evident, at least in area 17, than in the geniculate, and of the cells that show colour-opponent responses, most are of the simple or concentric type, and gathered together in 'blobs'.

It is important to appreciate that these various classifications of specificities amongst cortical cells are to a large extent arbitrary and artificial; as was emphasized in Chapter 4, if an experimenter finds any response at all from a cell, it must necessarily be to a stimulus that he has chosen beforehand. Recent examinations of cortical visual cells suggest a richness of variety that is not well conveyed by conventional descriptions in terms of 'simple cell', 'complex cell' and so forth.

Orientation-specific responses appear to be functionally grouped in *columns* perpendicular to the cortical surface, the cells in a particular column sharing the same preferred orientation. This orientation

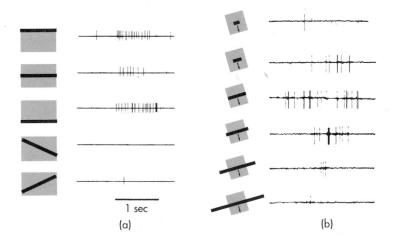

FIG. 7.53 Complex cells. **(a)** Responses of a complex cell to a dark bar within its receptive field (shaded): it responds if the bar is horizontal, wherever it is within the field, but not if the bar is tilted. **(b)** Responses of an end-stopped ('hypercomplex') cell to a moving bar of optimum orientation but different lengths: there is clearly an optimum length for evoking maximum activity. (After Hubel and Wiesel, 1965)

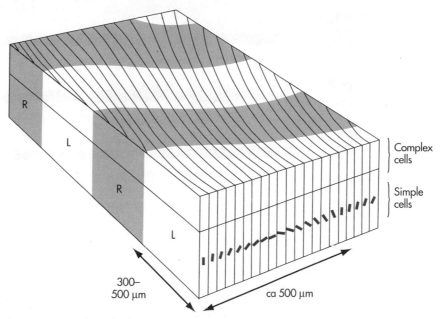

FIG. 7.54 Highly stylized representation of a slab of visual cortex, showing its organization into 'columns', narrow strips in which cells share a common preferred orientation, and roughly perpendicular dominance bands, preferentially driven by one or other eye. Preferred orientation usually changes systematically (as shown) in passing along a set of columns. An analogous 'columnar' organization is found in other neocortical regions.

changes in a systematic way as one moves across the cortical surface (Fig. 7.54), such that after half a millimetre or so we are back to the first orientation. Thus the visual cortex is traversed by a series of bands, within each of which every possible orientation is represented. But columns can differ in another way too, related to the fact that we have two eyes. We saw that in the geniculate the inputs from each eye are strictly segregated. This segregation is maintained in the projections up to the cortex, with each column receiving fibres associated either with one eye or the other, but not both. A column receiving right eye fibres is called right eye *dominant*, and columns having the same dominance form a second series of bands at right angles to the first. Together they create a sort of chequerboard, with both eyes and all orientations being represented in a patch about one millimetre by a half, called a *hypercolumn*; each hypercolumn typically also contains two colour blobs.

Although the simple cells in layer IVc of a column will normally be driven by one eye only, the complex cells on each side are normally found to be binocular, driven by both eyes. Some of these neurones have receptive fields that are identically situated with respect to the fovea of each eye, others have pairs of fields that do not exactly correspond in the two eyes: this retinal *disparity* is undoubtedly an important

source of information about the distances of visual objects from the plane of fixation, and is later discussed in the context of depth perception, on p. 163.

So here are cells coding a wealth of information about the visual world, looking for spots and edges and lines of a certain orientation, of a particular length and moving in a particular direction. Where do we go from here? Clearly once you see the principle of what is sometimes called *feature extraction*, it could go on like that for ever. One could join line detectors together to make special detectors for squares, for numbers, for letters of the Russian alphabet, for teacups ... and so on. Is there perhaps a special cell for everything we see? For *porcelain* teacups, for *18th century French porcelain* teacups? For *my grandmother's* 18th century French porcelain teacup? It is not at all clear whether, even with the huge numbers of neurones at our disposal, we could actually do something like that. Nevertheless, what can be demonstrated are visual cells that code for particular objects of outstanding behavioural significance. The information from area 17, passing outward into areas 18 and 19 and beyond, seem to form two streams, broadly corresponding to complex localization (to posterior parietal areas; Fig. 7.50) and to complex recognition (infero-temporal regions, areas 20 and 21). In the temporal lobe, cells have, for instance, been described in the monkey that respond

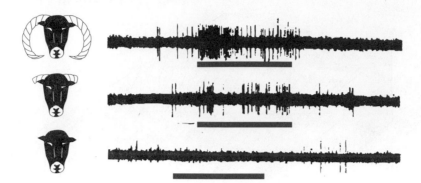

FIG. 7.55 Responses of a single cell in the temporal cortex of a Dalesbred (horned) sheep when presented with the three sheep faces shown. (After Kendrick and Baldwin, 1987)

to objects as closely defined as particular faces or the appearance of the monkey's own hand. In sheep, similar cells seem to identify other sheep, and classify the degree of threat they pose, and their place in the social hierarchy (based on the length of their horns: Fig. 7.55). Lesions of these areas in the monkey can give rise to visual defects that are more subtle than those associated with lesions in the occipital lobe, such as difficulty in recognizing or appreciating the significance of visual objects. These findings are further discussed in Chapter 13.

Box 7.3 Responses of visual neurones

Receptors

Circular uniform fields, tonic

Bipolars

Circular concentric +/− fields, essentially tonic

Ganglion cells

Many types, all with circular fields: mostly phasic: X cells: sustained, simple; Y cells: transient, complex; W cells: slow, may be complex. Some cells show colour-coding (R/G, Y/B), and in some species there can be responses to movement in specific directions. A small number of cells show tonic responses to light level over a wide dynamic range

Lateral geniculate

Essentially similar to ganglion cells. Little response to diffuse light

Visual cortex

The first level at which binocular cells are found; in primary cortex, colour less common than in the geniculate. Many types, some circular, mostly linear. No response in absence of pattern. Simple: linear +/−, localized. Complex: linear, often directionally selective; larger response area. Hypercomplex: linear, generally directionally-selective, end-stopped. In inferotemporal cortex, more specificity and more colour (including responses showing colour constancy). Towards parietal, more response to movement

Superior colliculus

Small uniform fields in centre, larger in periphery. Uninterested in shape or colour

Pretectum, pons

Very large fields, directional selectivity when detail in field moves as a whole; firing rate reflects the velocity

COLOUR VISION

This is a convenient point to consider another factor that contributes specifically to visual recognition, namely *colour*. Different objects reflect different amounts of light at different wavelengths, which is another way of saying that albedo is wavelength-dependent. A red apple can be seen against green leaves, even though its overall albedo is identical, because in some parts of the spectrum its albedo is different. So when we say one object is a different colour from another, what we mean is that the shape of the corresponding spectrum is different. But we are actually very bad at determining this shape. Whereas the ear is capable of analysing mixtures of pure tones into their components – so that a competent musician can listen to a chord played by an orchestra and say which instruments are playing which notes – not even the most perceptive and experienced observer can say by looking at a coloured light exactly what wavelengths are present in it. The reason is that although we have millions of cones in our retina, from the point of view of wavelength they fall into one of only three classes, responding essentially to long, medium and short wavelengths: to red, to green and to blue. Information about the spectral composition of a light can only be conveyed by the relative degree of activity in each of these channels: the system has only *three degrees of freedom*, a condition known as trichromacy. It is rather as if we tried to classify people using only the three parameters of weight, height, and size in shoes: although this would enable us to discriminate quite well between particular pairs of people, it clearly could not reflect the rich variety of human forms that actually exists.

One result of this fact is that it is possible to 'fool' the colour system in a way that cannot be done with the ear. If we sound two pure tones simultaneously, they sound like what they are, a mixture of two frequencies. If we shine two monochromatic lights on a screen, the result is a new colour that often bears no obvious relationship to its components – red and green, for example, making yellow – and does not even look like a mixture. All that is needed for us to accept two colours as a match is for the red content of the first to equal that of the second, the green the green and the blue the blue. It is this fact that enables artists to paint with only a small number of pigments on their palette, and makes colour printing and colour television a practical possibility. And in fact a good deal may be learnt about how the colour system works by investigating experimentally the rules that determine the results of such mixtures.

Colour mixing

Imagine a creature with only two types of colour receptor, red and blue, with spectral sensitivity curves as shown in Figure 7.56a. It is clear that any single wavelength within the total range will make the units fire at certain rates, say f_R and f_B. If we now increase the intensity of the light without changing the wavelength, f_R and f_B will both increase, but the ratio f_R/f_B will remain the same. The ratio, in fact, depends only on the wavelength, which is precisely why it is a measure of colour: experience tells us that altering the intensities of coloured lights does not – within limits – affect their perceived colours: an orange still looks orange whether brightly or dimly lit. Colour can almost be defined as that property of a light that is independent of its brightness. So our creature certainly enjoys colour vision, since it can *distinguish wavelengths independently of their intensities.*

But what will happen if two wavelengths are presented simultaneously? Suppose we shine on this eye an extreme red and extreme blue light (R,B), each of unit intensity: the ratio f_R/f_B will then be unity. But a precisely identical response could have been achieved by shining a light of single wavelength (Y) on the eye, such that the two types of receptor were equally stimulated. In other words, R and B together here produce the same neural response as (and must therefore match) another wavelength, Y; and in general, any pair of wavelengths whatever will look the same as some other single wavelength. We can derive rules to predict what wavelength they will look like quite easily from the two spectral sensitivity curves by means of a diagram showing the 'response space' of the two channels (Fig. 7.56b). Here the two axes show frequencies of firing in the R and B channels, and so every point in the figure corresponds to a particular pair of frequencies and hence to a unique sensation. Lines like OA, OB join points for which the ratios of these frequencies are constant, and therefore correspond to lights having the same perceived colour (*chroma* or *hue*). The distance of a point along such a line from the origin corresponds to its intensity. The thick line shows the way in which f_R and f_B vary if a light of fixed intensity is varied in wavelength. If more than one light is present, the result of the mixture can be deduced at once from the diagram; if the channels are linear, the total activity in each will be the sum of the activities generated by each component separately. Thus if we simultaneously present two lights J and K of different intensities and wavelengths (Fig. 7.56c), the result will be the vector sum of the two (which may be found by constructing the familiar parallelogram of

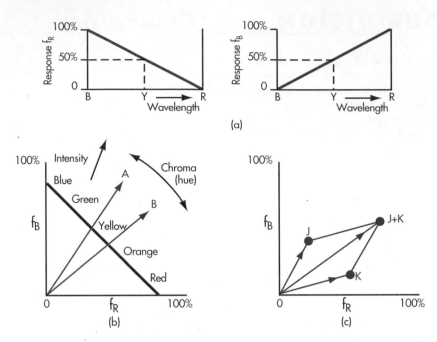

FIG. 7.56 Colour vision in a hypothetical dichromat. **(a)** The spectral sensitivities of the two types of receptor, B (blue) and R (red). **(b)** The colour response space: the axes show the degree of activity of each of the two channels, and any particular colour will result in a particular point in the diagram. The thick line indicates how the B and R responses vary as a light of constant intensity is varied in wavelength, while lines such as OA, OB represent stimuli of constant wavelength but variable intensity: in each case the ratio of B and R activity is constant, and they are thus of constant hue or chroma. **(c)** J and K represent two stimuli of different intensity and wavelength. If they are added together, the resultant response is given by the vector sum (J + K) of each separate response.

forces as shown), and the position of the resultant point will indicate the perceived colour of the mixture. It is clear that any colour can be matched exactly by using appropriate proportions of any two other given wavelengths (with the proviso that the apparent wavelength of the result must lie between the wavelengths of the two components) and this is what is meant by dichromatic vision. It follows that if we want to be able to produce any colour by mixing two others, we must choose an extreme red and an extreme blue in order to encompass the entire range of possible wavelengths. These may then be called *primary* colours, stimuli from which all other hues can be made by mixture.

Now although there are many dichromatic animals, and some colour-blind humans, for whom the above provides an adequate description of their colour sense (except that the shapes of the sensitivity curves in Figure 7.56 are overidealized), it is the normal human eye with which we are concerned, and it has not two but *three* classes of receptor with respect to wavelength sensitivity, and hence three degrees of freedom. Plate I (top) (opposite page 150) shows the spectral sensitivities of the three types of human

cone. It is clear that we cannot match a colour such as Y by using only two others together (such as B and R): although we may get f_R and f_B right, the value of f_G will in general be wrong and we cannot correct f_G without messing up one of the other channels. In fact we now need three colours to match any other, to take care of the three degrees of freedom involved: a pair of colours will only match if f_B for one is equal to f_B for the other, and so on for the other channels. Because of this, the diagram of the response space corresponding to Figure 7.56b now has to be *three-dimensional* rather than flat; and because the individual sensitivity curves do not have the simple form of Figure 7.56a, the locus of a light of fixed intensity whose wavelength is altered is no longer the simple straight line of Figure 7.56b but one having a twisted three-dimensional shape (Plate I, middle).

This looks awkward to use; but a simplification can be made. As before, the *distance* from the origin to a particular point represents *brightness*, whereas its *direction* represents *colour* (Fig. 7.57). If it is only the latter quantity that interests us, we can reduce the whole diagram to a two-dimensional form by the following simple expedient. Suppose we set up an equilateral triangle whose vertices are at equal distances along the three axes: then the point where the line joining the origin to a particular light intersects the plane of this triangle will depend only on the light's colour and not on its intensity. This triangle is called the colour triangle (Plate I, bottom) and each point on it corresponds to a different colour. Its centre, W, corresponds to white light that stimulates each type of receptor equally and lines radiating from this point are lines of equal chroma. Along such a line, the nearer a point is to W the more unsaturated it is, i.e. the more it is diluted with white. Thus pink and red

lie on the same line of chroma but pink is nearer the centre. The thick line represents the locus of a light whose wavelength is varied over the visible range: it therefore represents colours that are of maximum saturation. The fact that this locus does not reach the G vertex reflects the fact that there is no wavelength that can stimulate G alone without at the same time stimulating R or B or both, as can be verified in the spectral sensitivity curves of Plate I. The edge RB of the triangle represents saturated violets and purples that are not in the spectrum, but can be formed by mixtures of deep red and deep blue.

The rules for colour mixture can now be stated simply, and were described in this form by Newton in 1704. To find the result of mixing two colours J and K (Fig. 7.58, top), join JK with a straight line: all the colours on that line can be made by mixing J and K in different proportions, and the more J is used, the nearer the resultant will lie to J. In general it can be seen that the effect of mixing two colours is to produce a new one of intermediate chroma but less saturated, i.e. nearer to W: such mixtures are therefore

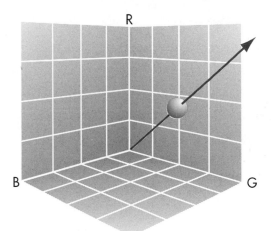

Different intensities

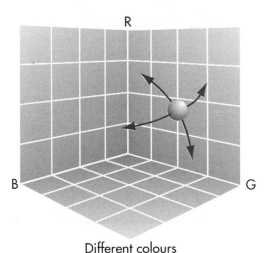

Different colours

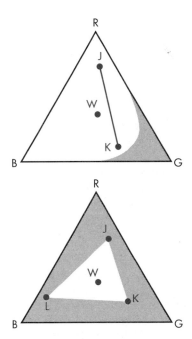

FIG. 7.58 The laws of colour mixing. Above, by mixing two colours (J, K) in different proportions we can form any of the colours lying on the line JK. Below, with three colours (J, K, L) we can form any colour lying within the triangle JKL. If this triangle encloses the white point (W), then any hue can be formed by mixing them in suitable proportions, though not with full saturation.

FIG. 7.57 Trichromatic colour space. The effect of varying just the intensity of a given colour is to move it along the line joining it to the origin, without affecting its direction (above). Changing just the colour, on the other hand, affects the direction but not the distance (below).

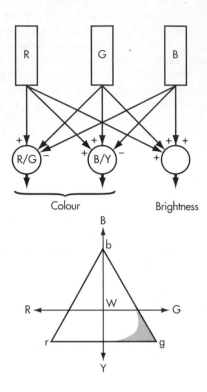

FIG. 7.59 Above, how information from the three receptor channels (R, G, B) is neurally recoded into a red-versus-green channel (R/G), a yellow-versus-blue channel (B/Y) and a brightness channel. The resultant form of colour space, based on R/G and B/Y axes, is shown below with the colour triangle superimposed.

paler than pure spectral colours. If JK happens to pass through W, J and K are said to be *complementary*: by mixing them in suitable proportions, pure white can be made. By mixing *three* colours (J,K,L) we can produce any colour lying within the triangle JKL; so long as this includes W, this means that any chroma can be mixed from any three colours (Fig. 7.58, bottom). Obviously, the bigger the triangle JKL is, the more saturated are the colours that can be mixed but even if we use pure spectral wavelengths as our primaries, there will be certain colours (notably saturated blue-greens or yellow) that cannot be matched. In practical colour mixing, as with colour film or colour television, one tries to choose primaries that make the triangle JKL as large as possible but one's choice is limited by the dyes or phosphors actually available. The reason why colour television in particular is often unsatisfactory can be seen by looking at the position of the primaries used – they are in fact close to the JKL of Figure. 7.58: the result is that blue-greens and purples are rather desaturated, though grass-greens and flesh tints are relatively

good. The only practical solution to this sort of problem is to use more than three primaries, and high-quality colour printing – for example, of

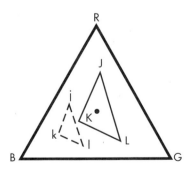

FIG. 7.60 Effect of coloured illumination. A picture whose range of colours falls within the triangle JKL under white lights is illuminated instead with blue. The effect is to shift the triangle as shown, to jkl; however, the perceived changes of colour will generally be very much smaller than this, because of the effect of chromatic adaptation: the sensitivities of the R and G channels increase, and that of B decreases.

reproductions of paintings – may use six or more to get as close as possible to fully saturated mixtures.

The essential point, then, about colour vision is that although there are three degrees of freedom, the sensation of colour itself is two-dimensional – it can be described by the two variables of chroma and saturation – and the third quality, intensity, is not essentially a colour attribute at all. That is not to say that it doesn't contribute to the popular idea of 'colour': the colour brown, for example, is only an orange of low intensity. The way in which the two dimensions of colour are abstracted from the signals in the three receptor channels is by making a comparison of the red and green activity, and of the blue and yellow (Fig. 7.59). Amongst retinal ganglion cells, the majority are not interested in colour because their function is to provide information about localization and shape. But some are colour-sensitive, and they behave as if they were excited by one colour channel and inhibited by another, a situation called *colour opponency*; the same is found in all subsequent levels of colour processing. Some cells are excited by blue and inhibited by yellow or vice versa, some show similar antagonism between red and green; the majority pay no attention to wavelength at all, and appear simply to add the signals from three channels together.

What one might call psychological colour space thus has two perpendicular axes, one being blue/yellow and the other red/green. The fact that yellow, on such a representation, is on a par with red, green and blue although it has no corresponding cone type is probably the explanation for the fact that yellow behaves in many ways like a subjective primary colour: it doesn't, for example, look in the least like a mixture of red and green in the way that corresponding mixtures of red and blue or blue and green do. Evolutionarily, it seems that the blue/yellow axis is the more fundamental one: it is essentially a division of the spectrum into short wavelengths versus long. The red/green axis seems to have evolved later (though the evolutionary history of colour vision is complex and shows many anomalies), and it has been suggested that it was the need for primates to distinguish between the reds and greens of ripe and unripe fruit that led to the split of the original yellow cone into red and green varieties.

Chromatic adaptation

Just as adaptation is important in helping the visual system to register the albedo of an object independently of the intensity of the light that falls upon it,

so *chromatic* adaptation – the independent adaptation of the individual colour channels – can help the visual system make allowance for the colour of the illumination. Suppose we have a painting whose full range of colours falls within the triangle JKL of Figure 7.60 under white light. If we now illuminate it with blue light, the effect will be to reduce the signals in the red and green channels relative to those in the blue, and the result will be a distorted triangle (jkl) and hence misperception of hues. But the red and green channels will respond to their reduced stimulation by increasing their sensitivities, which will have the effect of restoring the total range of colours perceived to something like its original extent. In fact the eye is surprisingly tolerant of changes in the spectral composition of the illuminating light, and the sensation of colour is much more closely related to an object's relative albedo for short, long and medium wavelengths than it is to the actual spectral composition of the light reaching the retina. This kind of behaviour – colour constancy – is demonstrable in the responses of many colour-sensitive cells in the more temporal regions of the visual cortex, which can respond to an object of a particular colour even when the spectrum of its retinal image is quite different because of changes in the colour of its illumination.

These adaptational changes can easily be demonstrated by means of *successive contrast* or coloured after-images. If the coloured spots of Plate IIa (opposite page 151) are fixated for about 20 seconds in a good light, and the gaze then transferred to the blank area next to them, striking after-images of the complementary colour will be seen that are due to distortion of one's colour space because of adaptation: what was originally a white that fell in the centre of the colour triangle now falls to one side, in a direction opposite to the adapting colour. The same explanation probably underlies *simultaneous contrast* (Plate IIb): an area of pale colour lying next to a strong one tends to take on the complementary tinge.

Disorders of colour vision

If one of the three channels were inoperative, vision would become dichromatic, and the colour triangle would collapse into a single dimension (Fig. 7.61). One would then be able to match any colour in the spectrum by mixing blue and red in suitable proportions. Defects of this kind are often seen: loss of the red mechanism is called *protanopia*, of the green, *deuteranopia*, and of the blue, *tritanopia*. Probably because the division of a single yellow mechanism into red versus green came relatively late in evolution,

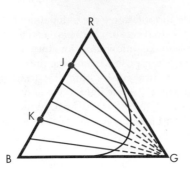

FIG. 7.61 Effect of lack of one channel on colour perception. Colours lying on a line such as GJ or GK differ only in the amount by which they stimulate the G channel. If, in a colour-blind subject, this channel were inoperative, such colours would all look identical: lines like GJ, GK can then be called lines of confusion. Consequently such a subject could match any colour by using only mixtures of deep red and deep blue light, in appropriate proportions.

the first two deficiencies are much commoner than the last and give rise to what is commonly called red–green blindness: the resulting confusion of red with green forms the basis of clinical tests such as simple matching (Plate IId) or the Isihara test in which coloured dots are made up into figures that are read differently with different deficiencies. Some 8 percent of males are thus affected but a much smaller percentage of females: the gene in question is sex-linked and recessive. Tritanopia is much less common, though in normal subjects the central fovea appears to lack blue cones and is tritanopic, as can be seen from the demonstration in Plate IIc. More severe defects involving the functional loss of more than one channel – for example, the rod monochromat, whose retina contains only rods – are also found. Colour deficiencies might be due to a loss of one or more types of pigment, to lack of development of adequate neural connections or possibly to a mixing of pigments or connections, so that discrimination is lost. Studies using retinal densitometry (see p. 133) have shown that in some dichromatic subjects, at least, one of the cone pigments appears to be missing. One might wonder if it was possible to know what the world actually looks like to a colour-blind person. Thanks to a very rare condition indeed, in which only one eye is colour-blind, the answer is probably yes: such a subject seems to see everything in terms of blue and yellow with the affected eye so that the spectrum appears deep blue at one end, fading to white in the middle, and then passing through progressively deeper shades of yellow to the long wavelength end. This is exactly what would be expected if colour space has simply been collapsed down to the yellow/blue axis.

Less severe than actual colour-blindness are the various colour *anomalies*. A protanomalous subject, for example, is trichromatic but if asked to match a particular yellow by means of red and green will tend to use more red than a normal subject; deuteranomolous subjects use more green. It is likely that such defects are due to imbalance in the amounts or spectral sensitivities of the cone pigments.

Finally, disorders of colour vision can arise with damage to specific temporal cortical areas and can take many forms; in some cases colour constancy may be impaired so that colours appear to change under coloured illumination more than would be experienced by a normal observer.

VISUAL LOCALIZATION

There are two components to localization, *direction and distance*. Of these, distance is the more difficult feature to extract from visual information; clearly the spatial organization of the retina provides immediate information about the relative visual angles between different visual objects, since the retinal subtense between two receptors that are stimulated is directly proportional to the angle between the corresponding stimuli in the outside world. It is convenient to deal with direction first.

Direction: the colliculus

Computation of visual direction is a function associated particularly with a primitive visual integrating area high at the back of the brainstem, the *superior colliculus (tectum* in lower animals). It is basically organized in two layers, the upper layer receiving visual information from the retina, the LGN and visual cortex, and the lower layer being motor in character, projecting down to areas of the brainstem and upper spinal cord concerned with the generation of eye movements and head movements (Fig. 7.62). Neurones in the upper layer do not show orientation specificity and have large, overlapping and roughly circular fields: they are interested in *where* an object is but don't mind in the slightest *what* it is. Some are also responsive to targets moving in particular directions, especially moving away from the fovea. The cells are arranged in an orderly way on the surface of the colliculus, forming a map of visual space, and one

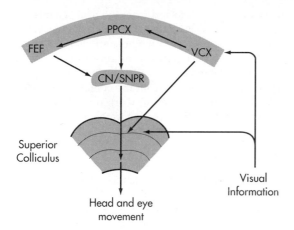

FIG. 7.62 Simplified scheme of the colliculus and its afferent and efferent connections.

interesting feature of this map is that electrical stimulation of deeper layers of a region corresponding with a particular part of the visual field often initiates an eye movement or head movement which is of the right size and direction to bring that part of the visual world onto the fovea. This suggests that one of the functions of the colliculus might be to move the eyes to objects of interest in the visual field. (In primates, lesions of the colliculus have surprisingly little effect on such eye movements, suggesting that this func-

tion has in the course of evolution come to be taken over by some other region, perhaps cortical.) Eye movements that are made to look at a visual stimulus are called *saccades*. These are very fast steplike movements in which the eye moves suddenly from one position in the orbit to another. They are also seen when a subject tries to look at a target that is moving: during visual tracking of this kind the oculomotor system moves the eye smoothly at a rate that ideally matches that of the target (smooth pursuit), with occasional saccades to correct any errors of position that still remain (the various types of eye movements are listed on p. 194).

Saccades are generated by special neural circuits in a region of the brainstem that lies near the motor neurones for the eye muscles, called the *prepontine reticular formation*. These circuits are normally held in check by inhibitory *pause cells* in the brainstem that are tonically active but stop firing briefly during a saccade. The superior colliculus sends inhibitory fibres to these pause cells, and a burst of activity in such a fibre appears to trigger a saccade to a particular target. Now, of course, there are many objects in the outside world which we might want to look at, and although the colliculus is well adapted to determining where they are and to initiating appropriate eye movements, what it cannot do is decide whether any particular object is worth looking at: this requires recognition. Consequently, we would expect to find

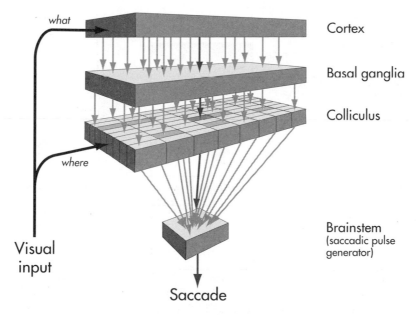

FIG. 7.63 Selection of saccadic targets. Although the colliculus has sufficient information to convert information about the location of one saccadic target into a command to the saccade-generating circuits of the brainstem, only the higher levels (cortex and basal ganglia) can decide which of various competing targets should be selected as a saccadic goal.

that the colliculus is itself under tonic inhibition from higher levels of the visual system, and only permitted to act when a possible target is recognised as being interesting. Such a descending inhibitory system to the deeper layer has recently been demonstrated in the form of a group of neurones in the substantia nigra (part of the basal ganglia: see p.238). They fire continuously, keeping the colliculus in check, but pause briefly in response to a visual stimulus, well in advance of the subsequent saccade that is made to look at it. Thus, through a curiously bureaucratic cascade of inhibitory neurones, the substantia nigra (driven by higher structures in the basal ganglia) allows the colliculus to give its permission to the brainstem to do its work of moving the eye to a certain position. They in turn appear to be controlled by areas of the cerebral cortex – notably the posterior parietal cortex – that are concerned with the identification and localization of objects that might be of interest.

The motor system needs to know about the position of objects relative not to the eye but to the body as a whole. We shall see in Chapter 11 how knowledge of the position of objects relative to the eye is combined with information about eye position derived from the commands that are sent to the eye muscles (*efference copy*: see p. 193) in order to compute the position of objects relative to the head; and how in turn this information, combined with signals from the vestibular system and from the neck, enables the motor system to calculate the position of objects both relative to the body as a whole, and also to absolute frames of reference such as the direction of gravity. The deeper layers of the colliculus receive copies of the efferent commands from the oculomotor system, and use this information to work out where targets are in space as well as relative to the eye.

Distance

The sense of distance is a little more complex, relying more heavily than the sense of direction on what might be called 'high-level' cues. Some of these cues derive from information about differences in the retinal images of the two eyes (*binocular* cues), while some are essentially *monocular*. The use of one eye rather than two substantially reduces the accuracy with which judgements of distance can be made but does not abolish it altogether. It is convenient to consider the monocular cues first.

The simplest, though probably the least important, is *accommodation*. For objects within a metre or so of the eye, the amount of effort of accommodation needed to focus an object certainly contributes to our sense of its distance, though in isolation this source of information is rather inaccurate. More important is information derived by moving the head: objects that are close to us then move more rapidly relative to the

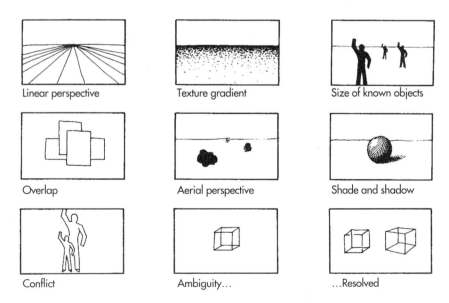

Linear perspective   Texture gradient   Size of known objects

Overlap   Aerial perspective   Shade and shadow

Conflict   Ambiguity...   ...Resolved

FIG. 7.64 *Illustrating schematically some of the monocular depth cues. The third row illustrates first how conflict may arise, in this case between size and overlap; and secondly, how it is possible to construct figures that may be interpreted in more than one way (in this case, as a cube viewed either from above or below). Addition of extra depth information (overlap, linear perspective) resolves the ambiguity.*

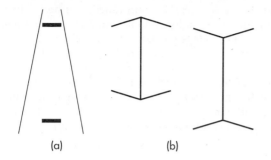

(a)   (b)

FIG. 7.65 Illusions that probably result from false depth inter-pretations. **(a)** The Ponzo illusion: the lower bar looks smaller than the upper, probably because it is perceived to be nearer (the sloping lines being perceived as parallel but receding into the distance). **(b)** Müller–Lyer illusion: the upright in the right-hand figure looks larger than the other, perhaps because the figure is interpreted as the far corner of a room or box, whereas the left-hand figure is taken as the near corner.

horizon than those that are far away (as can be seen on looking out of a train window) and this *movement parallax* can provide very accurate and absolute infor-mation about distance. It can often be seen when a cat is preparing to leap onto a ledge and needs to know its distance: it pauses first, moving its head up and down to generate motion parallax.

The other monocular cues are those that require some prior knowledge of the real world, and are the ones used by artists in portraying depth: painters have a particularly difficult job in trying to do this because accommodation, movement parallax, and the binocular cues combine together to tell the view-er that the picture is really flat. Some of these higher-level cues are illustrated in Figure 7.64. They include *overlap* (nearer objects tend to obscure further ones), *size of known objects* (if we know the actual size of an object and the angle it subtends at the retina we can deduce its distance), and various miscellaneous cues that are really special cases of 'size of known objects'. These include *linear perspective* (for example, the apparent convergence of parallel lines) and *tex-ture gradient* (that the spatial frequencies of a pattern or texture get higher the further away it is). Finally, *shadows* can give useful information about three-dimensional shape, and at great distances *aerial perspective* – the fact that distant objects are fuzzier and bluer than near ones – may be used. It is possi-ble to create artificial situations in the laboratory in which these cues are contradictory, and work out from subjects' response to them which cues are given more weight by the visual system than others. Many well-known illusions occur because assumptions about the distance of an object affect one's estimate of

its size – demonstrating that, of all the cues to depth, linear perspective is probably the strongest (Fig. 7.65).

What extra information is available if we use two eyes rather than one? Because we now see the visual world simultaneously from two different points of view, there are bound to be differences in the images that fall on each retina that will be more marked the closer an object is to the eyes. Imagine the two eyes fixating a point A in the middle distance (Fig. 7.66). The image of A will fall on the fovea of each eye (F, F'), and points like B that are as far away as A will be at the same angular distance from A as seen by each eye, and their images will therefore fall on points that are at the same distance and direction from the fovea in each retina: such points are called *corresponding points*. However, a point like C that is at a different distance from the eye will form images in the two eyes that are at different positions relative to the fovea: these are called *disparate images*. Now it turns

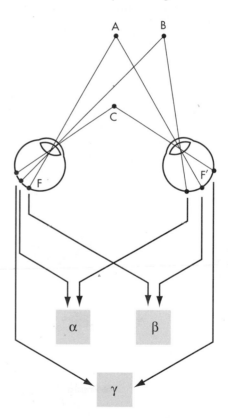

FIG. 7.66 Retinal disparity and disparity detectors. When binocularly fixating A, targets such as C that are at a different distance give rise to disparate images on the two retinae. Of neurones in the visual cortex that respond to signals from both eyes, many are stimulated by corresponding points in each reti-na (α, β) but some are connected to disparate points (γ).

out that if we examine the visual fields of cortical cells that have a binocular input (p. 152), although many of them are connected to corresponding areas in the two eyes, others are connected to disparate regions of the retina, and may be called disparity detectors (Fig. 7.66). So with the eyes both fixating A, a unit like α will be responding to the image of A, a unit like β with zero disparity will be responding to the image of B, and a unit like γ with marked disparity will be looking at the image of C. Thus even with the gaze fixed on one point in space, some cortical units will be 'looking' at points lying in planes either in front of or behind the target, and will thus provide immediate information about depth. Subjectively, there is indeed an area around the plane of fixation, called *Panum's fusional area*, in which one is not aware of the double image normally perceived when an object is out of this plane; the disparity units seem in some way to have fused the two images back together again in one's perception.

It is important to emphasize that though this mechanism of disparity detection is a very sensitive one indeed, it can only provide information about the distance of an object *relative* to the plane of fixation. As in the case of direction perception, we need further information about the positions of the eyes, about their angle of convergence, before it can be used to compute absolute depth. Since it turns out that knowledge of the convergence of one's eyes – derived through efference copy – is rather imprecise, it follows that disparity, though highly accurate for determining *relative* distances, is not of great use for

absolute estimates: its main function is probably to provide information about the three-dimensional shape of objects (stereopsis). It is not clear what is in fact used to sense absolute depth: it may well be that the visual size of well known objects, particularly of parts of the body such as the hand whose distance can be checked by direct proprioception, provides the ultimate measure by which the rest of visual space – beyond one's own reach – is calibrated.

VISUAL PROPRIOCEPTION

The most important contribution of vision to proprioception is that of sensing the movement of the head in space. As with the sense of visual direction, this relies on knowledge of any movements of the eyes, provided by efference copy. But other assumptions are necessary as well. When two areas of the field move relative to one another, it is usually the larger area that is assumed to be stationary: on a cloudy night, the moon appears to sail through the clouds. Of course it is the moon that is stationary and the clouds that move, but the latter occupy so much more of the visual field that the visual system assumes that they are stationary.

The fundamental source of information about the movement of retinal images comes from *visual movement detectors*. Several different areas in the brainstem seem to be involved in sensing retinal image

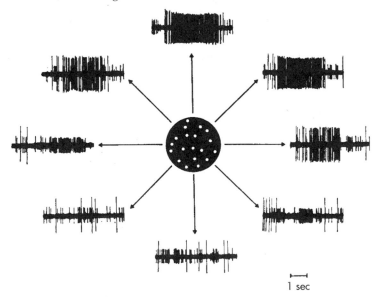

1 sec

FIG. 7.67 Pontine visual proprioceptive cell (cat), showing marked preference for movement of an extended, textured, field in a particular direction. (Baker *et al*, 1976)

movement of this kind, areas that are not very well defined and show considerable species variation. They include the pretectal nuclei and other nuclei at the very top of the brainstem, and groups of cells in the pons, but are best referred to collectively as the *visual proprioceptive system* (VPS). Neurones in the VPS typically have very large receptive fields indeed, and respond maximally when the field is filled with detailed pattern moving as a whole in a specific direction, precisely what happens if we move the head in natural surroundings (Fig 7.67): the rate at which they fire codes for velocity. Their information is sent to the vestibular nuclei and to the cerebellum, where it is added to information about head position derived from the vestibular apparatus, and generates compensatory postural reactions and eye movement. In the cerebellum it also appears to be used to calibrate the vestibular signals, bringing both sources of information about head movement into correspondence with one another; this function is described in more detail in Chapter 11. The fact that they adapt under prolonged stimulation gives rise to the striking *waterfall illusion*. If one stares for a minute or so at a surface that fills a substantial part of the field and is in continuous motion in one direction – like a waterfall – and then turns away to look at a stationary scene, one has the strong and persistent notion that it is moving in the opposite direction. Presumably the sense of visual motion depends on the balance between the rates of firing of movement detectors having opposite preferred directions: after adaptation an imbalance is caused by the depression of one set of these, leading to the illusion of movement in the opposite direction.

References

Aguilar, M. and Stiles, W. S. (1954) Saturation of the rod mechanism at high levels of illumination. *Optica Acta* 1, 59–65.

Baker, J., Gibson, A., Glickstein, M. and Stein, J. (1976) Visual cells in the pontine nuclei of the cat. *Journal of Physiology* 255, 415–433.

Baylor, D. A. and Fuortes, M. F. (1970) Electrical responses of single cones in the retina of the turtle. *Journal of Physiology* 207, 77–92.

Baylor, D. A., Matthews, G. and Yau, K.-W. (1980) Two components of electrical dark noise in toad retinal rod outer segments. *Journal of Physiology* 309, 561–591.

Blakemore, C. B. and Rushton, W. A. H. (1965) The rod increment threshold during dark adaptation in normal and rod monochromat. *Journal of Physiology* 181, 629–640.

Campbell, F. W. and Robson, J. G. (1968) Application of Fourier analysis to the visibility of gratings. *Journal of Physiology* 197, 555–566.

Dowling, J. E. and Boycott, B. B. (1966) Organization of the primate retina: electron microscopy. *Proceedings of the Royal Society B* 166, 80–111.

Fisher, R. F. (1973) Presbyopia and the changes with age in the human crystalline lens. *Journal of Physiology* 228, 765–779.

Hubel, D. H. and Wiesel, T. N. (1962) Receptive fields, binocular organisation and functional architecture in the cat's visual cortex. *Journal of Physiology* 160, 559–568.

Hubel, D. H. and Wiesel, T. N. (1965) Receptive fields and functional architecture in two nonstriate visual areas (18 and 19) of the cat. *Journal of Neurophysiology* 229–289.

Ikeda, H. and Sheardown, M. J. (1983) Functional transmitters at retinal ganglion cells in the cat. *Vision Research* 23, 1161–1174.

Kaneko, A. (1970) Physiological and morphological identification of horizontal, bipolar and amacrine cells in goldfish. *Journal of Physiology* 207, 623–633.

Kendrick, K. M. and Baldwin, B. A. (1987) Cells in temporal cortex of conscious sheep can respond preferentially to the sight of faces. *Science* 236, 448–450.

Kolb, H. and Nelson, R. (1984) Neural architecture of the cat retina. *Progress in Retinal Research* 21, 1081–1114.

Lamb, T. D. (1980) Spontaneous quantal events induced in toad rods by pigment bleaching. Nature 287, 349–351.

Lamb, T. D. (1984) Effects of temperature changes on toad rod photocurrents. *Journal of Physiology* 346, 557–578.

Marks, W. B., Dobelle, W. H. and MacNichol, E. F. (1964) Visual pigments of single primate cones. *Science* 143, 1181.

Normann, R. A. and Perelman, I. (1979) The effects of background illumination on the photoresponses of red and green cones. *Journal of Physiology* 286, 491–507.

Rushton, W. A. H. (1977) Visual adaptation. *Biophysics of Structure and Mechanism* 3, 159–162.

Rushton, W. A. H. and Powell, D. S. (1972) The rhodopsin content and the visual threshold of human rods. *Vision Research* 12, 1073–1081.

Van Ness, F. L. and Bouman, M. A. (1967) Spatial modulation transfer in the human eye. *Journal of the Optical Society of America* 57, 401–406.

NOTES

Vision There are many excellent books on vision in general, intended for readers with different interests. A selection: Bruce, V. and Green, P. (1985) *Visual Perception: Physiology, Psychology and Ecology* (Lawrence Erlbaum, London); Cornsweet, T. N. (1970) *Visual Perception* (Academic, New York); Davson, H. (1990) *Physiology of the Eye* (Macmillan, London); Walls, G. L. (1942) *The Vertebrate Eye* (Hafner, New York); Howard, I. P. (1982) *Human Visual Orientation* (John Wiley, Chichester); Hubel, D. H. (1988) *Eye, Brain and Vision* (W.H.Freeman, New York); Zeki, S. (1993) *A Vision of the Brain* (Blackwell, Oxford).

Page 126 Getting older The lens also starts to lose its transparency: if the tendency to cloudiness and yellowness goes too far we have *cataract,* with an inability to form proper retinal images. These changes are probably through a gradual accumulation of damage to cell protein and membrane disruption, and are accelerated by both short- and long-wave radiation.

Page 127 Astigmatism Astigmatism also results in different magnification in different meridians, and there has sometimes been speculation whether this might explain the distortions that some well-known artists seem to introduce into their paintings – El Greco is a good example. At first sight, there is an obvious logical flaw in this, for the artist would suffer the same distortion when looking at his canvas as well as at the model; but nevertheless there are optical defects that could account for it. This and many other ocular disabilities amongst artists are discussed in Trevor-Roper, P. (1970) *The World through Blunted Sight* (Thames and Hudson, London).

Page 127 Poorly-designed optics Recall the saying of the great physicist and physiologist Hermann von Helmholtz: *'If an optician made me a lens as bad as the one Nature gave me, I would send it back'.*

Page 128 Large pupils reveal bad optics Presbyopes often complain that their eyes are weaker, in the sense that they need more light in order to read. The reason is not that their sensitivity is low but that with very bright illumination the pupil shrinks down and increases their depth of focus, enabling a tolerable image to be formed of an object considerably closer than the real near point.

Page 129 Emotional pupils Photographs retouched to make the pupils larger are generally judged more attractive and stimulating than the original. Curiously, the viewer's own pupils then dilate, suggesting a covert system of sexual signalling that would result in positive feedback in certain circumstances – possibly an explanation for 'love at first sight'.

Page 131 The retina Three classic accounts of retinal structure, of various vintages: Dowling, J. E. (1987) *The Retina: an Approachable Part of the Brain* (Belknap, Cambridge, Mass); Polyak, S. L. (1941) *The Retina* (University of Chicago Press, Chicago); Rodieck, R. W. (1973) *The Vertebrate Retina* (W.H.Freeman, San Francisco).

Page 133 Pigment regeneration 11-cis retinol is more familiar as vitamin A, and one of the consequences of vitamin A deficiency is incomplete regeneration and hence a condition known as nightblindness, cured by eating more carrots.

Page 134 Electrical responses A clear account of

this area is Lamb, T. D. and Pugh, E. N. (1990) Physiology of transduction and adaptation in rod and cone photoreceptors. *The Neurosciences* 2, 3–13.

Page 134 Black on white And of course the way text is ordinarily printed.

Page 137 Adaptation Useful articles in this area may be found in Hess, R. F. (1990) *Night Vision* (Cambridge University Press, Cambridge).

Page 138 Spontaneous isomerization It occurs at a rate of about one molecule per receptor every two minutes.

Page 138 Gain The gain of a system is simply the magnitude of the output divided by that of the input; so, for example,an amplifier that generates 100 mV for a 1 mV input has a gain of 100. In a linear system the gain is always constant, regardless of the size of the input.

Page 150 Optic radiation It is worth emphasizing that as we go from geniculate to cortex there is an enormous expansion in the neural *width* of the visual system. Whereas in the retina there are something of the order of 130 million receptors, the LGN has only 1.5 million cells – net convergence; yet in primary visual cortex we are back to something like 200 million. It is clear that cortical cells are elaborating rather than condensing the information that they receive.

Page 150 Stripe of Gennari Discovered in 1776 by Francesco Gennari while he was a medical student, studying histology: which goes to show that diligence in this area can bring you fame as well as immense intellectual satisfaction.

Page 159 Opponent processing Curiously enough, exactly the same system is used in colour television. The camera provides a red channel, a green channel, and a blue one; but these three signals are then recoded to provide a luminance signal plus two colour or chroma signals that are formed, as in the retina, by subtraction. Black-and-white sets simply ignore the chroma part of the signal.

Page 159 Colour constancy This topic (amongst many others) is intelligently discussed in Zeki, S. (1993) *A Vision of the Brain* (Blackwell, Oxford).

Page 159 Red v. green More recent sequencing has shown that the red and green cone opsins are more than 90% homologous, much more than in relation to blue.

Page 160 Foveal tritanopia This seems to have been realised empirically for a long time. Tritanopia causes yellow and white to be indistinguishable at a distance, and blue and black. The flags used for signalling at sea are designed such that tritanopia can never make one confuse one signal for another; similarly, the strict laws of heraldry forbid a yellow charge on a white field, or vice versa.

Page 162 Monocular distance cues These are the ones that artists have to use to create a sense of depth – a hard task, since the binocular cues, accommodation and motion parallax work against them. One trick is the use of the *peep-show*, in which the painted interior of a box is viewed through a small hole; this rather cleverly limits the viewer to monocular vision, eliminates parallax and reduces the effect of accommodation because of the small aperture. Some accounts of psychological and physiological aspects of artistic representation include Gage, J. (1993) *Colour and Culture* (Thames and Hudson, London); Kemp, M. (1990) *The Science of Art: Optical Themes in Western Art from Brunelleschi to Seurat* (Yale University Press, New Haven); and Wright, L. (1983) *Perspective in Perspective* (Routledge and Kegan Paul, London).

Page 163 Corresponding points Strictly speaking, as you can probably prove for yourself geometrically, points like B must lie on a circle that passes through the centres of the two eyes and also through A. Such a circle is called a *horopter*.

Page 165 The waterfall illusion First described by R. Addams, who wrote in 1834: '*During a recent tour through the Highlands of Scotland, I visited the celebrated Falls of Foyer on the border of Loch Ness, and there noticed the following phaenomenon. Having steadfastly looked for a few seconds at a particular part of the cascade, admiring the confluence and decussation of the currents forming the liquid drapery of waters, and then suddenly directed my eyes to the left, to observe the vertical face of the sombre age-worn rocks immediately contiguous to the waterfall, I saw the rocky surface as if in motion upwards, and with an apparent velocity equal to that of the descending water, which the moment before had prepared my eyes for this singular deception.*' *Philosophical Magazine* Series 3, Volume 5, 373–374.

NEUROLAB

Visual optics

Page 126–128

This shows a schematic eye and the way in which light is focused on the retina under different circumstances. You can choose to see what happens with white light or with red and blue (check box at bottom). The various controls are self-explanatory. There are radio buttons to select three possible target distances, and various conditions of refractive error. The slider bar controls the state of accommodation, and you can add spectacles with either positive or nega-

tive lenses. Experiment with various combinations of settings. Some things in particular that you might note: (1) that myopes see better with red light, hypermetropes with blue; (2) that a presbyope reads better (i.e. target distance 0.1 m) in very bright light, when the pupil is constricted; (3) a small pupil improves chromatic aberration. If you click on Demo, you can see a simple demonstration of the influence of chromatic aberration on apparent depth: the red elements appear to be closer than the blue, mainly because a slightly greater effort of accommodation is needed to focus them.

Blind spot

Page 130

This exhibit allows you to demonstrate your blind spot, and plot out its boundary. First decide which eye you are going to use; click on the corresponding radio button at bottom left, and keep the other eye covered. Then look at the red fixation spot, and move the cursor around within the window. You will be aware that within a certain area it disappears from view: this is the blind spot. While still fixating the red spot, try to trace the boundary of the blind spot with the cursor. Click whenever you think you are just on the edge, leaving a mark permanently on the screen. Go on doing this all round the edge, and you will end up with a tracing of the edge of the blind area. You can erase the marks with the Clear button. You may like to drag one of the two brightly coloured objects at bottom left on to the blind spot and demonstrate that they too are completely invisible. Finally, click on Pattern, and notice how the brain fills in the blind spot with the prevailing background pattern, so that you are not aware of a blank.

Photoreceptors

Page 134

This exhibit embodies a very simple model of the cascade of events between absorption of light by photoreceptors (toad rods), the activation of PDE, reduction in cGMP, and closing of sodium channels. If you press Sweep, a trace is initiated showing the stimulus (a brief pulse of light) in red, and the resultant photocurrent in green. You can set different background levels as well as different sizes of stimulus (radio buttons at right). Observe saturation with large stimuli, and also the way in which a steady background reduces sensitivity mostly by affecting calcium levels, which mediate adaptation by altering the rate at which cGMP is recycled. The Auto-zero check box makes every response start at the same level; if you want to examine steady states, turn it off. For easier comparison, sweeps are superimposed until the Clear button is activated.

Horizontal cells

Page 135

This very simple demonstration shows how horizontal cells can mediate the lateral inhibition seen in bipolar cells of the retina. Move the cursor on to one of the receptors (light blue) and press and hold the left button. The thermometers to the left of each neural element indicate membrane potential (down = hyperpolarization). If you have selected Hyperpolarizing bipolars (radio button at right), notice how the bipolar immediately connected to the receptor hyperpolarizes, while its neighbours show decreasing degrees of depolarization with distance, mediated by the horizontal cell (far right, hyperpolarizing).

⊙ Receptive fields

Page 137

This exhibit enables you to perform virtual experiments on different kinds of visual cell, determining their receptive field properties by using different kinds of stimulus. On the right are two sets of controls, for Stimulus type and Field type. Select Circle as your stimulus, and Simple large-field as the field type. When you click in the window at left, which represents the visual space for your experiment, you will see a white disc appear (or a black disc on a white background, if you have selected the check box Invert white/black). You can alter the size of the circle with the Size slider, and in the case of elongated stimuli, the Angle slider alters their orientation. When you click, the horizontal thermometer at the bottom will light up blue to indicate the degree of response of the cell, and if you have a sound card, you will hear simulated action potentials.

Explore all round the window, and try to estimate the extent of the receptive field, and its general characteristics (for example, do you get inhibition rather than excitation at any point?). You will find it actually responds only excitatorily, in a roughly circular area in the middle. You can confirm this by selecting the Reveal check box on the right. The two check boxes just above it determine whether the response is inverted (i.e. inhibitory rather than excitatory) and whether the cell is predominantly transient in its response. Try them. Then go on to look at more elaborate receptive fields, perhaps with other kinds of

stimulus. Don't forget to investigate movement sensitivity (drag the cursor within the field) as well as simple on/off (clicking).

⊥⊥ Linespread function and ⋀⋀ acuity

Page 141

The linespread function is to a very thin line stimulus what the pointspread function is to a very small point. This exhibit demonstrates how the linespread function is related to the appearance of various kinds of visual targets: single lines, edges, bars and pairs of lines (selected by the radio buttons on the right: the controls below them allow you to alter the spacing of the pair of lines, and the width of the bar, as well as selecting whether the stimulus is white on a black background or black on white). In the window we have, from top to bottom: first a representation of the stimulus itself; then (yellow) a plot of the distribution of light across the stimulus; and then (green) the distribution of light across its image. If you select Single line, you can see the linespread itself directly: the slider at bottom right alters its width. Select Two lines, and see for yourself how the image cannot be resolved if the lines are close together in relation to the width of the linespread. Select Single edge, and see how blur reduces the rate of change of intensity as you go from light to dark. Finally, select Single bar, start with a wide spacing and gradually make it smaller. You will see that at first the image also gets narrower, but there comes a point at which making the stimulus thinner does not reduce the *size* of the image: what it does is reduce its *intensity*. This is why measurements of how thin a line we can just detect are not essentially measures of acuity, since the dimensions of the retinal image do not alter.

⌐¬ ∿∿ Lateral inhibition

Page 146

This exhibit demonstrates some aspects of lateral inhibition; it was introduced in Chapter 4 (p. 88), where the more general demonstration in the left window was described: that part of the description is repeated here, since it is relevant to vision as well. The section which is more general is on the left, which shows a spatial stimulus (blue) and the spatial pattern of its response (green). The radio buttons choose as stimulus either a single line or point and edge or a pair of lines. The buttons just to the right generate either blur or lateral inhibition, and can be used repetitively to increase the effect: Restore returns to the original state. At top right, the slider called Completeness determines how much lateral inhibition is applied. Look first at an edge, blur it once, and then apply lateral inhibition once; do this for several settings of completeness. With full completeness, the steady DC component on each side of the edge is completely removed. Using a point stimulus, notice how lateral inhibition counteracts blur, at least up to a point. With a double stimulus, notice that if you add blur to the point where the two stimuli cannot be distinguished, lateral inhibition does not separate them again. In other words, strictly speaking, lateral inhibition does not improve acuity. These effects of blur and lateral inhibition are also shown more graphically in the centre window: if you click on the buttons below the picture, it will be processed by applying either one or the other. You will see that the general appearance of a blurred picture can be improved with a certain amount of lateral inhibition, but that detail can be irretrievably lost. Notice that very complete lateral inhibition leads to a kind of outline drawing in which only edges and high spatial frequencies appear.

Two visual illusions related to lateral inhibition are also shown: click on Cornsweet illusion or Strip illusion. In the *Cornsweet* illusion, a central perturbation is introduced into an otherwise uniform field: from left to right, it consists of a gently increasing luminance followed by a sudden drop in luminance, and then a further gentle increase back to the original level. When looking at the whole field, especially at a little distance, what is seen is two more or less uniform fields side by side, brighter on the left and darker on the right. This is presumably because lateral inhibition enhances the sudden transition at the expense of the more gentle luminance gradient, so that the former dominates the overall perception. In the *strip* illusion, a perfectly uniform strip is seen against a background that changes systematically from dark on one side of the screen to light on the other. Because of contrast effects mediated by lateral inhibition, the strip does not appear uniform at all, but graded in brightness the opposite way round.

Cortical regions

Page 151
A simple map of functional cortical areas, for self-testing. Click on one of the radio buttons designating an area of cortex, and the name and Brodmann number will appear in the box at right. Alternatively, click on the pull-down button at the right of the box to display the whole list, and click on an 'item: the corresponding radio button will be selected.

Colour

Page 157
This exhibit demonstrates some aspects of colour mixing, and some contrast phenomena. Note that it will not work properly, or at all, if your computer display is not set to at least 256 colours. On left, for reference, the colour triangle (this is displayed using only 16 colours, so that the gradations are not very satisfactory). At top right, a small foreground patch of colour is shown against a background of a different colour. You can alter the red, blue and green components of foreground and background with the sliders. You can prove to yourself (in case you didn't believe it) that red and green make yellow and you can see how the appearance of the patch is modified by the colour of the background: simultaneous colour contrast. Below the patch and background is a strip showing all the colours lying along the line joining the foreground and background colours on the colour triangle, representing the range of colours that could be mixed from the two colours chosen. Below it, a small patch shows the complementary colour to the foreground, the colour which would create white if mixed with it. The Blackout and Whiteout buttons enable you to see successive contrast and after-images. Stare at the central patch, and then press Whiteout. The whole field will go white, and you will see an illusory patch at the centre having the complementary colour to the original patch; it is also in effect a negative after-image. If instead you select Blackout, you will see a positive after-image.

⌐_ Adaptation

Page 165
Most of this exhibit has already been introduced (Chapter 3, p. 70)., but it also contains a specifically visual demonstration of the effects of adaptation, the waterfall illusion (click on the button). Click on Adapt, and fixate the centre of the figure. The stripes move steadily inward, stimulating visual motion detectors, which then begin to adapt. After some 10–20 seconds, click on Test, stopping the motion. The stripes will now appear to be moving backwards, although they are in fact stationary; the adaptation has upset the balance between units signalling motion in different directions. The effect is also very pronounced if after adaptation you look away at other objects around you.

Smell 170   Taste 179

All neurones in the brain respond to chemical transmitters, so chemosensitivity is hardly a specialization of function at all. We shall be concerned here only with chemical stimuli that originate outside the body, with *olfaction* (smell) and *gustation* (taste). The chemoreceptors that monitor the composition of the blood, and are used in the regulation of autonomic and hormonal functions are discussed in other volumes in this series.

SMELL

Receptors

Those readers who have had the privilege of dissecting a human head will be aware that the nose has an internal complexity that is quite startling in comparison with its rather drab exterior. The surface area of the nasal cavity is enormously inflated by the presence of three *conchae* on each side, highly vascular organs covered with erectile tissue whose function is primarily to moisten and warm the incoming air, and conversely to limit the loss of heat and water in the air that is expired (Fig. 8.1). The olfactory receptors form part of the *olfactory epithelium*, tucked away in the olfactory cleft right at the top of the cavity, and in normal quiet breathing only a very small proportion of the air actually reaches the olfactory epithelium However, in sniffing, turbulences are set up round the conchae, and an appreciable fraction of the air gets to the olfactory receptors. This fraction is critically dependent on the state of the conchae: if you have a cold, they tend to become engorged with blood, hindering the passage of air to the higher regions and causing the familiar partial loss of smell.

Man is a *microsmatic* animal: smell plays a far smaller part in his sensory world and in the regulation of his actions than in the case of macrosmatic animals such as the dog, and his olfactory sensitivity

is in general correspondingly reduced. To some extent this is reflected in the small area of his olfactory epithelium: about 5 cm^2 in all, compared with some five times that in the cat, despite its very much smaller head. This epithelium has a number of easily recognizable features. It contains *Bowman's glands* of tubuloalveolar form producing a lipid-rich secretion that bathes the surface of the receptors; consequently,

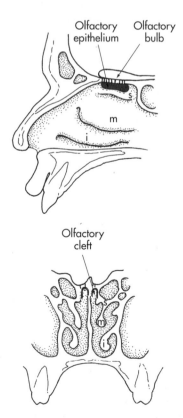

FIG. 8.1 The nasal cavity in humans; longitudinal and transverse section, showing the superior, medial and inferior conchae (s, m, and i) and the olfactory cleft.

to have an odour a substance must to some extent be lipid-soluble. Another characteristic is that one of the types of epithelial cells contains granules of *pigment*: the depth of colour in different species is often correlated with olfactory sensitivity, being light yellow in humans and dark yellow or brown in dogs. It has sometimes been suggested that this pigment may play some part in the mechanism of olfactory transduction, perhaps being involved in the absorption of some kind of radiation such as infrared: this idea is discussed later in the chapter. Finally there are the receptors themselves, of which there are some 10 million in humans. They are distinguished by a terminal enlargement above the surface of the epithelium, from which project some 8–20 *olfactory cilia* (Fig. 8.2). These cilia show the usual 9 + 2 fibril arrangement at the base but are not actively motile: they form a dense and tangled mat that covers the olfactory area. Vacuoles can also be seen in the terminal enlargement, and experiments have shown that they are actively pinocytotic: fluid is being continually taken in by the receptors and passed down the olfactory nerves into the brain. The significance of this surprising feature is unclear. A further curiosity of the olfactory receptors is their remarkably short life: after a month or two they degenerate and are replaced by new ones from below.

Olfactory bulb

Unlike many receptor cells, the olfactory receptors send their own axons to the CNS without an intervening synapse. These fibres, the *fila olfactaria*, make up the first cranial nerve: they are exceedingly fine and difficult to see with the light microscope. They pass through the *cribriform plate* in individual holes ('cribriform' = 'sievelike') and enter the *olfactory bulb* which lies just above the olfactory epithelium (Fig. 8.3). Here they synapse with dendrites of the large *mitral cells* (they are supposed to look like bishops' mitres) and *tufted cells* in specialized nexuses called glomeruli. In rabbits, which have been particularly well studied, each glomerulus receives information from some 26 000 receptors, and has an output to about 24 mitral cells: there are probably only some 2000 glomeruli in all. The fibres entering any one glomerulus come from a wide area of the epithelium, so that detailed information about any spatial patterns of activity must be largely thrown away; but ,as is the case for rods in the eye, this enormous degree of convergence must certainly enhance the nose's sensitivity by providing a mechanism by which the contributions of very large numbers of receptors can be added together. The final output of the bulb con-

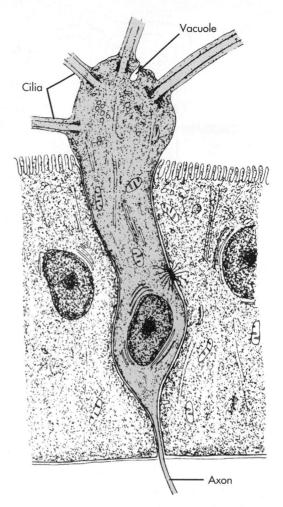

FIG. 8.2 Typical olfactory receptor, showing terminal enlargement with cilia and vacuoles projecting above the level of the surrounding epithelium. Note that the cilia are truncated in this picture: in practice they vary considerably in length, some being shorter than the receptor cell body, and some several times its length.

sists of the axons of the mitral and tufted cells, forming the *olfactory tract*: this has two divisions, lateral and medial, of which only the lateral one appears to be important in humans.

However, the olfactory bulb is not just a simple relay but has two other properties that we have already seen to be common to all the sensory systems examined so far, namely lateral inhibition, and negative feedback control of afferent information. The most prominent feedback path is formed by projections from the second-order mitral and tufted cells that synapse excitatorily with *granule cells* (Fig. 8.3) which in turn inhibit neighbouring second-order

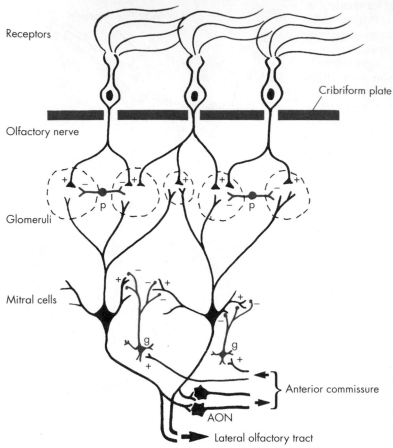

Receptors

Cribriform plate

Olfactory nerve

Glomeruli

Mitral cells

Anterior commissure

AON

Lateral olfactory tract

FIG. 8.3 Simplified representation of the cell types of the olfactory bulb, and their connections: p, periglomerular cells; g, granule cells; AON, anterior olfactory nucleus.

cells. An interesting feature of these synapses is that they are dendrodendritic (the granule cells have no axons), and reciprocal: excitation and inhibition occur simultaneously – in opposite directions – at the same synapse. Other collaterals of the second-order cells' axons synapse in the anterior olfactory nucleus with interneurones which also return and synapse with granule cells but in this case some of the interneurones project contralaterally in the anterior commissure to influence the opposite bulb in the same way. The significance of this mutual inhibition between the two bulbs is not clear: one possibility is that it may serve to enhance differences between the activities of the two bulbs – another kind of lateral inhibition – in a way that might perhaps be useful for localizing smells. Careful experiments have shown that even humans are capable of localizing odorous objects in a rather approximate way, presumably through slight differences in the timing or intensity of the stimuli in each nostril. Finally there are the *periglomerular cells*, which appear to subserve lateral inhibition at the level of the glomeruli through

reciprocal synapses with the second-order cells, and direct connections from the fila olfactaria. All this is strikingly reminiscent of the retina, where horizontal cells appear to carry out similar functions to periglomerular cells, and amacrine cells to granule cells, using similar kinds of synaptic mechanism.

Central olfactory projections

The central projections of the olfactory system provide something of an *embarras de richesses*, very different from the orderliness with which, for example, the optic tract projects to the lateral geniculate nucleus and thence to the cerebral cortex: indeed, olfaction seems to be unique in projecting straight on to cortical areas without relaying in the thalamus or any equivalent structure. One must bear in mind that the olfactory system is very much older than such senses as vision and hearing, and in more primitive animals a very much larger proportion of the brain is directly or indirectly concerned with olfaction (Fig. 8.4). The reason for this is not hard to see: simple

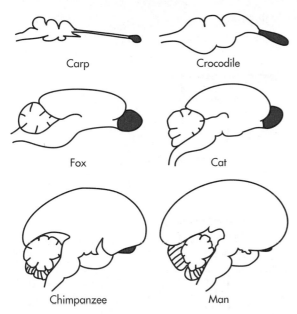

FIG. 8.4 Reduction in relative size of olfactory bulb (colour) with phylogenetic development of the brain. (Partly after Carpenter, 1976)

towards nutrients and avoid poisons, and to seek out mates by recognizing the chemical attractants they release. Their motivation – the drive that tells their motor systems what to do – is essentially olfactory.

Even in humans, the remains of this very basic system for chemical motivation and emotion (emotion being the sensory correlate of motivation) can still be seen in the central olfactory projections (Fig. 8.5). Many of these structures form part of the *limbic system*, a group of nuclei, cortical regions and connecting tracts of great evolutionary antiquity that appear to be concerned with precisely those kinds of function that one would expect in a primitive animal to be closely related to chemical stimulation: motivation, emotion, and certain kinds of memory. The limbic system and its functions are discussed more fully in Chapters 13 and 14; for the moment we may note, for example, that the septal nuclei and amygdala contain regions known as 'pleasure centres', in the sense that when electrically stimulated they seem to provide a kind of direct positive motivation. The hippocampus seems to be concerned with motivational memory, the ability to associate a previously uninteresting stimulus (like the bell in Pavlov's well-known conditioning experiments) with the promise of food or pleasure signalled more directly by olfactory stimulation, and to recognize such a stimulus in the future as a source of motivation in its own right.

What seems to have happened in the course of

animals depend much more immediately than we do on knowing directly from their senses whether food is in the vicinity, and their motor systems are likely to be more pressingly governed by the need to move

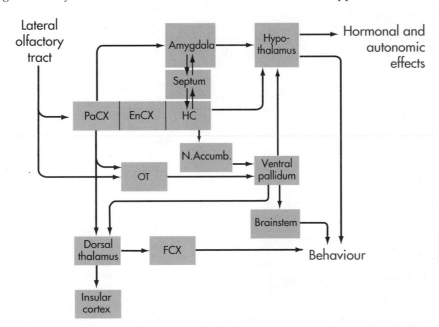

FIG. 8.5 Highly schematic diagram of areas of the brain directly or indirectly driven by olfactory stimuli: OT, olfactory tubercle; PaCX, periamygdaloid and prepyriform cortex; EnCX, entorhinal cortex; HC, hippocampus and subiculum; N. Accumb, nucleus accumbens; FCX, frontal cortex.

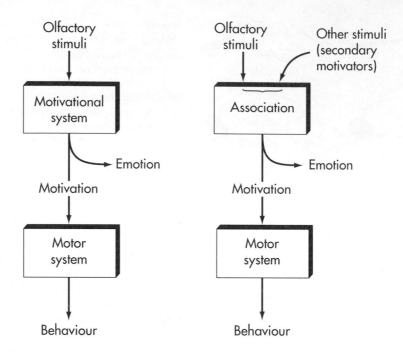

FIG. 8.6 Schematic representation of motivation through primarily olfactory stimuli in primitive organism (a), and in a more developed animal (b) through other stimuli (secondary motivators) that become potent through association.

Box 8.1 Examples of behaviour controlled by olfaction

Feeding
Hunting and finding food, eating and aversion, stimulation of digestive secretions

Sexual
Recognition of receptive females, triggering or suppression of ovulation, sexual attraction and arousal

Maternal
Recognition of offspring, triggering of maternal behaviour

Avoidance
Scenting of predators, response to alarm pheromones released by other herd members

Territorial
Recognition of urinal territorial markers, homing and recognition of breeding grounds

Social
Recognition of individuals and members of species or group, social dominance

evolution is that this kind of *secondary motivation* by stimuli that only acquire their meaning through experience and learning has steadily grown in importance relative to that of primary olfactory motivation (Fig. 8.6). For humans, money is perhaps the most obvious secondary motivation, and the most powerful of all: given the choice between a bag of crisps and a bag of £10 notes, unless one were exceptionally hungry there is no doubt which would cause the greater motivational drive!

For this reason, limbic structures that were originally subservient to olfaction are now not primarily olfactory at all; and the name *rhinencephalon* ('nose-brain') which is sometimes given to the *limbic system* is an inappropriate one in higher animals.

Finally, there are important connections between the limbic system and the hypothalamus (see Chapter 14, p. 281), providing routes by which olfactory stimuli can cause such obvious autonomic effects as salivation and other secretory responses to food smells, as well as influencing the choice of food: a single instance of a particular odorant associated with nausea, even some hours later, can condition an animal to avoid the substance for the rest of its life. Smell my also have much more widespread hormonal and behavioural effects, of which the best known are perhaps sexual arousal and modification of reproductive cycles, even abortion. Many creatures

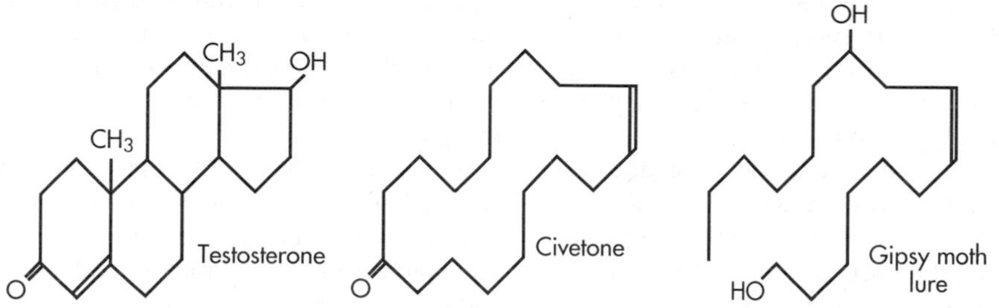

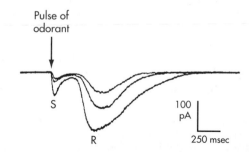

FIG. 8.7 The structure of testosterone and of two olfactory sexual attractants.

emit specific pheromones (air- or waterborne signals) that act as sexual attractants, often over large distances. A curious feature of some of these lures is that they often resemble, in species as different as the civet and the moth, the steroid reproductive hormones themselves (at least in overall shape: Fig. 8.7). Furthermore, some of them – such as civet oil and musk – are used in perfumery and so presumably act as lures for human males as well (curiously abundant also in church incense). There are said to be marked sex differences in the olfactory thresholds for some of these macrocyclic compounds, which may also vary with the phase of the menstrual cycle.

But it is not just the sex life of animals that is dominated by smell. Predators sniff out their prey; fish find their way back to their native streams – sometimes from hundreds of miles away – through smell. Pheromones in the urine or from facial glands may be used as territorial markers; herd animals use them to warn others of the approach of a predator and personal smells are an essential means by which many animals recognize their own social groups and mothers their young. It is natural to speculate whether we humans are influenced subconsciously in the same kind of way: if so, it would have the most profound psychological and sociological implications. Firm evidence is lacking, though pheromone sprays for men apparently sell well.

However, one striking indication of the psychological links between olfactory and limbic functions in humans is the very vivid way in which odours may call up – often with surprising intensity – recollections of past experience. It is interesting how often such evocations are not just of the objective circumstances of a particular event, but also of the mood or emotion that was felt at the time, in a way that is seldom experienced with purely auditory or visual stimulation. The direct penetration of the emotional areas of the brain by olfactory fibres seems exactly reflected by what we feel.

Recordings from olfactory cells

Perhaps because smell does not seem as useful or important to us as, say, vision or hearing, and also because of certain difficulties of experimental technique, our knowledge of the electrophysiology of olfaction is still somewhat rudimentary. As was mentioned in Chapter 3, we now know the initial transduction process is of the conventional indirect form, with cAMP acting as an intermediary. In those species where it has been possible to measure the time-course of the response, the transduction process is found to be extremely prolonged, extending over a second or more (Fig. 8.8). This, and the extraordinary olfactory sensitivity to be discussed later (with a very steep stimulus–response curve), suggests some kind of amplificatory cascade similar to what is found in photoreceptors: in the case of smell there has presumably been less evolutionary pressure to make

FIG. 8.8 Patch-clamped salamander olfactory receptor responding to brief puffs of odorant of different concentrations. The odorant was mixed with potassium to act as a marker to give the effective duration of the stimulus; the potassium generated the first, brief, phase of the response (S). The later, extended part of the response (R) is due to the odorant itself. (After Firestein and Werblin, 1989)

things happen fast. However, the nature of the initial interaction of odorant with receptor, and of the subsequent coding of the neural messages sent to the olfactory bulb, are not well understood. One of the difficulties is that whereas it is comparatively easy to stick an electrode into the optic nerve or auditory nerve and record the way in which single fibres respond to particular stimuli, it is rather hard to do the same thing in the case of smell: the olfactory fibres are exceedingly fine, rather short, and buried for much of their length in the cribriform plate. An electrode in the olfactory epithelium tends to pick up not spike responses from individual cells but an averaged slow potential from many of them together, the electro-olfactogram or EOG. The size and shape of the EOG often shows rather little obvious correlation with the kind of substance that is applied.

With care, one may be lucky enough to record spikes from individual fibres, usually with the EOG superimposed on top, but again there is generally no simple relation between firing frequency and the kind of stimulus applied. In fact, with a single-unit preparation of this kind one can draw up a list in two columns, showing for a particular cell which substances excite it and which inhibit it. Such lists turn out to be quite chaotic, with apparently similar substances like menthol and menthone (which smell identical to us) often on opposite sides. Even more perplexingly, if one moves the electrode to record from a different cell, one finds in general an entirely different list, with substances that were excitatory for one cell being now inhibitory for the other, and substances that were on the same side of one list being on opposite sides of the other. In fact, there seems very little system in the way in which chemical stimuli are coded into patterns of firing of the olfactory nerve: each unit has its own assortment of molecular receptors, and thus its private idiosyncratic view of the olfactory world, like a spoilt child who likes baked beans but not bananas, fudge but not fish fingers, in a wholly arbitrary manner. The situation could hardly be more different from a sensory organ like the retina, with each of its units closely specified in terms of position, intensity and colour. Randomness of this kind is not necessarily a weakness in a sensory system; no information need be lost since, by looking at the pattern of response over the fibres as a whole, the nature of the original stimulus can still be reconstructed. Imagine a nursery of spoilt children seated at a dinner table and provided with push buttons with which they can register approval or disapproval of what is set in front of them: if these buttons were connected to an array of lights on a screen, it is clear that although any individual child's preferences may be quite idiosyncratic and quite unlike any other's, nevertheless any particular dish will result in a perfectly characteristic and reproducible pattern of lights by which it may be recognized.

Recordings from the olfactory bulb show a reduced degree of chaos: Figure 8.9a shows in graphical form the responses of a large number of units in the olfactory bulb of a monkey, and it can be seen that a small proportion of the cells responded to just one of the eight chemicals used as stimuli, and most showed excitation or inhibition to at least three. This increased specificity is undoubtedly the result of the *lateral inhibition* via periglomerular and granule cells that occurs early on in the bulb. Just as in the skin, where lateral inhibition reduces functional overlap between receptors by emphasizing differences in spatial firing patterns, here too – in a more abstract sense – it is reducing overlap between receptors not literally in space but in 'odorant space'. Of more central areas little is certain: responses to olfactory stimulation can be recorded from wide areas of the

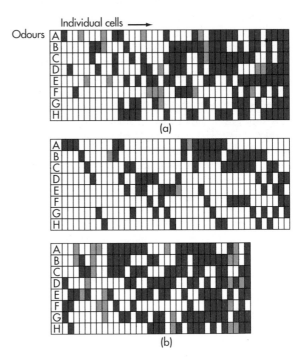

FIG. 8.9 Graphical representation of responses of neurones in the olfactory system of a monkey to each of eight different odours (A–H). Black = excitation, grey = inhibition. **(a)** 40 different units in the olfactory bulb; **(b)** 73 units in prepyriform cortex and amygdala: a larger proportion of the more central units respond to a smaller set of the stimuli applied. (Data from Tanabe *et al.*, 1975)

brain, not just in the limbic system but as far afield as the basal ganglia as well. One region that has been studied in more detail is the *prepyriform cortex*: here units show properties that suggest that the chaos characteristic of preceding levels of the olfactory system is beginning to be sorted out, and a significantly larger proportion of units respond to just one of a series of chemicals (Fig. 8.9b). On the whole there is a tendency for a larger proportion of units to respond to 'meaningful' smells like food or urine than to such things as the smell of mothballs.

Psychophysics of smell

The sense of smell shows a number of interesting and unusual features, which shed light on one's understanding of sensory processes in general as well as accounting for some of the peculiar experimental difficulties of studying olfaction.

The *sensitivity* of olfaction in many species is astonishing: just as the rods in the eye respond to single photons, and the ear to subatomic vibrations of the air, so the olfactory receptors are very near the theoretical limit of their sensitivity, and can apparently respond to the absorption of one or two molecules. Tests on tracker dogs have shown that they can respond to one millilitre of butyric acid (an ingredient of stale sweat) in some 10^{11} litres of air. This means that each sniff contains only about 200 000 molecules, and since the dog has roughly 200 million receptors, it follows that the absorption of *two molecules at the most* must be enough to excite an individual receptor. Sensitivity of this kind makes for considerable difficulty in experimentation, for when one measures an apparent response to one particular substance A, unless A is quite exceptionally pure, one can never be quite certain that what one is measuring is not the response to some other substance B present in exceedingly small amounts as a contaminant.

Another characteristic of olfactory sensitivity is that adaptation, though not particularly rapid, is usually absolutely complete. Thus men working in uncommonly smelly environments such as sewers or gas works soon become quite insensitive to the smells around them, and people are in general unaware of their own body odours. Professional food evaluators have to take special precautions to avoid adaptation of this kind. Wine tasters, aware of this danger, may nibble a piece of cheese between sips to restore the keenness of their palates (and with intriguing symmetry, Scottish cheese tasters take a nip of whisky after each sample, ostensibly for the same reason). This may perhaps be why the olfactory epithelium does not lie on the path of the incoming air in normal breathing: in sniffing, a sufficient change in odour concentration may be set up that overcomes unwanted adaptation.

The most fundamental way in which smell differs from the other special senses is in the lack of a systematic method of classifying and analysing different types of odour. To some extent this is because we ordinarily pay little conscious attention to smell, having enough to do in coping with the flood of more interesting information pouring in from our eyes and ears. Helen Keller, the writer who was blind and deaf from an early age, was able to develop her olfactory discrimination to an extraordinary degree through not being distracted by her other senses; she could, for example, recognize people she met and places she visited solely through their characteristic odours.

Part of the trouble is undoubtedly our lack of a proper *vocabulary* for describing smells: if we want to convey to someone what a eucalyptus smells like, we are literally at a loss for words. The difficulty is that there exists no objective, physical way of *classifying* smells systematically in the way that we can, for example, order colours into a spectrum or tones into a scale. In the case of vision our system of classification leads us to formulate simple rules using the colour triangle that enable us to predict the result of mixing colours in certain proportions to produce other colours, but in the case of smell this is quite impossible. We can never predict in advance what the result of mixing two odours together will be, and the results of doing so are frequently quite paradoxical. For example, the smells of iodoform and of coffee, individually strong and characteristic, are said to cancel each other out if appropriately mixed; other examples of cancellation of this kind have sometimes been exploited commercially to produce specific deodorants. Worse still, many odours smell quite different at different concentrations. Indole, which is a major component of dog excreta, and smells like it when concentrated, has a pleasant floral smell when very dilute and has actually been used in cheap perfumes! Many of the organic sulphides smell appalling at close range, but in small quantities turn out to be mainly responsible for the appetizing smell of foods such as roast beef and onion. Conversely, without special training, the nose is usually unaware whether a particular smell is pure, in the sense that only one kind of molecule is present, or a mixture. Many natural odours that seem perfectly unitary and pure, like that of raspberries, are in fact composed of dozens of components, many of which taken by themselves are rather unpleasant, and cannot be detected for what they are in the whole ensemble.

For all these reasons, although in the past strenuous

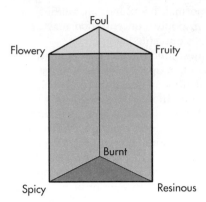

FIG. 8.10 Henning's prism: an attempt to divide olfactory stimuli into six 'primary' classes.

efforts have been made to try to classify smells into primary odour classes, like the nineteenth-century six-fold classification shown in Figure 8.10, no classification is ever really satisfactory because it does not enable one to predict the results of making mixtures in the way that the colour triangle does for colours. There is no such thing, in fact, as a *primary* odour. The explanation for this unsatisfying state of affairs lies in the chaotic way in which individual receptor cells respond to particular chemicals, which in turn is presumably a function of the apparently haphazard way in which they are allocated different types of molecular receptors. If we have two substances A and B which each produce characteristic patterns of activity in the olfactory nerve as a whole, then the response to A and B together will not be simply the sum of the responses to each separately: it will be a new pattern altogether. Thus the number of 'primary odours' will be of the order of the number of types of receptor, which is likely to be very large.

Transduction mechanisms

Though we know in a general way that the firing of olfactory nerve fibres is a consequence of a non-specific increase in ionic permeability, mediated by cAMP, how odorant molecules actually trigger this change remains something of a mystery. Presumably there are receptor sites that recognize particular molecules or classes of molecule but the basis of this recognition is not as straightforward a matter as one might imagine. A simple concept that has been around for some time is due to Amoore (1963). He suggested that either on the receptor membrane or possibly inside, there are hollow receptacles of molecular proportions which accept or reject odorant

molecules according to how well they fit the site (Fig. 8.11). In his theory he chooses just seven types of site, and each site has its corresponding odour quality – floral, minty, and so on – and two of the sites are for electrophilic and electrophobic molecules. In general terms the theory is plausible enough, except for the very small number of primary classes that is envisaged: we have already seen that a classification with only a few primary odours is quite insufficient to describe the richness and complexity of the real olfactory world. Another problem is that in practice there is often a striking lack of the expected correlation between a molecule's overall shape and what it smells like. Camphor and hexachlorethane smell practically identical to us, yet one could hardly imagine two molecules more different in size and

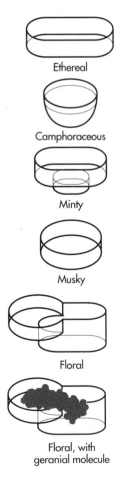

FIG. 8.11 Five of the receptor sites proposed by Amoore, and (bottom) the floral site occupied by a molecule of gerianol, a constituent of the smell of roses. (After Amoore, 1963; copyright Macmillan Journals Ltd)

structure (Fig. 8.12). Again, optical isomers – molecules having the same structure but mirror images of one another – generally have identical smells: it is difficult to see how the same site could fit both forms.

A second theory that was devised partly to get round this problem of lack of consistency between molecular shape and odour quality is the infrared vibrational theory developed by Wright (1964). The basic notion here is that while odour must ultimately be determined by chemical structure – the structure after all defines what the chemical is – overall shape is by no means the only property of a molecule that is determined by its structure. All molecules undergo mechanical vibrations, and the frequencies of these vibrations lie mostly in the infrared region, and depend in a rather complex way on the molecule's structure. In principle one could certainly imagine a sensory system that analysed the spectrum of these frequencies of vibration, perhaps through receptor sites tuned to different frequencies. In such a case one might well find two substances with similar shape but different smells because their frequencies of vibration were different; or conversely, substances sharing particular vibration frequencies and thus smelling similar, but of very different overall shape. There are a number of examples of the latter phenomenon that lend some support to the theory: nitrobenzene, benzonitrile and alphanitrothiophen, all of which smell of bitter almonds, happen to have many of their vibrational frequencies in common but have widely differing shapes. Optical isomers necessarily have identical vibrational frequencies, and usually smell identical as well. But while the theory has a certain plausibility in the more primitive parts of the animal kingdom, in the case of warmblooded animals there is a grave physical objection: it is very difficult to see how an olfactory system working with infrared radiation could function with such exquisite sensitivity – responding to single odorant molecules – in the presence of the inevitable background 'noise' generated by the body's own heat. It might conceivably be that the pigmentation of the olfactory epithelium could play some role in the absorption of radiant energy, and its presence is otherwise somewhat puzzling. But few physiologists would care to accept the infrared theory as the explanation of olfaction in higher animals.

It may very well be that Amoore's theory is basically correct, but with many hundreds of different receptor sites rather than just seven, whose affinity for different molecules is determined by something rather more sophisticated than simply their overall shape (perhaps vibrational frequency, inducing resonance in some kind of receptor molecule, might come into it as well). Finally, it is interesting in this context that many otherwise normal people show specific anosmias – 'blindness' to particular smells (that of freesias being a common example) – that are inherited as single recessive genes, suggesting perhaps the loss of a single receptor protein. More than 60 such specific anosmias are known, suggesting that the number of fundamental receptors – equivalent in a sense to 'primary' smells – must be at least this large. An extension of a genetic approach might well hold the key to a further understanding of the basic transduction process.

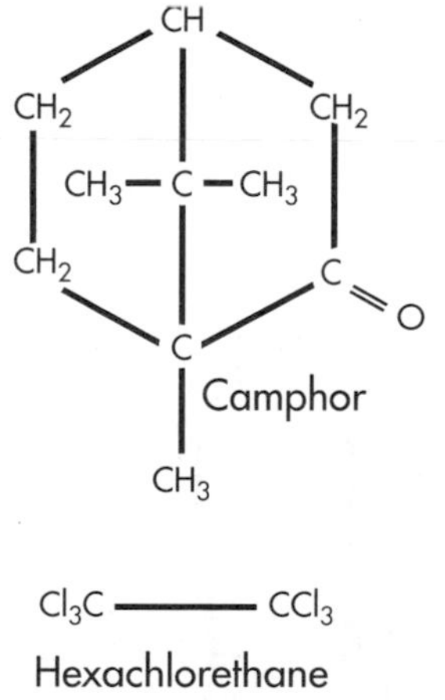

FIG. 8.12 Two substances whose smell is extremely similar though their molecular shapes and chemical properties are entirely different.

TASTE

The receptors and central pathways

What the man in the street means by taste is actually very largely *smell*, with purely somatosensory contributions such as texture, temperature and even pain (as in pepper) playing a part as well. People with anosmia, perhaps as a result of a cold, find their sense of taste profoundly disturbed: apples taste like onions, vintage port like blackcurrant syrup. In fact the human tongue appears to have only four modalities of taste apart from ordinary cutaneous sensation: *salt, sour, bitter* and *sweet*. These four qualities have obvious physiological significance: sweet things are on the whole sources of metabolic energy; bitterness is usually associated with poisons; sourness

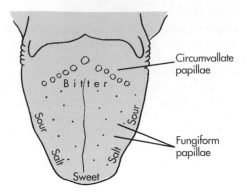

FIG. 8.13 Human tongue, showing regions where the four components of taste are most readily evoked, and the approximate distribution of two kinds of papillae. (After Moncrieff, 1967) The distribution of the different sensations actually overlap more than this figure implies.

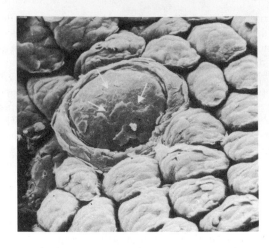

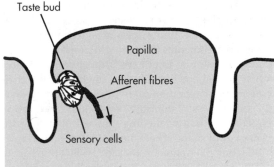

is simply a measure of acidity, and salt essentially of sodium chloride. To some extent taste thresholds and preferences are under the influence of the body's state of physiological need: salt-deprived rats show a preference for drinking salt solutions instead of water, and will tolerate strong saline solutions that other rats will refuse to drink. Coal miners, who sweat a lot, often used to put salt in their beer, though to others it tasted revolting.

If one stimulates the tongue with solutions applied locally through small pipettes, it is evident that certain areas are more sensitive than others to particular stimulus modalities (Fig. 8.13), and

FIG. 8.14 (a) Scanning electron micrograph of circumvallate papilla; the arrows show the openings of taste pits or buds on the surface of the papilla. (Kessel and Kardon, 1979; copyright W. H. Freeman and Co) **(b)** Schematic section of such a papilla, showing the sensory cells lying within the tastebud.

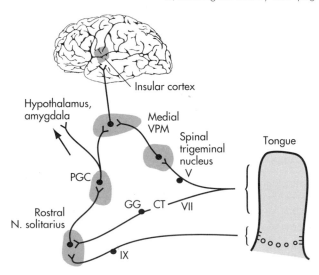

FIG. 8.15 Simplified scheme of the main afferent gustatory pathways (V, VII, IX, cranial nerves; CT, chorda tympani; GG, geniculate ganglion; VPM, ventral posterior medial thalamic nucleus; PGC, pontine gustatory area).

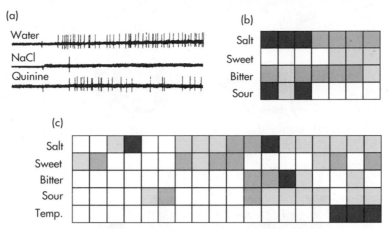

FIG. 8.16 Responses of gustatory neurones. **(a)** Records of activity of a single fibre in the chorda tympani of a cat, showing discharges in response to water and quinine (bitter), but not to salt. **(b)** Diagrammatic representation of the responses of seven individual taste receptors in the rat to four different stimuli, showing the varieties of stimulus preference. **(c)** Similar representation for 18 taste units in monkey thalamus (colour indicates size of response). (Data from Cohen *et al.*, 1955; Kimura and Beidler, 1961; Benjamin, 1963)

furthermore that the sense of taste is confined to special structures on the tongue called the *papillae*. In humans, three main types of papilla have been described: one of these, the *filiform* papilla, is not concerned with taste at all but is specialized for rasping and particularly well developed in meat-eaters like the cat. *Circumvallate* papillae, associated with sour and bitter taste, are found at the back of the tongue and consist of a sort of dome surrounded by a moat (Fig. 8.14), and in the walls of this moat one can find sensory cells with microvilli arranged in pitlike invaginations together with accessory cells, 30–50 in all, forming *tastebuds*. Similar buds are found in the *fungiform* papillae, which respond to salt and sweet and lie more towards the edge of the tongue. Unlike the olfactory receptors, these do not send their own axons to the CNS but are innervated by fibres of cranial nerves VII and IX, whose cell bodies are in the geniculate ganglion and glossopharyngeal ganglion respectively; the tongue is also innervated by the trigeminal nerve (V), providing ordinary somatic sensibility. The afferent taste fibres go to the rostral part of the *nucleus solitarius*, which projects via a pontine relay to the medial part of the ventral posterolateral area of the thalamus, whence fibres ascend to a small area of the *insular* cerebral cortex (Fig. 8.15), where they are joined by a part of the olfactory projection. On the whole the anatomy of the gustatory system is much more like that of ordinary cutaneous sense than is the case for olfaction, though gustatory projections to the periamygdaloid cortex, hypothalamus and other limbic areas exist as well.

One branch of the lingual nerve passes rather conveniently in the chorda tympani, where it is relatively accessible for recording. Single units show almost the same chaotic properties seen in the olfactory fibres (Fig. 8.16); instead of responding strictly to just one of the four modalities, they tend to respond to a random assortment of them (and often to water as well, which in many species should really be thought of as a fifth gustatory modality). Once again, each unit seems to have its own viewpoint of the gustatory world, and stimuli are encoded in the spatial pattern with which the ensemble of afferent fibres discharges. At the thalamic level (Fig. 8.16) the situation seems hardly less chaotic, although there may be more of a tendency for units to be selective for one type of stimulus.

Transduction mechanisms

For two of the modalities of taste, salt and sour, the complexities so characteristic of olfaction seem to be absent: sourness depends in a simple way on pH (though not all solutions of equal pH are equally sour, and the anion contributes), and saltiness is a function mostly of the sodium ion concentrations, though to some extent of lithium as well. The transduction of both these modalities seems relatively straightforward: in the former case, hydrogen ions appear to reduce the permeability to potassium, either directly or via cAMP, while the response to sodium seems simply through its direct entry through passive sodium channels (Fig. 8.17). One can also show that the neural response to salt solutions is

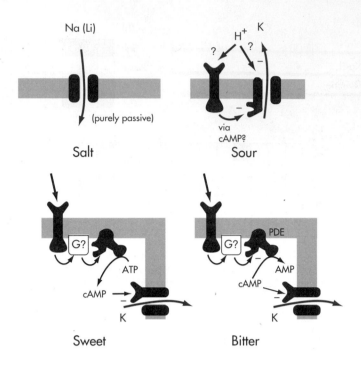

FIG. 8.17 Probable transduction mechanisms for the four taste sub-modalities.

modified by salt deprivation in the way that would be expected from behavioural observations.

But in the case of sweet and bitter, the situation is much more like that in the nose: once again we find a distinct lack of correlation between overall molecular shape and taste, as for example in the well-known artificial sweeteners, whose thresholds are vastly lower than the actual sugars for which the receptors were presumably intended. But the fact that we are dealing here with only two classes instead of indefinitely many simplifies things considerably, and it is now clear that there are specific receptor proteins which in some cases have been extracted and found to bind to sweet or bitter substances, and are 'fooled' by false stimuli like saccharin in the same way that we are ourselves. Bitter substances appear to increase cAMP and generate a depolarization through a decrease in P_K; the sweet receptors – which respond to some amino acids as well as sugars and sweeteners – probably also work via cAMP (Fig. 8.17). These findings give some confidence to the idea that olfactory transduction might also be mediated by specific receptor proteins, although necessarily with an enormously greater repertoire of types of binding site. Here and in the case of olfaction, there are also certain parallels with immunological mechanisms that may suggest a common origin.

References

Amoore, J. E. (1963) Stereochemical theory of olfaction. *Nature* 198, 271–272.

Benjamin, R. M. (1963) Some thalamic and cortical mechanisms of taste. In *Olfaction and Taste*, ed. Y. Zotterman. Pergamon, London.

Carpenter, M.B. (1976) *Human Neuroanatomy*. Williams and Wilkins, Baltimore.

Cohen, M. J., Magiwara, S. and Zotterman, Y. (1955) The response spectrum of taste fibres in the cat: a single fibre analysis. *Acta Physiologica Scandinavica* 33, 316–332.

Firestein, S. and Werblin, F. (1989) Ionic mechanisms underlying the olfactory response. *Science* 244, 79–82.

Kessel, R. G. and Kardon, R. H. (1979) *Tissues and Organs: a Text-Atlas of Scanning Electron Microscopy*. W. H. Freeman, San Francisco.

Kimura, K. and Beidler, L. M. (1961) Microelectrode studies of taste receptors of rat and hamster. *Journal of Cellular and Comparative Physiology* 58, 131–139.

Moncrieff, R. W. (1967) *The Chemical Senses*. Leonard Hill, London.

Tanabe, T., Iino, M. and Takagi, S. F. (1975) Discrimination of odours in olfactory bulb, pyriform-amygdaloid areas, and orbito-frontal cortex of the monkey. *Journal of Neurophysiology* 38, 1284–1296.

NOTES

Page 170 The chemical senses are under-represented in the literature. Three useful sources are: Cagan, R. H. (1989) *Neural Mechanisms in Taste* (CRC Press, London); Davis, J. L. and Eichenbaum, H. (1991) *Olfaction* (MIT Press, Cambridge, Mass); Finger, T. E. and Silver, W. L. (1987) *Neurobiology of Taste and Smell* (Wiley, New York). Moncrieff, R. W. (1967) *The Chemical Senses* (Leonard Hill, London) has a great deal of detailed information relating to the psychophysics, especially in relation to perfumery, but is otherwise out of date.

Page 170 The outer nose is not without neurological interest: see Critchley, M. (1979) *Man's attitude to his nose*, in *The Divine Banquet of the Brain* (Raven, New York).

Page 170 Air not normally reaching the olfactory cleft In 1882, the Viennese physiologist E. Paulsen performed an elegant but somewhat macabre experiment to establish this point. Having cut a human head down the middle, he placed tiny squares of red litmus all over the nasal cavities; then, sticking the two halves together again, he drew air laden with ammonia from a bottle held under the nose by appropriate manipulation of a pair of bellows attached to the trachea. On opening the head he could see what course the air had taken by the pieces of litmus which had turned blue : very little reached the receptor region. (See the description of this and other similar experiments in Finger, S. (1994) *Origins of Neuroscience: a History of Explorations into Brain Function* (Oxford University Press, Oxford).

Page 170 Man relatively indifferent to smell Aldous Huxley: *'Man's sense of smell is relatively poor and this apparent handicap has proved to be an actual advantage to him. Instead of running round like a dog, sniffing at lamp-posts and becoming deeply agitated by what he smells on them, Man is able to stand away from the world and use his eyes and his wits relatively unmoved.'* Quoted in McCartney, W. (1968) *Olfaction and Odours* (Springer , New York).

Page 172 Olfactory localization The experiments were conducted by von Békésy, of auditory fame: see von Békésy, G. (1964) Olfactory analogue to directional hearing. *Journal of Applied Physiology* 19, 369–373.

Page 174 Permanent olfactory aversions See for instance Garcia, J. and Ervin, F. R. (1986) Gustatory-visceral and teloreceptor-cutaneous conditioning: adaptation in internal and external milieus. *Communications in Biology* A1, 389.

Page 175 Olfaction and sexual attraction Recall Nelson's apocryphal message to Lady Hamilton: *'The fleet's in: don't wash!'*. Conversely, in one experiment (Kirk-Smith, M., Booth, D. A., Carroll, D. and Davies, P. (1978) Human social attitudes affected by androstenol. *Research Communications in Psychological Psychiatry and Behaviour* 3, 379–384) photographs of men were rated as more attractive when the air was scented with an extract from male armpits.

Page 175 Olfaction and behaviour in general Two excellent books by Stoddart review this field very well: Stoddart, D. M. (1980) *The Ecology of Vertebrate Olfaction* (Chapman and Hall, London) and Stoddart, D. M. (1990) *The Scented Ape: the Biology and Culture of Human Odour* (Cambridge University Press, Cambridge). Doty, R. L. (1976) *Mammalian Olfaction, Reproductive Processes and Behaviour* (Academic, New York) is another useful book in this area. Social aspects of smell are also discussed in Bedichek, R. (1960) *The Sense of Smell* (Michael Joseph, London) – with many entertaining anecdotes – and in Burton, R. (1976) *The Language of Smell* (Routledge and Kegan Paul, London).

Page 177 Helen Keller *'Smell,'* she wrote, *'is a potent wizard that transports us across thousands of miles and all the years we have lived. The odours of fruits waft me to my southern home, to my childhood frolics in the peach orchard ... The sense of smell has told me of a coming storm hours before there was any sign of it visible. I notice first ... a slight quiver, a concentration in my nostrils. As the storm draws near my nostrils dilate, the better to receive the flood of earth odours which seem to multiply and extend, until I feel the splash of rain against my cheek. ... I know the kind of house we enter. I have recognized an old-fashioned country house because it has several layers of odours, left by a succession of families, of plants, perfumes and draperies.'* Keller, H. (1903) *My Life* (Hodder and Stoughton, London).

Page 177 Changes of character on dilution Robert Boyle (1627–1691), describing an odd encounter of this kind: *'An eminent professor of mathematics affirmed to me, that, chancing one day in the heat of summer with another mathematician to pass by a large dunghil that was then in Lincoln's-Inn Fields, when they came to a certain distance from it, they were both of them surprised to meet with a very strong smell of musk, which each was for a while shy of taking notice of, for fear his companion should have laughed at him for it; but when they came much nearer the dunghil that pleasing smell was succeeded by a stink proper to such a heap of excrements.'* Quoted in McCartney, W. (1968) *Olfaction and Odours* (Springer , New York).

Page 178 Amoore's theory See for instance Amoore, J. E. (1964) Current status of the steric theory of odour. *Annals of the New York Academy of Sciences* 116, 456.

Page 179 The infra-red theory Support for this idea has also come from a study of the curious way in which male moths are attracted by candles. It turns out that candles have characteristically spiky infra-red spectra, and that a number of the emission lines coincide with the vibrational frequencies of the female moth's pheromone: other sources such as hurricane lamps that emit as much infra-red but lack the spikes are much less powerful attractants. So it seems that the suicidal fascination of the candle for the moth is a sexual one: the candle is the flamme fatale of mothdom! See Callahan, P. S. (1977) Moth and candle: the candle flame as sexual mimic of the coded infra-red wavelengths from a moth sex scent (pheromone). *Applied Optics* 12, 3089–3097. The infra-red theory is forcefully argued in Wright, R. H. (1982) *The Sense of Smell* (CRC Press, London).

Page 179 Molecular recognition See for instance Reed, R. R. (1990) How does the nose know? *Cell* 60, 1–2.

NEUROLAB

Olfactory recognition

Page 176

This very simple exhibit shows how a lack of specificity for particular odorants amongst receptors can easily be overcome by a subsequent stage of lateral inhibition. On the left, you can select an odorant (A–J) with a radio button. Each receptor (middle) is labelled with the odorants to which it responds, and any particular odorant will cause several of them to fire; the coding at this stage is by spatial pattern rather than by labelled lines. The second-order neurones (right) receive excitatory connections (red) from some receptors, and inhibitory (blue) from others. As a result, overlapping between patterns is eliminated, and each second-order neurone codes for one specific odorant. (Because there are more odorants than second-order neurones, some are not encoded at all.)

PART

3

MOTOR FUNCTIONS

9 TYPES OF MOTOR CONTROL

Difficulties in studying motor systems 187
Motor control and feedback 189

The hierarchy of control 195

Motor systems – unfortunately – are intrinsically rather more complex than sensory ones, and our knowledge of them is correspondingly more rudimentary: it may be helpful to begin a consideration of the principles of motor control by asking why this should be so.

DIFFICULTIES IN STUDYING MOTOR SYSTEMS

We need to go back to fundamentals. The brain's job is to turn patterns of stimulation, S, into responses, R. How it does it is clear, in principle at least. The brain consists of a sequence of neuronal levels, layers of neurones projecting onto one another (Fig. 9.1), in which incoming sensory information S is transmitted from level to level, and modified at each stage until it becomes a response R at the output. This network is able to generate specific patterns of response to particular patterns of input because, on a smaller scale, each of the neurones that make up a particular level is itself a sort of miniature computer, and responds only to a particular pattern of activity amongst the neurones of the level immediately in front of it. By joining together billions of units that are each quite intelligent, we end up with something that is very intelligent indeed: it is a commonplace that similar 'neural' networks embodied in computers can carry out such apparently high-level tasks as face recognition and 'intuitive' decision-making with rather little difficulty.

Though any one neurone may only be influenced by a tiny fraction of all the activity taking place in the previous level, nevertheless, because of the convergence implicit in the transfer of excitation from level to level, as one penetrates further and further into the model one finds neurones that can respond to more and more complex and wide-ranging aspects of the sensory world. We have already seen this happening in the case of the visual system. Receptors in the eye

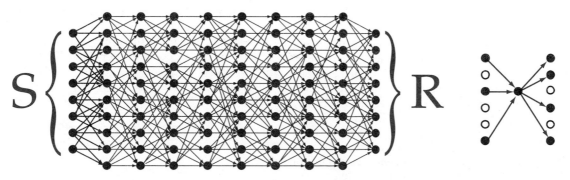

FIG. 9.1 Left, representation of the nervous system as a series of neuronal levels, through which sensory patterns (S) are converted to patterns of response (R). Each neurone itself responds to a particular pattern amongst the neurones of the preceding layer (right).

convey information about only a minute part of the retinal image; but after a few levels have been passed, in the visual cortex, we find units that are able to respond to a specific type of stimulus, such as a moving edge, over wide areas of the visual field. We shall see later that as one gets to the deepest levels of the brain, there seems to be an increasing tendency for neurones to be multimodal, responding not just to one kind of sense such as vision but to others, such as sounds and stimulation of the skin, as well. And of course if we consider the final level of all, the muscles that move our bodies, it is clear that they are utterly multi-modal, in the sense that we can learn to activate any particular muscle in response to any pattern of sensation, involving any or all of our sensory modalities.

To understand the details of the way in which such a system carries out this conversion of input patterns into patterns of response, we need to know how individual neurones at any particular level respond to different patterns of activity in the preceding level. Now in the case of sensory systems – that is, the left-hand half of Figure 9.1 – this presents the experimenter with relatively few problems of procedure. All we need do is to record from a selection of single units at the level we are interested in, perhaps the visual cortex, whilst applying a variety of visual patterns. We will then discover which kinds of patterns the neurones do or do not respond to, and can then hope to deduce the nature of their functional connections. This task is made easier for us because we have a pretty good idea in advance of what sort of patterns to try, namely those that actually occur commonly in real life. Thus in the visual system it is not unreasonable to start with things like straight lines and edges: there would be little point in searching for units in a cat's cortex that specifically responded to letters of the Greek alphabet.

But when it comes to the right-hand side of Figure 9.1, the motor system, the problem is turned inside out. We now have to *stimulate* the neurones individually, and see what patterns of movement are generated as a result. The difficulty now is that to get any response at all, we have to provide a pattern of stimulation that will be recognized at the next level down the chain and result in activation of the muscles. Quite apart from the extreme technical difficulty of actually generating any such pattern in the first place, there is the further difficulty of knowing what patterns are 'physiological' in the sense that they are likely to occur in real life and therefore be capable of arousing a response in the next layer. Unlike the situation in sensory systems, we do not have the patterns that we see in the outside world as a guide.

Consequently, when trying to stimulate the motor system, particularly in its more central regions, single unit stimulation seldom produces any effects at all, many areas that are certainly 'motor' are apparently incapable of responding to electrical stimulation with motor responses, and when movements are achieved, they are usually the result of using such large currents spread over such large areas that the specificity of the neurones is swamped, resulting in responses that are diffuse and unphysiological. For these reasons, electrical stimulation has not proved to be a very helpful way of studying motor systems.

A more fruitful approach is an extension of the sensory method, applying 'real' stimuli to the senses and tracing the resultant activity deeper and deeper through the levels of the nervous system until they emerge again at the motor end. In systems as complex as those controlling, for example, the human hand, this is not yet technically feasible. But where the number of levels is much smaller, as in more primitive brains like those of insects or in simpler subsystems of the mammalian brain (like those controlling eye movements, which may have as few as three neuronal levels between input and output), the problem is more tractable.

A second difficulty in studying the motor system is that whereas sensory systems by and large form a straightforward progression from level to level, a characteristic of motor control is that every action necessarily results in sensory *feedback*. If we raise our hand, there is an immediate influx of sensory activity from the skin, from muscle and joint receptors, from vision and the other special senses as well. So the effects of stimulating a particular region of the motor system are additionally complex: any movement that may result from it also generates new patterns of afferent activity. Coming up from behind the level at which we are stimulating, this messes things up by altering the pattern of stimulation we are trying to apply.

Though a nuisance from the experimenter's point of view, this feedback from the effects of motor responses is fundamentally important in the control of movement. A good way to begin a study of the motor system is to consider just how this sensory information may be used to improve motor performance.

MOTOR CONTROL AND FEEDBACK

Of course, one can have a motor system with no feedback at all. A spermatozoon, for example, gets along by flagellating its flagellum in a way that pays no regard to its orientation: if it is pointing the wrong way, that is just hard luck. Blind behaviour of this kind is not a monopoly of simple organisms: it can often be seen in animals with much more sophisticated motor systems. A classic example is the nest-building behaviour of the brown rat, described by Lorenz. When a brown rat decides to build a nest, it performs a characteristic series of actions: it runs out to get nesting material, drags it back to the centre of the nest, sits down and forms it into a sort of circular rampart, pats it down and smooths it, and then runs out to get more material; and so on until the nest is finished. This certainly looks like intelligent and purposive behaviour; yet a simple experiment shows it to be nothing of the kind. If a naive rat is not given enough to make a nest, it still runs out to grab the (non-existent) material, goes through the motions of dragging it back, forming it into a rampart and patting and smoothing it, even though in reality there is nothing there! And of course we ourselves have all experienced occasions on which we have absentmindedly carried out some equally complex series of actions – perhaps putting tea in the kettle instead of the teapot – in wholly inappropriate circumstances.

Besides, there are many circumstances when our motor systems are forced to act blindly because for one reason or another they are deprived of normal sensory feedback; any *throwing* action comes into this category. When I nonchalantly toss something into a waste-paper basket, I have actually been obliged to work out beforehand the precise sequence of motor commands necessary in order to produce the correct pattern of muscular contractions that I need to achieve my goal, and it is clear that once the object has left my hand, no amount of sensory feedback about its trajectory is going to enable me to modify its

flight. Motor acts of this type are called *ballistic* – a word meaning 'thrown' – and their control can be represented schematically by a diagram like Figure 9.2. Unfortunately, to talk about control systems such as this, one needs to get to grips with a certain amount of jargon. Here we start with the *desired result*, in this case the presence of the object in the basket. This is translated by a *controller* into an appropriate pattern of *commands*, drawing on a library of motor programs suitable for different acts; and these commands produce the *actual result* through their effect on what engineers call the *plant* – in this case, the body's muscles. If the controller is functioning properly, then the actual result will equal the desired result. A well-known example of such a system is the control of ballistic missiles. Here the operator decides which particular portion of the globe he wishes to destroy, and makes the necessary computations to determine where to point the missile and how large a thrust is required at take-off but once it is launched he takes no further action – the missile is in any case no longer under his control – beyond hoping that his calculations were in fact correct.

Ballistic control is in a sense conceptually simple but it has a fatal defect: it is extremely vulnerable to what systems engineers call *noise*. Noise is any kind of unpredictable disturbance that makes the actual result different from what the controller expects. In this case, the inevitable existence of noise in the outside world means that a particular set of motor commands will never produce quite the same result twice in succession. A given pattern of innervation will produce different movements of a limb on different occasions, depending partly on the load to be moved but also on a host of internal factors such as body temperature, fatigue, amount of energy available, and so on. Or again, our ballistic missile, if the wind happens to be blowing the wrong way, may land on Aberdeen instead of Moscow.

One way of dealing with noise is to have some kind of sensor that will monitor the noise before it affects the system, and use this information to modify the parameters of the controller to allow for it.

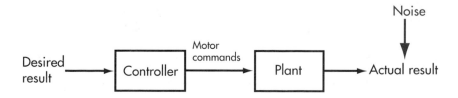

FIG. 9.2 A ballistic control system.

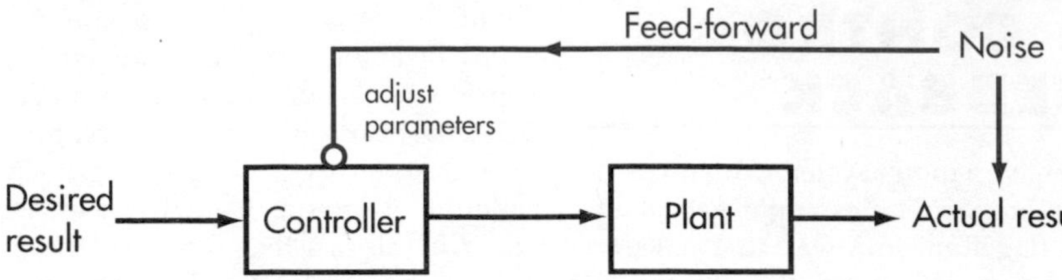

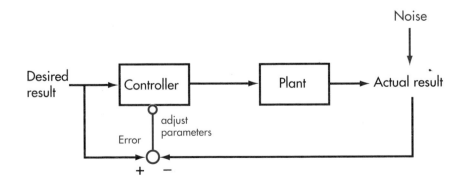

FIG. 9.3 A ballistic system with feedforward, altering the parameters of the controller in response to noise.

Modification of the controller's parameters in this way is called *parametric feedforward* (Fig. 9.3). As we shall see, there is evidence that the neural circuits that control muscle length use information from force detectors in the skin and tendons that monitor load to modify the commands sent to the muscles.

But even this approach is doomed to failure, for there are in general infinitely many things that might cause unpredictable perturbations, and the brain clearly cannot monitor and respond to them all. Instead of trying to anticipate absolutely everything that might possibly occur, one solution is to take a more pragmatic approach, with a system that learns from its own mistakes, using not feedforward but *parametric feedback* (Fig. 9.4). Two new pieces of jargon are needed: a *comparator* compares the actual result with the desired result by subtracting one from the other, and generates an *error signal* which is simply a measure of how well the system is doing. This error signal is then used to modify the controller's parameters as before, the difference being that this time the system is not particularly interested in what kind of noise is causing the problem. If there are no errors, then nothing changes; if it keeps on making a mess of things, then the commands are gradually adjusted until it gets it right. Such a system does not have to have stored programs ready in advance for any conceivable kind of action: by starting with rather simple, all-purpose programs, one may refine, through trial and error, what is needed for the tasks that are actually encountered.

It goes without saying that this kind of behaviour – using error information from one attempt to improve performance on the next – is highly characteristic of the way in which our motor systems learn to execute complex actions. In playing darts, a novice may at first use pre-existing programs developed perhaps from his experience of throwing other objects such as cricket balls (and ultimately from throwing rattles out of his pram) but as he practises, the feedback from each throw, though obviously arriving too late to use immediately, is used to reduce future errors, and in the end he may gradually evolve very accurate programs specifically for dart-throwing. A great deal of the learning of motor skills can usefully be thought of as a parametric feedback of this kind, in which errors are used to modify one's stored motor programs.

A specific example, discussed in more detail in Chapter 11, is the vestibulo-ocular reflex. When we move our head, the resultant signals from the semicircular canals are used to move the eyes by an equal and opposite amount so that they maintain their direction of gaze and the retinal image of the outside world remains relatively fixed. This is clearly a ballistic system. But it is obviously very important to

FIG. 9.4 Parametric feedback, modifying the controller's parameters in response to errors in performance.

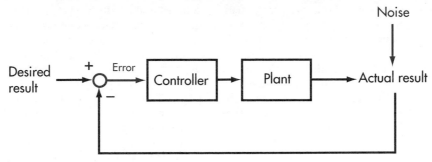

FIG. 9.5 A direct feedback system.

ensure that the eye movements really are exactly matched to the size of the head movement, and it turns out that the reflex is being continually adjusted to ensure that this is so, using parametric feedback from neurones that respond to any movement of the image across the retina.

Though parametric feedback and feedforward can vastly improve the performance of ballistic systems, they are still not perfect. In the first place, the calculations that are needed before the action takes place are in general extremely complex – even throwing something in a waste-paper basket requires, in effect, the solution of a set of partial differential equations with countless variables – and it is not altogether plausible that the brain could actually have at its disposal a library of such routines so vast as to be able to deal with all the possible motor tasks it might ever encounter during its lifetime. The controller needs to have acquired knowledge about how the plant will behave in response to any kind of command sent to it, and keep this information up to date. So it needs memory as well as intelligence. In addition, parametric feedback only corrects *after the event*, by which time it may be too late. But there is another approach, much simpler and often better: *direct feedback*.

Here we start as before with a desired result (Fig. 9.5) which we compare at every moment with the actual result. But now the error signal, instead of being used to tweak the parameters, is used directly as the input to the controller, generating motor commands whose function is essentially to reduce the difference between the desired and actual result. The computation of these correcting commands is in general very much simpler than the calculations needed in a ballistic system. Guided missiles are controlled by systems of this type: here the error signal might be something like the angle between the direction in which the missile is pointing and the direction of its target.

In such a system, instead of calculating what to *do*, all you have to specify is what you *want*. Like a well-trained servant, the system does all the rest by itself: such control systems are often called *servo systems*. Thus in another familiar example, a domestic central heating system, the thermostat acts as the comparator of Figure 9.5, and generates an error signal which consists very simply of one of just two possible messages: either that the actual temperature is below what is wanted or that it is above it. The subsequent computations of the motor commands could hardly be simpler: in the former case the boiler is switched on, in the latter case it is switched off. Another, physiological, example also illustrates this essential simplicity of guided systems. If we instruct a subject to look at a small light such as A, Figure 9.6, and then suddenly move it closer to his nose as at B, we find that his eyes converge smoothly and quite quickly in such a way that in the end the image of the light still falls exactly on the fovea of each retina. The velocity of the convergence movement is quite high at first, but declines exponentially as the eye gets closer and closer to its target. This is rather what would be expected of a guided system, in which the eyes are essentially driven by an error signal. It turns out that this is indeed what is happening, and that it is disparity between the two retinal images, presumably sensed by disparity detectors of the kind described in Chapter 7, that provides an error signal which moves the eyes so that their velocity is at all times proportional to the size of the error. As the eyes reach their goal, the error gets smaller, and so the rate of movement correspondingly declines to zero. One can see in Figure 9.6 how the velocity of the eye relates to the degree of disparity in human subjects, and hence how simply the correcting commands may be derived from error signals in guided systems.

The overwhelming advantage of guided systems, however, is perhaps not so much their simplicity but rather the fact that they are almost immune to the effects of noise. For if something unexpected happens that upsets the normal relationship between command and performance – if in the house with the central heating system someone leaves all the windows open – this fact will be noticed at once (because it will result in a new error) and appropriate commands to achieve the desired result despite the existence of the disturbance will be automatically generated: the thermostat will sense the sudden drop in temperature, and the boiler will automatically be switched on until the temperature once more reaches the desired level. The power and elegance of such a system is thus that it will guarantee to achieve what it has been designed to achieve, even in the presence of types of interference that could not have been anticipated by its creator; it is capable of producing results that look intelligent even though – in sharp contrast to the ballistic system with its library of programs for different occasions – it knows very little (only the size of the error) and remembers nothing.

Its weakness is that its proper functioning depends critically on the fast and reliable transmission to the comparator of information about the progress of the action. In physiological systems, where both the sensory receptor processes and the transmission itself may be rather slow, this can be a serious problem; delay of this kind 'round the loop' will mean that instead of responding to the error as it actually is, the system will be responding to the error as it was however many milliseconds ago it takes for the information to get back to the brain.

For example, we know that the visual receptors are rather slow, and that the shortest reaction times for any kind of visual task are of the order of 200 milliseconds. Consider a batsman in a game of cricket; one might think that he could use a system like that of Figure 9.6 to bring his bat up to the ball under visual guidance, using error information about the distance between bat and ball. But the existence of this large visual delay means that any such information is hopelessly out of date: if the bowler is delivering at 90 mph, the ball will travel half the length of the pitch in the 200 milliseconds it takes for

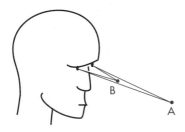

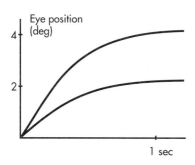

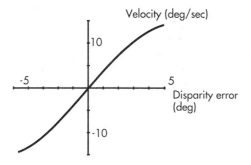

FIG. 9.6 Vergence occurs (top) when a subject looks between two objects at different distances from the eyes; its time-course (middle) shows a slowing towards the end, as the disparity error approaches zero. Bottom, observed relation between disparity error and the velocity of the eye movement. (Data from Rashbass and Westheimer, 1961)

Box 9.1 Basic types of control system

Ballistic

The desired result is translated into a command, issued regardless of whether an error has occurred. However, subsequent commands may be modified in the light of errors that have been made (parametric feedback) or can be anticipated (parametric feedforward)

Guided (direct feedback)

The desired result is compared with the actual result at every moment, and any error results immediately in an alterationof the command so as to reduce the discrepancy

Internal feedback

As direct feedback, except that a prediction of the result is used rather than its actual value. The commands that are sent out are monitored and used to calculate what result they ought to achieve, using a model of the way the system normally behaves. Any discrepancies between the predicted and actual result cause the model to be updated (parametric feedback)

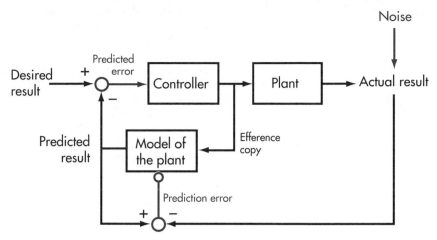

FIG. 9.7 A system using internal feedback, the model of the plant being adjusted so that its predictions match what actually happens.

any visual information about its position to be of use. Thus the last useful visual fix on the ball is when it is still more than 10 metres away; clearly the bat cannot in any sense be guided on to it.

The final type of control system to be considered is at its best in this sort of situation. Though similar to parametric feedback in that it involves modification of behaviour through experience, it has closer affinities with the guided system of Figure 9.6 than with a ballistic one, and uses *internal feedback*. The notion here is that if it is difficult to obtain feedback about actual results sufficiently quickly for them to be of use during an action, nevertheless it may be possible as the result of experience to *predict* what the result of a particular motor command is going to be, before the actual result is known. From a general knowledge of the mechanical properties of one's hand and arm, and information about the kinds of loads that are present, one can form an estimate in advance of what position the limb is going to adopt in response to any particular pattern of motor commands that is sent to it. Since this estimate is formed entirely within the brain, it may well be available long before any feedback from the actual movement has found its way back from the periphery. When things are happening fast, such an estimate – one may call it the predicted result – will at least be better than no information at all. Thus in an internal feedback control system (Fig. 9.7) the desired result is compared not with the actual result but with this predicted result, which is in turn derived by sending a copy of the motor commands (an *efference copy* signal) to a neural model of the mechanical properties of the body, which is used to predict the probable result. A final refinement of this basic system is that the actual result may also – later – be compared with the predicted result, and any errors used to correct the model itself: another variety of parametric feedback, that continually improves the accuracy of the predictions.

One excellent example of a physiological system that seems to work in this way is in the control of saccadic eye movements. Saccades are the eye movements made when a subject shifts his gaze from one target to another at the same distance from him but in a different direction. Large saccades are made with virtually constant velocity – which may be as much as 900° per second – whatever the distance between the targets; thus the duration of a large saccadic movement is a nearly linear function of its size (Fig. 9.8). At first sight, one might think that the eye was simply moving off towards the new target at a constant rate, and that as soon as the visual system senses that the target has been reached, the brakes are applied and the eye comes to rest. But it is easy to calculate – as in the case of the batsman and cricket ball – that this cannot possibly be the true explanation. Because the movement is so extremely rapid, few saccades last more than 100 msec, and most are between 20 and 40; since visual processes in general take considerably longer than this, by the time the brain had recognized that the target had been reached, the eye would have grossly overshot. Thus a simple feedback loop like that of Figure 9.7 cannot possibly be used. However, the control of eye movements is an almost ideal example of a case where internal feedback can be profitably employed: unlike our limbs our eyes are not subject to varying loads, and consequently we can form a very good idea of where the eye is pointing from knowledge of the commands we send it. Thus the internal model of Figure 9.7 is not difficult to conceive in neural terms, and in fact we

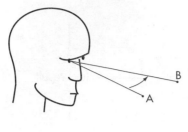

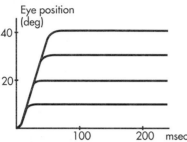

FIG. 9.8 A saccade is made in looking between two objects at the same distance. Below, the time-course of saccades of different amplitudes, showing the approximately constant velocity of the movements.

shall see later that there is good evidence that efference copy is indeed the means by which we normally sense the position of our eyes. In the saccade, efference copy information can be used in this way to deduce what angle the eye has moved through, and

when this calculated eye position is equal to the desired new position previously requested by the visual system, the drive to the muscles is in effect switched off, and the eye comes to rest on the new target; a system, in fact, precisely of the type shown in Figure 9.7, and embodied for the most part in neural circuits in the brainstem.

Oddly enough, the various types of eye movements exemplify each of the different kinds of motor control that have been presented here, and they are summarized in the box below.

On the face of it there is perhaps no obvious advantage in using internal feedback rather than ballistic control with parametric feedback. But because the model of the body that is embodied in the former system is essentially a general one, not tied to any particular type of action, it means that experience in carrying out one kind of skilled motor function will benefit the performance of other ones in a rather more direct way than was the case for something like Figure 9.4, particularly when, as in the case of the eye, the expected result can be computed relatively easily from the motor commands. Learning motor skills then becomes a matter of learning to predict the behaviour of one's own body.

The existence of parametric or internal feedback obviously makes the interpretation of the results of experimental stimulation or lesions no easy matter. For instance, it is not obvious what the effect would

---

Box 9.2 The main classes of eye movements

Gaze-holding: maintaining the direction of gaze in space.

    Conjunct:

Optokinetic (OKR)	direct feedback
Vestibular (VOR)	ballistic, parametric feedback from vision

Gaze-shifting: foveation of visual targets.

    Conjunct:

Saccades	probably internal feedback
Smooth pursuit	ballistic/direct feedback

(Small moving targets are tracked with a mixture of saccades, to move the eye to the right position, and smooth pursuit, to match the target velocity)

    Disjunct: vergence

        Disparity-driven: direct feedback
        Blur-driven: ballistic

Spontaneous: micro- or fixational movements.

Drift	probably central noise
Microsaccades	saccades correcting for drift
Tremor	probably peripheral noise

be of artificially stimulating the parametric feedback system of Figure 9.4 at the 'modify' input. Equally, we would anticipate that lesions in such regions as the library of motor programs, or the neural model inside the internal feedback system of Figure 9.7, would result in complex and subtle effects: not just simple paralysis but perhaps loss of quality of performance, of the ability to modify responses through experience, and perhaps the appearance of rigidly stereotyped patterns of behaviour not properly adjusted to their objects. Defects of just these kinds are indeed characteristic of many types of clinical derangement of the higher levels of the motor system.

THE HIERARCHY OF CONTROL

Finally, another factor that makes both the anatomy and the physiology of motor systems alarmingly complicated is the way in which it has developed in the course of evolution. Whereas the behaviour of the very simplest organisms can be largely described in terms of simple local segmental mechanisms at a peripheral level – as, for example, the co-ordination of a centipede's legs when it walks – in ascending the evolutionary tree we find more and more domination of the special senses, and as a consequence of this, a corresponding degree of *encephalization:* control by higher centres grouped near these sense organs, in the head. It is important to appreciate that by and large this has been a process of *accretion.* Simpler mechanisms are not in general displaced by more recent ones: they are left essentially intact, but supplemented and controlled from above. They are, after all, carrying out useful functions. Human walking movements are in essence not so very different from the centipede's, and associated with rather similarly stereotyped sequences of muscle actions mediated by spinal mechanisms of the same general character: such sequences can often be evoked from spinal preparationsof animals in which the higher levels of control have been surgically disconnected. It would clearly be foolish for the brain to build its own neural circuits that merely duplicated what the spinal cord was already doing perfectly well, and it is important not to underestimate what the cord is capable of. Classic examples include the spinal dog wagging its tail after defecation or the wiping reflex in the frog: if a small piece of filter paper is moistened with acid and placed on its back, it will quite accurately use the nearest leg to wipe it off the skin; if that leg is held down, after a short delay another leg is used! It is clear that one should not think of the spinal cord merely as a sort of speaking-tube down which the brain shouts its orders to the muscles: rather, it provides a repertoire of fragments of action, 'party pieces' that can be called on when necessary by the higher levels.

The main difference, in fact, between the spinal cord of a 'higher' and 'lower' animal is that the former in a sense expects to receive more in the way of commands from above; consequently, when isolated from the brain in a spinal preparation, it may appear less responsive. This phenomenon is known as *spinal shock:* immediately after making the cut that separates cord from brain, spinal reflexes are depressed or absent, because the usual 'permission' from above is not there. But after a period of time the cord becomes more lively, and may in the end actually show a greater degree of responsiveness than before the operation. This period of time depends markedly on the degree of encephalization: in humans it may take many months; in a dog, days; and in a frog perhaps only a few minutes, reflecting the differing degrees of control normally descending from the brain. In the end, one can never be sure that a spinal animal is really exhibiting all the things that the cord could do if the brain were intact: we always tend to underestimate what the spinal cord is capable of.

Experiments of this kind lead naturally to the idea of a hierarchical organization of the motor system into a series of functional *levels* (Fig. 9.9), the higher levels having more diverse kinds of sensory information at their disposal and therefore able to plan and anticipate more effectively than the lower. Because of their ability to store experience through memory, they can also be more flexible in their responses and learn to conform to the outside world in a way the spinal cord cannot. It follows, therefore, that as well as being able to stimulate the spinal cord to generate particular patterns of output, these higher levels must also exert a tonic inhibitory influence on lower levels. Brain and cord may well often have conflicting ideas about what is the right thing to do in a particular situation, and this conflict needs to be won by the brain. Consequently the effects of lesions in higher levels of the brain are usually two-fold: first a *loss* of function, particularly of the more flexible and integrated kinds; and secondly the *new appearance* of abnormal and more primitive modes of response. The latter phenomenon is often described by neurologists as *release:* the lower centres are released from the restraining influences of the higher, like schoolboys when the teacher is called from their class.

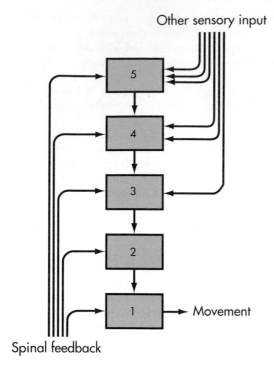

Other sensory input

Spinal feedback

FIG. 9.9 Schematic representation of hierarchy of levels in the nervous system. Higher levels have more access to information from diverse sources, lower ones have more immediate feedback. On the whole, levels act by controlling those immediately beneath them, rather than by generating movements directly.

An understanding of the concept of hierarchical control is essential if one is to make sense of the clinical effects of lesions of the motor system, and analogies with man-made hierarchies are often useful in thinking about them. In an army, for instance, if a general decides on invasion, he doesn't himself give detailed orders about how many pairs of boots to order, where the latrines are to be dug, and so forth. What he does is to indicate the outline of the overall strategy that is required to his immediate subordinates, who elaborate them a little and pass them on to their subordinates, and so on until detailed patterns of activity are eventually carried out by the men themselves. The general has the advantage of having integrated information available to him from a wide variety of sources, which he can use to develop wide-ranging strategies: the men have the advantage of immediate and detailed experience of local conditions, with which they can modify their individual behaviour. In the same way, a well-written computer program will typically consist of simple subroutines that do very small tasks, called by other subroutines which are in turn called by other subroutines, and so

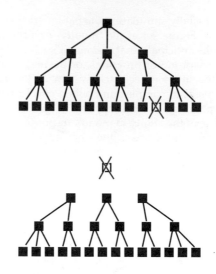

FIG. 9.10 Different consequences of lesions at different levels in a hierarchy.

on. A computer game might have one routine to draw a single dot on the screen, called by another routine that displays a set of dots to form a small pattern, called by another that draws a single object, called by another that displays an entire scene. Clearly, at the level at which the programmer is thinking about the general organization of the game, he does not want to be bothered with the repetitive detail of exactly how each dot in a picture is to be sent to the display.

The existence of a hierarchical organization carries very important implications for what happens if part of the system goes wrong. In military terms, the effects of blowing up a platoon are very different from those of shooting a general (Fig. 9.10). In the first case, the defect is obvious, immediate, and limited: very specific jobs no longer get done: there is a clear correlation between the 'lesion' and the 'symptoms'. In the second case, at first nothing may appear to be wrong at all: the army still functions. But gradually more subtle defects may begin to show themselves, such as a lack of long-term planning or co-ordination. At the same time, new patterns of activity may start to become apparent as the general's subordinates begin to put their own ideas into practice without restraint: symptoms, in other words, of 'release'.

These are precisely the kinds of disorders commonly described after damage to higher motor regions of the central nervous system. A classic example is the *Babinski sign* or 'up-going big toe'. If the foot of a normal adult is firmly stroked, the immediate response is an involuntary flexion of the foot

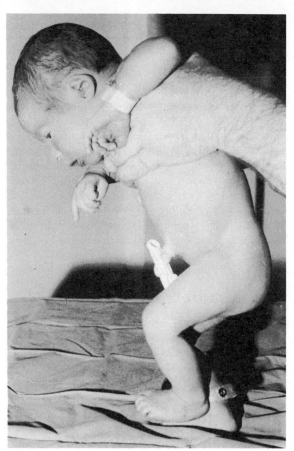

FIG. 9.11 A newborn child walking: this ability will be suppressed within a few days by the developing brain, even though adult walking patterns will not appear until a year or so later.

and toes: but in certain kinds of brain damage, as also in newborn children, the reaction is the exact opposite: the toes curl upwards. It is clear in this case that cord and brain have different ideas about what to do when the foot is stroked; in the adult, the brain wins. Another example is the co-ordination of walking movements. A newborn infant is actually able to walk after a fashion (Fig. 9. 11), so long as its weight is supported. But one of the first things that the developing brain does is to suppress this primitive response, many months before it develops its own much more sophisticated patterns of walking that make better use of integrated sensory information.&

With this notion of hierarchical control in mind, it is appropriate to begin the motor system by considering what the lowest level of all, the spinal cord, can and cannot do, and the ways in which descending pathways from the brain may control and modify its activity.

References

Rashbass, C. and Westheimer, G. (1961) Disjunctive eye movements. *Journal of Physiology* 159, 339–360.

NOTES

Page 187 Neural networks A readable account of neural networks is Levine, R. and Drang, D. (1988) *Neural Networks: The Second AI Generation.* A more technical source is McClelland, J.L. and Rumelhart, D.E. (1988) *Parallel Distributed Processing* (MIT Press, Cambridge, Mass). A stimulating, biologically-oriented but controversial book is Edelman, G.M. (1989) *Neural Darwinism: the Theory of Neuronal Group Selection* (Oxford University Press, Oxford).

Page 189 Lorenz For examples of similarly complex but apparently ballistic behaviour, see Lorenz's *Studies in Animal and Human Behaviour* (1965; English translation 1970).

Page 189 Control systems Good books on specifically biological aspects of control systems that are not too technical are hard to find. The appendix to Carpenter, R. H. S. (1989) *Movements of the Eyes* (Pion, London) may be pitched at about the right level. Milsum, J.H. (1965). *Biological Control Systems Analysis.* (McGraw-Hill, New York) and Stark, L. (1968) *Neurological Control Systems.* (Plenum, New York) are both excellent but long out of print. Fairly technical introductory accounts, intended mainly for engineers, are Balmer, L. (1991) *Signals and Systems: an Introduction.* (Prentice Hall, New York) and DiStefano, J.J., Stubberud, A.R. and Williams, J.J. (1990) *Feedback and Control Systems.* (McGraw-Hill, New York).

Page 191 Disparity vergence Two classic papers describing the relation between vergence and disparity: Rashbass, C. and Westheimer, G. (1961) Disjunctive eye movements. *Journal of Physiology* 159, 339–360; Westheimer, G. and Mitchell, A. M. (1956) Eye movement responses to convergence stimuli. *Archives of Ophthalmology* 55, 848–856.

Page 193 Visual control of batting See, for instance, Bahill, A. T. and LaRitz, T. (1984) Why can't batters keep their eyes on the ball? *American Scientist* May-June, 249–254, and Lacquaniti, F., Carrozzo, M. and Borghese, N. (1993) The role of vision in tuning anticipatory motor responses of the limbs. In *Multisensory Control of Movement*, ed. A. Berthoz (Oxford University Press, Oxford).

Page 193 Internal model for prediction A system of this type is the Smith Predictor, originally developed to control the thickness of the finished product in steel rolling mills: since there was inevitably a certain lag between the steel leaving the rollers and the point where it had cooled enough for the thickness to be meaningful, an ordinary direct feedback system would have lead to unstable oscillations. See Smith, O. J. M. (1959) A controller to overcome dead time. *ISA Journal* 6, 28–33.

Page 194 Brainstem saccade circuits See, for example, Fuchs, A.F., Kaneko, C.R. and Scudder, C.A. (1985) Brainstem control of saccadic eye movements. *Annual Review of Neuroscience* 307–337, or Keller, E.L. (1992) *The brainstem.* In *Eye Movements*, ed. R.H.S. Carpenter (Macmillan, London).

Page 194 Eye movements General accounts of eye movements include Carpenter, R.H.S. (1989) *Movements of the Eyes* (Pion, London); Carpenter, R.H.S. (ed.) (1992) *Eye Movements* (Macmillan, London); good sources of information on clinical aspects are C Kennard, C. and F C Rose, F.C. (eds) *Physiological Aspects of Clinical Neuro-Ophthalmology* (Chapman and Hall, London) or Leigh, R.J. and Zee, D.S. (1991) *The Neurology of Eye Movements* (F.A. Davies, Philadelphia). Doucet, P. and Sloep, P. B. (1992) *Mathematical Modelling in the Life Sciences* (Ellis Horwood, Chichester) is a more general account of modelling that may also be consulted.

Page 195 Cleverness of the spinal cord The 19th century physiologist Charles Flourens has left a characteristic account of decerebrating a chicken: *'I removed the two cerebral lobes from a healthy chicken. The animal, thus deprived of its cerebrum, survived ten whole months in a state of perfect health and would in all probability have lived longer if I had not been obliged to leave Paris. I had scarcely removed the brain before the sight of both eyes was suddenly lost; the hearing was also gone and the animal did not give the slightest sign of volition, but kept itself perfectly upright upon its legs, and walked when it was stimulated – or when it was pushed. When thrown into the air, it flew; and swallowed water when it was put into its beak. It seemed entirely to have lost its memory, for when it struck itself against anything, it would not avoid it, but repeat the blow immediately.'*

Page 197 Newborn walking Figure 9.11 was very kindly supplied by Dr N. R. C. Roberton, Department of Paediatrics, Addenbrooke's Hospital, Cambridge. For a dissident view, that the loss of this stepping is due more to changes in body weight in relation to leg strength, see Thelen, E., Fisher, D. M. and Ridley-Johnson, R. (1984) The relationship between physical growth and a newborn reflex. *Infant Behavior and Development* 7, 479–493.

NEUROLAB

 ## Neural network

Page 187

Click in the boxes on the left; the input pattern is transformed as it passes from layer to layer, ending up on the right as a count of how many boxes have been checked. This is not a true neural net, in the sense that it learns for itself; it has been programmed to do it. But it shows how a network of simple neural elements (each has a threshold and fires when the number of active inputs exceeds that threshold) can perform quite a complex function. If you press Learning, you can experiment with a neural network that really does learn: it is described on p. 272

Parametric feedback

Page 190

This exhibit shows the functioning of parametric feedback in the vestibulo-ocular reflex. To understand it, you need to know something about the vestibular control of eye movements. See the description in Chapter 11, p. 225.

Control systems

Page 193

A demonstration of the different varieties of control system described in the text. Click on the buttons and check boxes at the left to select the kind of system you want to look at. On the right you can alter some of the characteristics of the control: Gain means how sensitive it is, Bias is a constant signal added to the output, Proportional means that the controller output is simply proportional to the input, Proportional + rate means that it is also partly proportional to the rate of change of the input, and Proportional + integral means that it is partly responsive to accumulated errors. In addition, you can add your own perturbations with the Noise slider, and alter the gain of the plant.

Press Sweep to see how the actual output y (green) responds to the desired output x (blue), a simple repetitive waveform. See for yourself how with parametric feedback or feedforward, the controller gain and offset adjust themselves automatically to improve performance, and in response to perturbations of the plant or external noise.

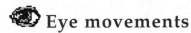 Eye movements

Page 194
Select a type of eye movement with the buttons at the left, then press Sweep. Note that the time and amplitude scales vary for the different types of movement. Notice that the saccades are stereotyped in form and very fast but occur with a rather random latency. Their ballistic behaviour is obvious in their response to closely spaced target movements: compare this with what happens in vergence. In pursuit, the target is tracked by a combination of smooth pursuit (to match the velocity) and saccades (to get the position right). As time goes on, the oculomotor system learns to improve the accuracy of the smooth pursuit, through parametric feedback: consequently, fewer saccades are made.

The demonstrations of vestibular, optokinetic and fixation movements are described more fully in Chapter 11, on p. 225.

Motor neurones 200
Descending pathways 201
Sensory feedback from muscles 205

MOTOR NEURONES

The final output from the central nervous system to the muscles of most of the body is from the *motor neurones* in the ventral horn of the spinal cord, cells whose large size reflects the length of their axons. Each controls a scattered group of individual muscle fibres called a *motor unit*: a unit may comprise as few as a dozen fibres in some of the muscles of the middle ear and in eye muscles, or as many as 1500 in large and crude muscles such as gluteus maximus. In the cat's leg, a single unit is capable of exerting a maximum force of some 10 g. Gradations of force are brought about partly by changes in the firing frequency of individual motor neurones, and partly by a process of recruitment, in which more and more units are brought into play as the required muscle tension increases, normally the smallest neurons, innervating the most 'tonic' and least fatiguable muscle fibres, being the first recruited. Although individual units may sometimes fire at very low frequencies, this does not normally cause discrete twitching of the muscles because different units fire out of synchrony with one another. One of the functions of the Renshaw cells mentioned in Chapter 3 is probably to provide a kind of lateral inhibition between motor neurones that discourages synchronization of this kind.

Motor neurones have an orderly and systematic arrangement within the cord, in clumps not quite well enough defined to be called nuclei, that reflects the topology of the muscles they serve (Figure 10.1). Medial neurones innervate the muscles of the trunk, the most distal parts of limbs are governed by the most lateral neurones, and flexors and extensors tend to be under the control of the more dorsal and ventral groups respectively. On these cells terminate all the afferents from interneurones, and in some cases receptors, that serve the various spinal reflexes and responses, as well as certain of the descending paths from higher levels. Because these cells represent the ultimate funnel through which all nervous excitation must pass whenever a motor act is made, whatever its source, together they form what is sometimes called the *final common path*. The quantity of information that thus converges on a single ventral horn cell is enormous, and is reflected in the huge size of its dendritic tree, which may often extend over a large part of the grey matter of the cord (Figure 10.1).

It is those afferents whose origins, perhaps via one or more interneurones, are sensory fibres that enter the dorsal roots that give rise to spinal *reflexes*. It is never easy to define exactly what is meant by a reflex. Any response that can be elicited from a spinal animal is certainly a spinal reflex. But we have already seen that although a response may be essentially a spinal one, in the sense that its neural circuitry lies entirely within the spinal cord, yet one may not be able to elicit it in the spinal preparation because the usual facilitating, permissive influences descending from the brain are absent. It is not quite enough to describe a reflex as an automatic, reproducible response that is independent of the will, as one may readily influence one's own spinal reflexes by willed inhibition or facilitation from above. For example, there is a mechanism in the cord called the withdrawal or flexion reflex that causes a rapid flexion when the skin is touched by a hot object or other noxious stimulus: yet we all know from personal experience that in cases of necessity – when carrying a plate that proves to be hotter than we thought when we picked it up – we can (up to a point!) inhibit the reflex completely. We shall see later on that what at first sight appears the simplest and most automatic spinal reflex of all, the monosynaptic stretch reflex, is

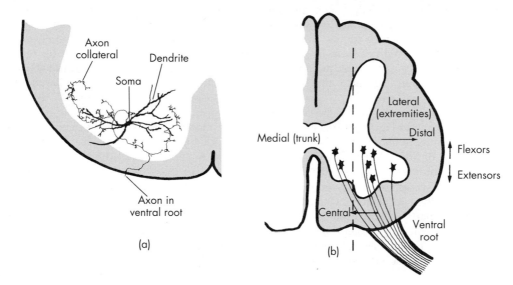

FIG. 10.1 (a) Golgi preparation of a single ventral horn cell, showing the enormous extent of its dendritic field. (After Scheibel and Scheibel, 1960) **(b)** Schematic representation of localization of motor neurones corresponding to various groups of muscles.

actually under almost total control from other, mainly descending influences. In fact, when we look at the mode of termination of the tracts descending from the brain, we find that the great majority of them end not on the motor neurones themselves but rather on the interneurones that form part of these reflex arcs. Descending control is not so much of muscles as of actions, amounting to a selection from the cord's repertoire: the brain plays on the spinal cord not as one plays a piano but rather as one selects a disc from a juke box.

DESCENDING PATHWAYS

There are five important tracts that descend from brain to spinal cord; four of these come from closely neighbouring parts of the brain, in the brainstem and medulla. These are the *reticular formation*, the *vestibular nuclei*, the *red nucleus*, and the *tectum*; the fifth origin of descending fibres is the *cerebral cortex* (Figure 10.2). The reticular formation ('rete' = net) is one of the most important and oldest structures in the brain, a direct descendant of the nerve nets controlling creatures like the sea anemone: in protochordates such as Amphioxus all descending influences from the brain have to be relayed via the reticular formation. Although it is a somewhat diffuse structure, comprising both cell bodies and connecting fibres, it is possible to make out certain condensations in it that are effectively nuclei. It stretches from the superior cervical spinal cord up to the intralaminar thalamic nuclei with which it merges at the top. Two areas in particular send

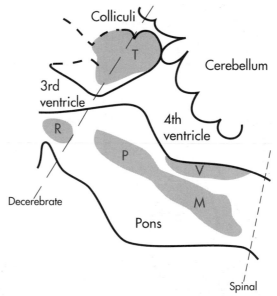

FIG.10.2 Sagittal projection of structures in the brainstem of the cat, showing reticular nuclei (P, pontine; M, medullary, including gigantocellularis), and other areas that are sources of descending tracts: R, red nucleus; T, tectum; V, vestibular nuclei. The dashed lines show the approximate positions at which cuts are made in the spinal and decerebrate preparations.

important tracts down to the cord: they are the *medullary* reticular formation, especially the nucleus gigantocellularis (the largeness of its neurones reflecting, of course, the length of their axons) that gives rise to the *lateral reticulospinal tract*; and the *pontine* reticular formation, giving the *medial reticulospinal tract.*

The positions of these tracts within the cord are shown diagrammatically in Figure 10.3: as is typical of the older tracts, both are mainly homolateral with only a little crossing of fibres. Most of the fibres terminate diffusely on interneurones rather than on the motor neurones themselves, except for certain fibres of the lateral tract; they influence muscles of the trunk and proximal parts of limbs rather than the extremities. It is difficult to generalize about their function, except to say that on the whole they are concerned not with the fine or fast control of skilled movements under voluntary control but rather with basic, instinctual reactions such as the startle reaction – the dramatic tensing of the whole body seen in response to a sudden stimulus like the sound of a gunshot – and also some of the postural mechanisms that will be described in Chapter 11.

In the course of evolution, areas of the reticular formation concerned with particular sources of sensory stimulation have tended to condense together as nuclei, and migrate together towards their common source of excitation. The vestibular nuclei seem to have emerged in this way under the influence of afferent fibres from the vestibular apparatus, which as we saw in Chapter 5 are concerned with sensing movements of the head and the direction of gravity.

At least four nuclei make up the vestibular complex, of which the medial and lateral (Deiter's) nuclei are the origin of an important descending motor tract, the *vestibulospinal tract* (Figure 10.3b). As might be expected from the reticular origin of the vestibular nuclei, the course of this tract is similar to those of the reticulospinal tracts: virtually all the fibres are uncrossed, most end on interneurones, but some excite motor neurones monosynaptically. A medial vestibulospinal tract also exists, projecting bilaterally mainly to cervical and upper thoracic regions. The functions of these tracts are essentially to maintain posture and to support the body against the force of gravity; consequently they are mostly concerned with the control of extensors rather than flexors. The vestibular nuclei are also closely associated with the cerebellum, one of the largest and most important higher motor areas, and the descending tracts may provide one way in which the cerebellum may control the spinal cord: it has no direct projections of its own.

The third descending pathway is the *rubrospinal tract*, which is derived from the red nucleus (Latin 'ruber', red), a well-defined region lying above the pons in the midbrain (Figure 10.2). This area, being highly vascular, is pinkish in fresh specimens, giving it its name. Like the vestibular nuclei, it forms an important output relay from the cerebellum but is not associated with any particular sensory modality; it also receives descending fibres from the cerebral cortex. In animals it is more prominent than in humans, and projects mainly to caudal rather than cervical parts of the cord, terminating on interneurones; it produces flexion rather than extension

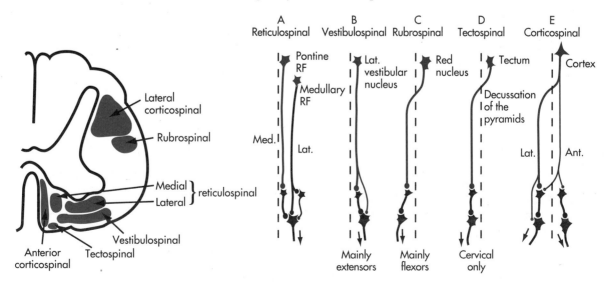

FIG.10.3 Left, section of cord showing the approximate positions of the major descending tracts. Right, diagrammatic representation of arrangement of the descending fibres in the major motor tracts. RF, reticular formation.

when electrically stimulated. Its fibres cross at a high level and then descend laterally, as shown in Figure 10.3c. Its functions are something of a mystery.

The fourth motor tract is the *tectospinal tract* (Figure 10.3d). 'Tectum' is Latin for roof, and anatomically the tectum is simply the roof of the fourth ventricle, comprising the superior and inferior colliculi in mammals. These are integrating centres for vision and hearing respectively, although as one ascends the evolutionary tree one finds their functions increasingly taken over, or at least supplemented, by the cerebral cortex. They seem to be concerned in particular with orientating responses, as for example in turning to look at the source of a sudden sound. In the superior colliculus one finds neurones that are responsive to visual stimuli in precise locations in the visual field, and which also respond to electrical stimulation by causing the eyes to execute a saccade to the very same part of the field (p. 160) As one might expect from such orientating responses, the tectospinal tract projects no further than cervical segments. The fibres are crossed, and end on interneurones.

Finally we come to a tract that has been investigated to a degree perhaps somewhat out of proportion to its real importance: the *corticospinal* or *pyramidal tract* (Figure 10.3e). Its neurones are some of the longest in the body, since they run from the cerebral cortex in the top of the skull all the way down into the cord. In humans, some 80 per cent cross in the medulla (in other species the proportion is greater: 100 per cent in the dog), and as they lie on the extreme ventral surface (the pyramids of the medulla, hence 'pyramidal'), the decussation can generally be seen with the naked eye. The crossed fibres descend as the lateral corticospinal tract, and the uncrossed ones as the anterior corticospinal tract. Both are relatively recent pathways, their development following that of the cerebral cortex itself, and consequently there is a good deal of species variation as to their size and disposition. In humans, they may form 30 per cent of the white matter of the cord: in the dog, 10 per cent. Only in humans and some primates do any fibres terminate on motor neurones; in many species they project no further than cervical segments, and in any case form a relatively small component of the total white matter of the cord. Their clinical importance is, however, very great indeed, since at the upper end, where in ascending from medulla to cortex the fibres fan out into a sheet called the internal capsule in order to squeeze past the thalamus and basal ganglia, they are peculiarly susceptible to damage from vascular accidents, resulting in the well-known form of paralysis called

stroke. The functions of the corticospinal tract will be considered in more detail both later in this chapter and also in Chapter 12; it predominantly controls the extremities and by and large it is concerned with fine, skilled, voluntary movements, and particularly with manipulation.

Decerebrate and related preparations

Some of the tonic actions of these various centres, and their interrelations, can be deduced from classic experiments involving lesions in the brainstem that effectively disconnect them from the spinal cord or from each other. Despite what might at first seem to be the crudity of the techniques, it is nevertheless possible to come to quite firm, if general, conclusions from them. The *spinal* preparation has already been mentioned; this is one in which all the tracts are cut, so that the cord is completely isolated from the brain (Figure 10.2). The result of this is a floppy or *flaccid* paralysis, in which there is loss both of voluntary movement and of muscle tone. Whereas a normal person's muscles fire tonically, excited by a steady level of motor neurone activity, and offer resistance to any movement imposed on the limbs from outside, in flaccid paralysis they are relaxed and offer no resistance at all: thus one may be able to pick up such a patient's arm and fling it in his face, something that cannot be done to a normal conscious subject.

Another frequently studied preparation is the *decerebrate* preparation, classically produced by a cut at the level of the colliculi (Figure 10.2). The effect of such a transection, once the animal is allowed to recover, is utterly different from the floppiness of the spinal preparation. The animal now has muscles that, far from being flaccid and relaxed, are tonically hyperactive (especially extensors), and the general picture is one of stiffness - decerebrate *rigidity*. The increased tonic activity of the decerebrate animal as compared with the spinal animal must presumably be interpreted as a release phenomenon of the kind discussed in the previous chapter, and due to unopposed activity originating in some structure that lies between the levels of the two cuts. A feature of decerebrate rigidity is that the pattern of stiffness in the legs depends markedly on which way up the animal is (Figure 10.4), and it seems therefore very likely that the tonic overactivity is essentially due to the influence of sensory stimuli from the vestibular apparatus, normally held in check by centres lying above the brainstem: the rigidity is abolished by lesions in the lateral vestibular nuclei.

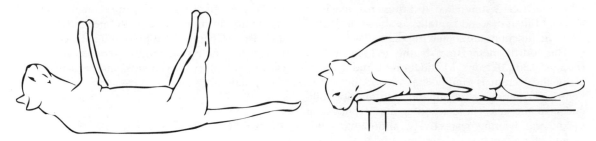

FIG.10.4 Tone in the limbs as a function of head position in the decerebrate cat. (Bell *et al.*, 1961)

A kind of rigidity may also be produced by destruction of the cerebral cortex (giving a *decorticate* preparation) rather than decerebration: but in this case lesions of the vestibular nuclei have relatively little effect. This second kind of rigidity – it differs in other ways as well, and is often called *spasticity* – is thought to be due to a tonic excitatory influence from upper areas of the reticular formation, which are disconnected from the cord in decerebration, and presumably normally inhibited by the cortex (Figure 10.5). Direct confirmation of this has come from electrical stimulation of the upper reticular formation, which results in a general facilitation both of spinal reflexes and of the effects of electrical stimulation elsewhere in the brain. In this respect, the lower or bulbar reticular formation is exactly the opposite: electrical stimulation causes not facilitation but depression of reflexes and evoked movements. The tonic relationships between these structures that may be deduced from such experiments are summarized in Figure 10.5; lesions and stimulation of the cerebellum and basal ganglia also influence rigidity, but these effects are more complex and will be described later on. A striking fact about the relation between the higher motor levels and the cord is that the two largest areas of all, the basal ganglia and cerebellum, have absolutely no direct projections to spinal levels: all that they do must be achieved by indirect relay through one of the five tracts described above. Furthermore, these tracts themselves act for the most

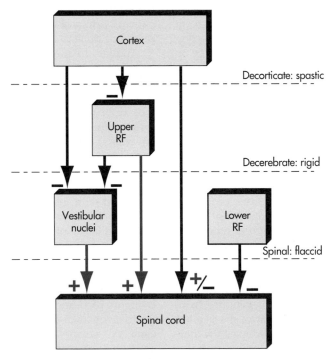

FIG.10.5 Simplified scheme of apparent tonic facilitatory (+) and inhibitory (-) influences between various central regions, and their relationships to the levels of section in different experimental preparations. RF, reticular formation.

part only indirectly, influencing spinal reflexes rather than motor neurones, underlining once again the essentially hierarchical nature of the motor system.

The rest of this chapter will be concerned with one particular spinal reflex, the stretch reflex, which probably plays a more important part than any other in the control of movements, and illustrates something of the way in which the brain can make use of indirect control of this kind.

SENSORY FEEDBACK FROM MUSCLES

In the previous chapter, we saw that there is an intimate involvement of sensory feedback at every level of the nervous system, and examined some of the ways in which this feedback might be used to improve motor control. Here we shall be concerned with the very lowest level of this feedback, that from the muscles themselves. Figure 10.6 shows what an enormous quantity of this information there is. In this particular instance, compared with the 150 or so fibres that are truly motor, innervating extrafusal muscle fibres, there are some 150 sensory fibres, and another 100 or so γ-fibres, which as we saw in Chapter 5 modify sensory signals from the muscle spindles rather than directly causing contraction of the muscle itself. In other words, some 250 fibres are concerned with afferent information, and only 150 are strictly motor.

Of the two types of sensory receptor within muscles, the spindle and Golgi tendon organ, the functions of the latter are less well understood. We saw in Chapter 5 that being in series with the main contractile elements, it acts as a *force* transducer; what is not altogether clear is how this information about muscle tension is actually put to use. One reflex for which it is probably responsible is the *clasp-knife* reflex; if you take hold of someone's hand and then push on it in such a way as to bend his elbow – having told him to push back as hard as he can to resist you – there will come a point (assuming that you are the stronger!) at which the force he exerts suddenly seems to give way, and the arm folds up like a clasp-knife. This reflex is thought to be brought about by some such neuronal circuit as in Figure 10.7, in which the incoming tendon organ fibres inhibit their parent motor neurone through an interneurone, with some kind of threshold. It is usually claimed that this reflex is protective in function, preventing damage to tendons by pulling on them too hard; if so, it is not very good at its job, since athletes do of course frequently 'pull' their tendons despite the existence of the reflex. It is difficult to believe, in fact, that this is all the tendon organs do, and a role for them in the control of muscle movement is suggested later in this chapter: it is the spindles with which we are mainly now concerned.

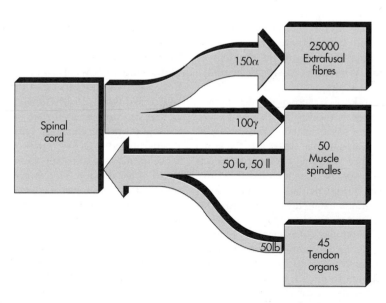

FIG.10.6 Flow of information to and from a typical cat soleus muscle, showing some 250 efferent fibres and 150 afferents; of the total number of fibres, 250 are concerned with sensory information from the muscle, and only 150 are directly responsible for muscle tension. (Data from Matthews, 1972)

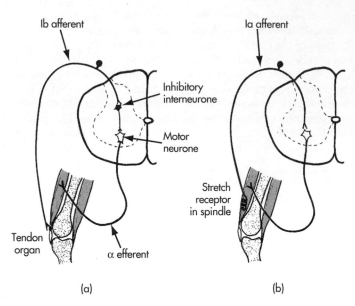

FIG.10.7 Schematic representation of the neural circuits thought to underlie two spinal reflexes. **(a)** The clasp-knife reflex: excessive muscle tension, sensed by the Golgi tendon organs, results in reflex inhibition of the muscle's motor neurones. **(b)** The monosynaptic phasic stretch reflex: rapid stretch activates the Ia fibres, which monosynaptically excite the motor neurones.

Spindle reflexes

We saw in Chapter 5 that spindles essentially signal both muscle length and also – especially in the case of the Ia fibres – rate of change of length, and that the messages they convey are also modified by the activity of the γ-efferent fibres to the intrafusal fibres: to a first approximation, their response is a function of the amount of external stretch plus the amount of internal stretch caused by γ-activity. Or to put it another way, they signal γ-activity *minus* the degree of muscle contraction. What do these signals actually do?

One of their best known actions comes about because the Ia afferents monosynaptically excite motor neurones of the same muscle (Figure 10.7), forming the classic monosynaptic reflex arc, the simplest imaginable kind of neuronal circuit that could link a stimulus to a response. The result is that any stretch of the muscle, but particularly a brief, phasic one that will preferentially excite the rate-sensitive Ia fibres, will stimulate the motor neurone and cause a rapid contraction of the muscle. An easy way to elicit such a response is in the familiar *tendon jerk:* tapping a muscle's tendon produces just the right sort of fast-rising stretch to elicit a brisk reflex contraction. The patellar tendon is convenient, and gives an easily noticeable response, but other tendons such as the Achilles tendon will do just as well. Another effective way of stimulating the Ia fibres is by the use

of massage vibrators; much of their 'exercising' effect is due to the fact that they induce tonic reflex contractions. In the normal person, these reflexes are rather feeble, but in certain experimental preparations – and pathological states – they are much increased, which is why they may often be valuable in clinical neurological diagnosis. In the decerebrate animal one may demonstrate not just a phasic reflex of this kind but also a tonic component, in which the muscle responds to steady stretch with a steady contraction – the *myotatic* or *tonic stretch reflex*. A record of this kind is shown in Figure 10.8: in response to the 6 mm stretch shown by the upper line, the muscle responded with a steady tension of nearly 4 kg: some of this, but only a small part, was due simply to the muscle's intrinsic elasticity, which may be revealed if it is paralysed so as to suppress the reflex component. Since in this case a stretch of 6 mm generated about 3 kg of reflex tension, we can say that the *gain* of the reflex – the extra tension evoked per unit of stretch – was about 500 g/mm. The stretch reflex thus makes muscles appear stiffer – less elastic – than they naturally are. In fact it is easy to show that the stiffness of decerebrate rigidity is entirely due to overactivity of the stretch reflexes, probably through excitation of the γ-efferents, for if the dorsal roots are cut in such a preparation, preventing the Ia discharges from reaching the motor neurones, rigidity vanishes. Decerebrate rigidity might therefore be described as a sort of hyper-stretch-reflexia.

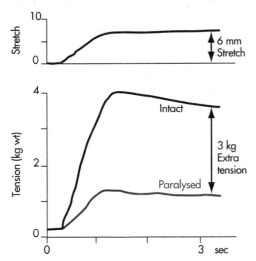

FIG.10.8 Tonic stretch reflex in decerebrate cat. The muscle was stretched with the time-course shown in the top curve, and the resultant tension was measured (black line below). The red line shows the result of the same experiment when the muscle was paralysed. (After Liddell and Sherrington, 1924)

The servo hypothesis

Thus the first notion about the function of muscle spindles that came to be accepted was that by acting through the stretch reflex, they were responsible for the generation of muscle *tone*, the constant muscular activity that is necessary as a background to actual movement in order to maintain the basic attitude of the body, particularly against the force of gravity. But tone is something that essentially opposes movement, that tends to keep muscles at preset lengths by making them resist any changes. Hence the idea arose that during movements one would have to alter the degree of tone in step with the movement if

there was not to be a degree of conflict between the two, and that the γ-fibres were ideally suited to doing just this. If every time a command was sent via the α-motor fibres (the ones innervating the extrafusal fibres) to make the muscle contract, the γ-fibres were simultaneously activated, then all would be well. The internal stretch generated by the intrafusal fibres would make up for the reduced external stretch, so that the stretch reflex would still function and there would be no loss of tone.

It then became apparent that one could carry this line of thought a stage further and envisage an even more active role for the γ-fibres than this. Imagine for a moment that the γ-fibres were stimulated without simultaneous direct activation of the α-fibres. What would happen? By shortening the intrafusal fibres of the spindle, such a stimulus would result in excitation of the sensory afferents just as if an actual stretch had occurred (Figure 10.9); consequently there would be a reflex activation of the α-motor neurones, and the muscle would contract automatically until the stretch receptors found themselves back at their original resting degree of stretch. In other words, γ-stimulation could in principle initiate contraction, in exactly the same way as direct α-stimulation. But would there be any point in such a roundabout way of making muscles contract?

The answer is that there would. We saw earlier that the sensory endings in the spindle are signalling something like the difference between the amount of γ-activity and the shortness of the muscle. If we think of γ-activity as telling the muscle how short it ought to be, then the spindle becomes a comparator generating an error-signal, 'error' here being the difference between the desired length of the muscle and its actual length. So if now we redraw the stretch reflex in a more formal way (Figure 10.10) it is immediately

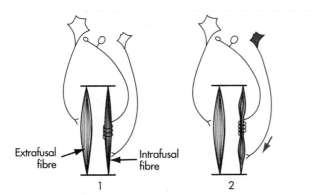
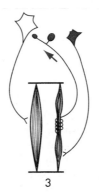
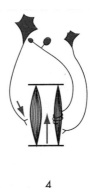

FIG.10.9 Reflex contraction via γ-fibre stimulation. 1, muscle at rest; 2, activation of γ-fibres stretches sensory endings in spindle, leading to (3) excitation of spindle afferents, which in turn (4) cause excitation of α-motor neurones and contraction of extrafusal muscle fibres.

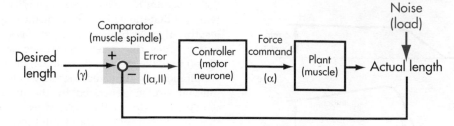

FIG.10.10 How the spindle might function as a comparator in a simple servosystem in which a muscle's length is automatically made to conform to the desired length signalled by the γ efferents (compare Figure 9.5).

apparent that what we have is a classic *feedback* or *servo system*. The γ fibres set the desired length; if this is shorter than the actual length, the spindle afferents stimulate the motor neurones to generate a force that makes the muscle contract. The advantage of such an arrangement, like all feedback systems, is that it automatically allows for noise, in this case the existence of unpredictable loads that have to be moved.

Consider for example the problem posed by holding out a cup while someone is filling it with tea: clearly, one's task here is to keep the various muscles concerned at a constant length, despite the fact that the force required to do this is continually increasing as the load – the amount of tea in the cup – gets bigger. Now, one could of course imagine the brain continually monitoring the situation, and deciding at every instant exactly how much direct α-excitation to send down into the cord to keep the hand steady. But how much simpler it would be just to send, once and for all, a message indicating not the force needed but the desired *position* of the hand, and leave the spinal cord to get on with the job of adjusting the force to the load automatically, by sensing the extent to which the actual position of the cup matches the brain's command. In other words, such a feedback system would provide load compensation, by acting as what is sometimes called a follow-up servo: the main muscles simply act as slaves that follow any length changes signalled to the intrafusal fibres.

The fundamental problem facing the brain in trying to control movement is that what it wants to achieve are limb positions and muscle lengths, but all it can *actually* do is alter the forces generated by muscles. So the problem is how to work out what force is needed to produce a certain position with a given load: the beauty of the simple servo model is that it saves the brain having to worry about such matters at all. It can think simply in terms of the desired effect, and leave the lower levels to get on with the humdrum task of working out how to achieve it.

Granted that the γ-fibres could in principle initiate movements of limbs on their own, is there any evi-

dence that they in fact do so? For certain types of movement, the answer is a clear yes. Figure 10.11 shows one such instance: we noted earlier that moving the position of a decerebrate cat's head causes reflex changes in the tone of its limbs; (a) here shows the discharge from a spindle afferent from the leg during such a stimulus, and it can be seen that the frequency of firing is modulated in time with the head movement. This in itself proves nothing, since it could merely be the result of changes in length of the muscle, rather than activation of γ-fibres. But if the dorsal roots are cut, preventing the stretch reflex from operating, two facts are immediately obvious. First of all, the limb movement is abolished, indicating that it must have been driven through the reflex rather than directly by descending pathways activating α-motor neurones. Secondly, the spindle discharge is still modulated by the stimulus. Since the muscle length is no longer changing, the only possible way in which this modulation can be taking place is by varying activation of the γ-fibres. In other words, it is quite certain in this case that the movement is indeed initiated by γ-activation of the stretch reflex servo and not by descending a commands. Of course, a decerebrate cat with its dorsal roots cut is hardly in a physiological condition; but other experiments in conscious human subjects have also demonstrated that γ-fibres may on occasion be used in voluntary movements.

But Figure 10.11b shows the results of another experiment, in which recordings were made in humans of activity in Ia fibres during voluntary movement of the wrist, together with the electromyogram from the muscle itself. It can be seen that although it is shortening that is taking place – which by itself would of course reduce Ia activity – nevertheless there is an increase in spindle discharge associated with the movement, implying that stimulation of γ-fibres must be taking place as well. However, experiments of this kind, though demonstrating that γ-activation occurs during voluntary movements, also reveal some disastrous discrepancies

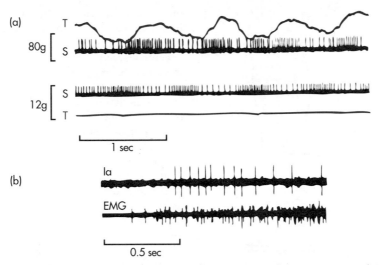

FIG.10.11 Demonstration that γ-fibres may be used to generate reflex movements. Above, tension (T) in decerebrate cat soleus muscle, and associated firing of a spindle afferent (S) during reflex contraction evoked by head movement. Below, after cutting the dorsal root, no contraction occurs, yet modulation of spindle discharge is much as before: this can only be through g-activation. (After Eldred *et al.*, 1953) **(b)** Records of Ia discharge and electromyogram (EMG) during voluntary human wrist movements; the Ia discharge clearly does not precede the muscle activity, as would be expected if the muscle were only driven by a servo-system like that of Figure 10.10. (After Vallbo, 1971)

with the notion that this activity is actually the cause of the movement. If the servo hypothesis were true, the sequence of events that we would expect to observe would be first activation of the γ-fibres, then the resultant Ia activity, and only then would we expect to see the discharge of the α-fibres and of the main muscle fibres themselves. But actual recordings of the relative timing of these events show that this is not what happens at all (Figure 10.11b): the Ia discharge actually occurs after the contraction has commenced, and therefore cannot possibly be its cause. So while γ-initiation seems to occur for certain postural responses, it is almost certainly not used for ordinary fast willed movements.

Further, there is a theoretical consideration that casts doubt on the possibility of driving real movements solely by means of γ-activation, and that is the size of the *gain* of stretch reflexes; 'gain' here means how much extra tension is generated by a given error in length. Returning to the problem of holding out the teacup, it is a relatively simple matter to work out what gain this reflex would need to have in order to perform adequately (Figure 10.12). From our definition of the gain, G, it follows that for every degree of error e (that is, for every value of the difference between actual and desired muscle length) there is a corresponding reflex force F that is developed by the muscle, where $F = e . G$. So when a muscle is supporting a load F, its actual length will be slightly greater than what is desired, by an amount $e = F/G$. In the

case of the muscle shown in Figure 10.8, this means that a load of 500 g would cause an error of 1 mm, the stretch required to generate the 500 g needed to sustain the load. Now most muscles, because of the way they are attached to their bones, work under a considerable mechanical disadvantage: in the case of the human biceps, every kilogram of load on the hand results in some 10 kg of tension in the muscle; and conversely, a muscle movement of 1 mm moves the hand by some 10 mm. If for the sake of argument the gain of the stretch reflex being used to hold the teacup was also 500 g/mm, then this means that every 50 g of load in the hand will cause a muscle extension of 1 mm, and the hand will move some 10 mm. In other words, the extra 300 g or so produced by filling the cup would be expected to make the hand droop by no less than 6 cm. It doesn't.

Somehow, the force generated by the system must be automatically increased in step with the changed requirements as the cup is filled, perhaps as the result of pressure receptors in the hand or by monitoring the tension in the muscle's tendons by means of the tendon organs. If, for instance, the force was always increased in such a way as to be proportional to the load, then the system would perform equally well, regardless of how big the load was. Experiments carried out in human subjects suggest that something of the sort does indeed occur. Here a subject was required to use his thumb to push a lever at a constant velocity against a fixed resistance: he was

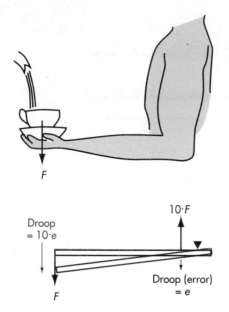

Fig.10.12 The problem of cup holding. Taking the mechanical disadvantage of the lever system in the forearm as 10, then a weight F in the hand must be balanced by a tension 10.F in the muscle. At the same time, an error e in muscle length will result in a descent 10.e by the cup. Thus if the static gain of the stretch reflex is G, the cup will fall by 100/G for each unit of weight.

provided with visual feedback from the lever to tell him how well he was doing. Recordings of his electromyogram (Figure 10. 13) show a steadily rising averaged activity during the course of the movement, as the muscle shortens. If now, without the subject's knowledge, a stop is introduced into the apparatus that prevents the lever moving past a certain point, one finds that after a short latency the EMG quickly rises, reflecting the subject's effort to overcome the unexpected obstacle. In fact the latency is too short to be due to a conscious decision of this kind, and a simpler explanation is that because of the stop there develops an increasing error between desired and actual thumb position – the former increasing steadily, and the latter having stopped – and this causes a stretch reflex. This reflex cannot be of the ordinary tendon-jerk kind, however, because its latency is considerably longer. What is found is that if the experiment is repeated with different degrees of resistance to the thumb movement – with different loads, in other words – the force generated by a given error increases with increasing load in any particular trial (Figure 10. 13b). That this change is caused by pressure receptors in the skin is suggested by the fact that if the thumb is anaesthetized the extra force drops nearly to zero (Figure 10. 13c).

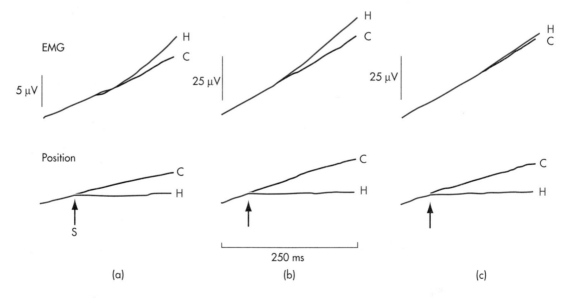

FIG.10.13 Evidence for variable forces produced by stretch reflex. (a) A subject moves his thumb (lower trace shows its position) against a steady load so as to track a uniformly moving target; the resultant steady increase in EMG is shown above (C = control). If a stop is now introduced at the point S, after a latent period the EMG starts to rise more rapidly (H = halt trial). (b) If the load against which the thumb is pushing is increased by a factor of 10, the EMG in response to the error also increases by nearly the same factor. (c) as (b) but with the hand anaesthetized, resulting in almost complete abolition of the stretch reflex. (Note the change in scale of the EMG in (b) and (c); each trace is an average of eight trials. (After Marsden *et al.*, 1972; copyright Macmilllan Journals Ltd)

Servo assistance

Consequently one is forced to conclude that in the control of movements there are two separate signals or commands that are sent to the spinal cord by the brain. One is a position command that indicates, via the γ-fibres, what the desired length of a muscle is to be; the other is a *force* command, an estimate of the load that is to be encountered. In the case of the teacup, the latter information could be obtained from receptors in the skin or, for that matter from Golgi tendon organs, but many tasks are more ballistic in nature and require anticipation in advance of what the load is likely to be. In such cases past experience and the more sophisticated use of special senses like vision may be brought into play as well. When we go to pick up a sack of potatoes as opposed to a sack of waste paper, or when we fling open a swing door with which we are familiar (too little force, and we walk into it: too much, and we smash it) we have clearly estimated beforehand what the likely load will be, and thus what force is required. This notion of simultaneous force and length command is sometimes called α/γ *coactivation;* if the estimate of force is an accurate one then the system behaves, in effect, ballistically, and there is no error for the spindles to have to correct. So the job of the stretch reflex is now simply to deal with any residual errors left over after

the estimated force is put into operation; it is not expected to provide the whole force necessary for the job, which we have seen it is too feeble to provide. A system of this kind is known as a *servo-assisted* system, and may be represented by an arrangement like that of Figure 10. 14: it is really a ballistic system with a safety net provided by a back-up guided system, a short-loop one through the spinal cord, and a long-loop one through the cerebral cortex. Thus a patient whose spindle afferents from the hand have been destroyed by disease may perform quite well in skilled movements where the loads are known in advance, but will come to grief as soon as any kind of unexpected resistance or variation in load is encountered.

In the servo assistance model the spindles play two distinct roles. In the first place, through the stretch reflex, they provide immediate correction of any errors in the estimate of force; in the second place, they may also supply parametric feedback that in the long term can make future corrections of the estimates themselves. We shall see later that there is reason to think that the origin of the force command may be the cerebral cortex, via the corticospinal tract, and that it may be the cerebellum, which is richly supplied with afferents from muscle spindles (unlike the cortex), that is the site of the motor program store. These ideas will be discussed later, in Chapter 12.

Finally, it is perhaps worth mentioning that the

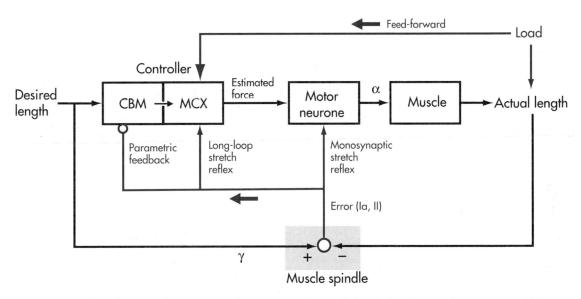

FIG.10.14 Hypothetical scheme of a servo-assisted control system for muscle length. Spindles provide an error signal (discrepancy between actual and desired length) that is used directly in the stretch reflex to correct the response, and also indirectly to modify the ballistic programs for future action. The brain signals to the cord not only desired length but also an estimate of the force needed to achieve that length, derived partly from stored programs embodying previous experience, and also partly from immediate information from sensory receptors about the load that is present.

muscles of the eye, though richly endowed with stretch receptors and γ-motor fibres, show no stretch reflexes whatever. It seems in this case that because of the predictable relation between force commands and resultant eye position emphasized earlier, errors arise so seldom that no short-term correction mechanism is needed. It seems very likely that the sole function of these spindle afferents is to provide parametric feedback in order that the essentially ballistic control of such movements as saccades may in the long run be performed accurately. Though ocular spindles fail to generate stretch reflex, where they do project in great numbers is the cerebellum, a region – as we shall see in Chapter 12 – known to be associated with parametric feedback and other kinds of motor learning.

References

Bell, G. H., Davidson, J. N. and Scarborough, H. (1961) *Textbook of Physiology and Biochemistry. Livingstone,* Edinburgh.

Eldred, E., Granit, R. and Merton, P. A. (1953) Supraspinal control of the muscle spindles and its significance. *Journal of Physiology* 122, 498–523.

Liddell, E. G. T. and Sherrington, C. S. (1924) Reflexes in response to stretch (myotatic reflexes). *Proceedings of the Royal Society B* 96, 212–242.

Marsden, C. D., Merton, P. A. and Morton, H. B. (1972) Servo action in human voluntary movement. *Nature* 238, 140–143.

Matthews, P. B. C. (1972) *Mammalian Muscle Receptors and their Central Actions.* Edward Arnold, London.

Scheibel, M. E. and Scheibel, A. B. (1960) Spinal motorneurones, interneurones and Renshaw cells: a Golgi study. *Archives Italiennes de Biologie* 104, 328–353.

Vallbo, Å. B. (1971) Muscle spindle response at the onset of isometric voluntary contractions in Man: time difference between fusimotor and skeletomotor effects. *Journal of Physiology* 218, 405–438.

NOTES

Page 200 Muscle Discussion of the functional properties of muscle itself is beyond the scope of this book. A clear and stimulating account is McMahon, T. A. (1984) *Muscles, Reflexes and Locomotion* (Princeton University Press, New Jersey).

Page 201 Reflexes Two classic accounts of reflexes in general: Creed, R. S., Denny-Brown, D., Liddell, E. G. T. and Sherrington, C. S. (1932) *Reflex Activity of the Spinal Cord* (Oxford University Press, Oxford), and Sherrington, C. S. (1906) *The Integrative Action of the Nervous System* (Yale University Press, New Haven, Conn).

Page 208 Thinking in terms of results A rather nice demonstration that broadly supports such a view is to have a subject first write their name and address in the usual way, with movement at the wrist, then (on a larger scale) with the wrist immobilized and using the elbow instead, and then finally with the whole hand and arm rigid, and the movement occurring at the shoulder. Despite the novelty of the second two tasks, and the fact that entirely different muscles are being used, the characteristics of the 'hand' writing are essentially retained.

Page 211 Deafferentation See, for instance, Marsden, C. D., Rothwell, J. C. and Day, B. L. (1984) The use of peripheral feedback in the control of movement. *Trends in Neuroscience* 7, 253–257. Taylor, A. and Prochazka, A. (1981) *Muscle Receptors and Movement* (Macmillan, London) is a useful account of the use of muscle feedback in general. Cole, J. (1991) *Pride and a Daily Marathon* (Duckworth, London) is a popular account of a patient with an unusually complete loss of afferent innervation who has to carry out consciously, under visual guidance, what most of us take utterly for granted: *'I'm going to buy a tin of beans in Sainsbury's. First, I have to pick a safe route down the aisle, because if someone brushes against me, and I haven't allowed for it, then I am thrown off balance. I reach the shelf and check my body position in space. I then lock my legs and focus on the tin. Then monitoring my arm movements all the time, I move it towards the tin. I grasp the tin – I don't know how much pressure to exert and I can't assess weight. The only way I know if something is too heavy is if I topple forwards.'* In addition, lack of sensory feedback can lead the person to feel alienated from the part affected, as brilliantly described in Sacks, O. (1993) *A Leg to Stand On* (Harper, New York).

NEUROLAB

Spinal tracts

Page 201

A simple self-testing exhibit covering the ascending and descending tracts of the spinal cord. Click on one of the buttons round the edge of the cross-section (ascending paths on the right, descending on the left).

The name of the corresponding tract will appear in the box at top right. Alternatively, click on the button to the right of the box to bring down a list of tracts: click on one, and its corresponding button will display.

Stretch reflex as a servo

Page 208, 212

This is a dynamic model of the stretch reflex that can be configured in different ways. On the left, a symbolic representation of extrafusal fibres (shown as a large hydraulic ram on the left) and intrafusal fibres (a smaller ram on the right, with a blue elastic ball representing the stretch-sensitive element) in parallel, supporting a load (purple square). One slider controls the size of this load, the other determines the size of the command sent to motor neurones. Radio buttons on the right select the mode of operation.

Select Alpha only, when commands are sent only to the a motor neurone, with no feedback. With a moderate load, try to set the muscle to a particular length: it is not easy, and any change in load immediately causes the length to change. Now select Gamma only. You can see for yourself how commands sent to the intrafusal fibres cause distortion of the stretch-sensitive endings, which in turn activates the α motor neurone. It is now much easier to set a particular length, though there is a tendency to overshoot, and although load has much less effect than before, it still has some. Now select Alpha/gamma. Information about load is now sent to the α motor neurone as well. As a result the system is much less affected by changes in load. It still shows a tendency to overshoot, which is because the spindle afferents in this model have not been given rate sensitivity.

11 THE CONTROL OF POSTURE

The importance of support 214
Vestibular contribution to posture 216
Visual contributions to posture 219

Neck reflexes 222
Posture as a whole 223

Movement begins and ends in posture: for most of the time, the motor system is not in fact concerned with moving the body at all, but rather with keeping it still. This is especially true in Man, his precarious twin supports needing constant motor commands to keep him upright against the force of gravity. At first sight one might perhaps think that this was merely a matter of keeping sufficiently rigid, once a stable balancing position had been found. But our centre of gravity is so high off the ground that this kind of passive stability is not enough: one need only compare the ease with which one can push over a tailor's dummy with the near impossibility of doing the same thing to a living person to realize that stability must involve *active* processes as well, that use proprioceptive feedback information.

THE IMPORTANCE OF SUPPORT

In physical terms, whether someone falls over or not is entirely a matter of the vertical projection of his centre of gravity relative to his supports (Fig. 11.1). If this line of projection lies within the area defined by the points of contact with the ground (the *support*

area), then all is well – small disturbances will result in a turning couple tending to restore the status quo. If it lies outside this critical area, then the system is unstable, and any further tilting will cause an ever-increasing couple that will make the person fall over. The support area is much smaller in humans than in four-footed animals, and maintaining an upright posture is correspondingly more difficult: a tilt of only a few degrees is sufficient to cause instability. Thus proper standing is *not*, as is often implied, just a matter of keeping upright: the man in Figure 11.2 clearly has an excellent upright posture, but is equally clearly about to experience a postural disaster because the vertical projection of his centre of gravity lies outside his region of contact with his support. Support is in every sense fundamental to posture, which must be controlled either by moving the centre of gravity relative to the feet or moving the feet relative to the centre of gravity.

Two sources of information enable us to do this. The first is the existence of *pressure* receptors in the feet themselves that provide information about the distribution of support. Knowledge of differences of pressure at different points of support tells us precisely what we need to know to determine our postural state, namely the position of the vertical projection of the centre of gravity relative to the body's

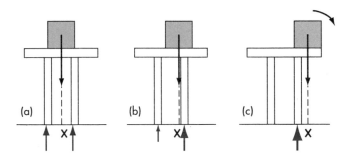

FIG. 11.1 A sufficient condition for postural stability is that the vertical projection of the centre of gravity on the floor (X) should lie within the area defined by the supports. The distribution of pressure between the supports (small arrows) provides sufficient information to determine the position of X.

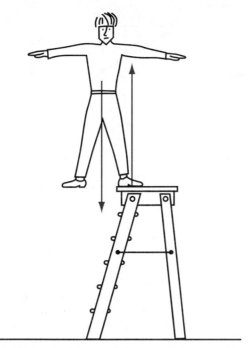

FIG. 11.2 A splendidly upright but nevertheless unsatisfactory posture.

supports (Fig. 11.1). The second source of information is in the head: those special senses that can tell us about the position and motion of the head relative to the outside world, the *vestibular* and *visual* systems. It is convenient to consider the use of information from the feet first, since this is a more direct process than the contribution of the special senses.

Responses to pressure distribution

Imagine that we had to design an automatic system for keeping a lunar module standing upright on uneven ground. One solution to this problem would be to equip each leg with a pressure transducer, and arrange things so that any leg that experienced more pressure than the others was automatically extended, while any that experienced less was shortened. The result would be a system that would always bring the vertical projection of the centre of gravity to the middle of the critical area defined by the points of support: if the craft leans in the direction of one particular leg, then that leg will experience more force and will respond by pushing it back. It is not difficult to demonstrate a precisely analogous mechanism in four-footed animals: if we suspend a decerebrate animal in the air with its legs hanging down, and push up on the sole of one of its feet, the animal responds by extending the corresponding limb. This tonic response is called the *positive supporting reaction*; there is also a transient component of the response called *extensor thrust*, and it is often accompanied by stiffening of the limb and arching of the back (Fig. 11.3). It is not difficult to see how this mechanism would act to increase postural stability, as for example when the animal is standing on sloping ground (Fig. 11.4). On the level, there is a roughly even distribution of pressure amongst the four feet, and hence no tendency for one leg to lengthen more than another. But if the animal is facing up a slope (Fig. 11.4b) the pressure on the back feet is greater than on the front, and consequently the positive supporting reaction will

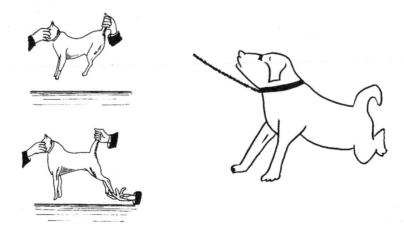

FIG. 11.3 Left, positive supporting demonstrated in decerebrate dog suspended in the air, on making contact with the back paws. (After Walsh, 1964) Right, typical 'buttress reaction' on trying to pull a dog forward and thus increasing the differential pressure on the front foot; note obvious front-leg extension. (From Rademaker, 1935)

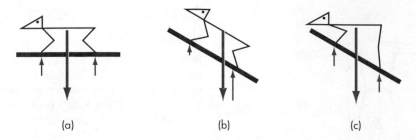

FIG. 11.4 How the positive supporting reaction results in good posture. **(a)** Animal standing on level ground, with projection of centre of gravity centrally placed between the supports. **(b)** Facing up a slope: the weight is now unevenly distributed between front and back legs, resulting **(c)** in front-leg flexion and back-leg extension, and a better position of the projection of the centre of gravity.

result in rear-limb extension and front-limb flexion: the final result will be that the body adopts a more horizontal posture, and the projection of the centre of gravity is brought more nearly to the middle of the points of support. The same mechanism may be seen at work in the *postural sway reaction*: if an animal's body is pushed from the side, the shift in pressure on the feet results in marked extension of the limbs on the opposite side, and retraction of the others, so that the animal in effect leans against the experimenter (compare Fig. 11.3). It seems likely that analogous mechanisms may be used when sitting, kneeling, lying down and so forth, involving information about differences of pressure on different parts of the body other than the feet. A blindfolded animal whose vestibular system has been destroyed (leaving cutaneous receptors as the only remaining source of postural information) will nevertheless right itself when laid on its side on the ground. But if a plank is laid on top of it that reduces the ratio of the pressures experienced by the two sides of the body, this body-righting reaction is inhibited, a phenomenon sometimes used by veterinary surgeons to help restrain an animal for operation.

The mechanisms described so far assume that some sort of support is already present: there are other types of response that may be used to *find* postural support. If for some reason the projection of the centre of gravity has moved outside the critical area, then automatic *stepping reactions* are elicited that in effect move the feet in such a way as to track the centre of gravity: if one happens to be standing on one leg, the result is a hopping *reaction*. One can demonstrate these responses quite easily to oneself by first standing upright and then trying to fall over deliberately by leaning over: at some point, however hard one tries not to, reflex stepping or *hopping* comes into play and actual falling is prevented. Incidentally, if you try to fall over backwards in this way, you will also observe an involuntary upward flexion of the

feet, as expected from the positive supporting reaction – though in these circumstances it is of no use whatever! It is also interesting to note that whereas in walking one is for most of the time in postural equilibrium – in the sense that one may 'freeze' at nearly any point of the walking cycle without falling over – this is not the case in running, when the centre of gravity is normally ahead of the support area. One can think of running as being a series of regular and almost unconscious stepping reactions in response to the bent-forward posture that the runner maintains.

Other responses, called *placing reactions*, are used for acquiring postural support when none is present. If a blindfolded animal is suspended in the air and brought up to a table until the edge touches the backs of its paws, it will bring them smartly up to rest on the top of the table, in turn evoking a positive supporting reaction: a similar response may be triggered if the animal's whiskers are brought to touch the table. These responses are, however, rather more complex then those described above, and probably involve the cerebral cortex: unlike the stepping and supporting reactions, they cannot be shown in decerebrate animals.

VESTIBULAR CONTRIBUTION TO POSTURE

The physiology of the vestibular apparatus was described in Chapter 5. We saw that it provided two separate types of information about the head: angular velocity from the semicircular canals, and attitude relative to the effective direction of gravity, from the otolith organs. From the point of view of the control of posture it is of course the *effective* direction of gravity rather than its 'real' direction that matters. What

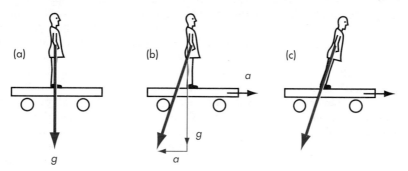

FIG. 11.5 Effective direction of gravity, and true vertical, defines a good upright posture. (a) Man standing on a stationary platform, with vertical acceleration *g* due to gravity. (b) If the platform accelerates horizontally, the effective direction of gravity, as sensed by his otolith organs, is the vector sum of *g* and *a*, the acceleration of the platform. (c) It is the projection of the centre of gravity along *this* direction that must now be brought between his feet if he is not to fall over.

determines, for instance, whether one falls over when standing in a bus that starts to accelerate is not the projection of the centre of gravity vertically relative to the critical area, but rather its projection in the direction of the vector formed by gravity and the horizontal linear acceleration acting together (Fig. 11.5), and this is what the utricle and saccule tell us. Each of these two divisions of the vestibular system gives rise to its own kinds of postural reactions, and so it is useful to distinguish between the *static* or *tonic* vestibular responses due to the otolith organs and the dynamic or phasic ones driven by the canals

The otolith organs produce on the whole rather less powerful postural responses than do the canals, particularly in higher animals. But in the long run they are the *only* source of information about the absolute position of the head in space, since the canals essentially signal only changes of position.

One of their main functions is in fact to keep the head upright despite changes in the position of the body, through appropriate changes in the tone of the neck muscles; these are the *head-righting reflexes*. If the head is forcibly tilted in different directions, so that the head-righting reflexes cannot operate, one can observe compensatory *static vestibulo-ocular reflexes* that similarly help to maintain the normal attitude of the eyes with respect to the outside world. In humans these eye reflexes cannot easily be demonstrated, and if the head is tilted to one side the resultant counter-rolling of the eyes is seldom of more than a few degrees and so cannot maintain the correct orientation of the retinal image. But in animals like the rabbit whose eyes essentially point sideways, tilting the head results in almost exact compensation over a wide range of angles (Fig. 11.6). While both these types of response obviously aid the sensory

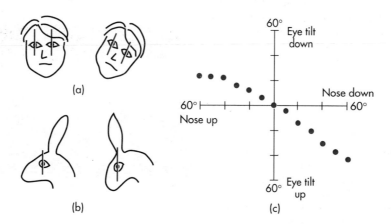

FIG. 11.6 Static vestibulo-ocular reflexes. Head tilt in humans (a) produces only a few degrees of ocular counter-rolling; in the rabbit (b), with its sideways-pointing eyes, vestibulo-ocular compensation is substantial over a wide range of angles (c). (Data from de Kleijn, 1921)

organs of the head by providing a stable 'platform' from which to operate, they are not of course strictly postural in the sense of contributing to the maintenance of equilibrium of the body as a whole.

Reactions which are truly postural in this sense may be quite easily demonstrated in conscious animals, and are called *tonic postural vestibular reflexes*. If an animal is suspended in the air, and its head and body tilted nose downwards (Fig. 11.7a), one observes extension of the front legs and retraction of the rear. Corresponding limb movements are found if the animal is tilted in other directions, for example to the side: in each case, there is extension of the limbs in the direction of downward tilt and retraction of the others. The function of this response is clear: if the animal is facing down a slope, this tonic vestibular response will assist the positive supporting reaction in shifting the centre of gravity backwards in relation to the feet, as may be seen in Figure 11.7.

Dynamic vestibular reactions

Because the canals are velocity-sensitive, they effectively give advance warning that one is *about* to fall over, possibly before the otolith organs have sensed that there is an actual error in head position. Perhaps for this reason, their responses are particularly fast, and generally bigger and more dramatic than the static vestibular reactions. The types of response they generate fall essentially into the same categories as the tonic ones: thus there is a dynamic component to the head-righting reflex that may be elicited by selective stimulation of the canals alone, and one may also demonstrate clear effects of canal stimulation on the eyes and limbs. If we seat someone on a rotating chair and record their eye movements (in the dark, so that there is no visual input to the oculomotor system), we find that the eyes move in the opposite direction to that of the head with a velocity that compensates almost exactly for the rotation, keeping the eyes stationary with respect to the outside world. Clearly this dynamic *vestibulo-ocular reflex* cannot go on indefinitely, since sooner or later the eyes are going to reach the limit of their rotation in the orbit: what in fact is observed is that the smooth counter-rotation in one direction is interrupted at more or less regular intervals by a quick flick in the other direction, giving rise to a sawtooth-like eye movement called *vestibular nystagmus* (Fig. 11.8). The smooth, compensatory movement is called the slow phase of the nystagmus, and the quick flick – which is essentially the same as an ordinary voluntary saccade – is called the quick phase; rather confusingly, it is the latter which is used in clinical practice to describe the direction of

nystagmus, so that a subject turning to the right produces what would be called a nystagmus to the right, even though the more important, functional component of the response is to the left. During rotation of this kind at constant angular velocity the response declines over a period of some 20 seconds or more on account of the natural adaptation of the canals (see Chapter 5), and so does the velocity of the slow phase. If the chair is suddenly stopped, so that the cupula is deflected in the opposite direction, a corresponding reversed nystagmus is seen which in turn declines with a time-course of some 20 seconds; these two types of nystagmus are respectively known as *per-rotatory and post-rotatory* nystagmus. Vestibular nystagmus provides a convenient means for clinical investigation of the functioning of the semicircular canals, since the eye movements produced by caloric stimulation (Chapter 5) of each of the two labyrinths may be examined separately to reveal imbalance of function on the two sides.

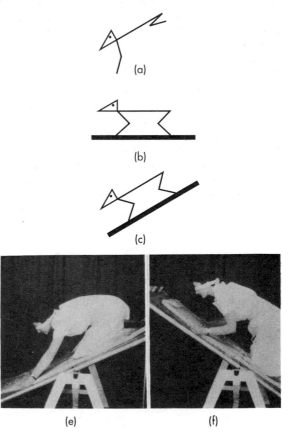

FIG. 11.7 Static vestibular righting reflexes. Tilting an animal's head and body nose-down (top) results in front-leg extension and rear-leg retraction; this response helps to produce a good posture when standing on a slope (b, c). Below, a human subject under similar conditions. (Martin, 1967)

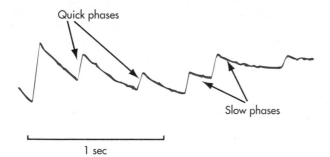

Quick phases

Slow phases

1 sec

FIG. 11.8 A record of human vestibular nystagmus, showing slow and quick phases.

Finally, dynamic *postural vestibular reflexes* exist, functionally equivalent to the static ones (head moving down gives front-leg extension, and so on), but much more powerful. In humans, unnatural stimulation of the canals may produce inappropriate postural responses that are vigorous enough to throw the subject to the floor – despite the action of all the other postural mechanisms in trying to keep him upright – as, for example,if one attempts to stand up after having been rotated in a revolving chair with one's head on one side for more than 20 seconds or so. The canals, because of their adaptation, then falsely signal that one is falling over: the consequent and extremely violent reflexes actually make one fall over, in the opposite direction.

VISUAL CONTRIBUTIONS TO POSTURE

The other receptors in the head that help maintain posture by providing information about head position are those of the retina. It turns out that there is a close parallel between the ways in which visual and vestibular information about head position are used in postural control, very probably because to a large extent they appear to share common pathways. One may again distinguish tonic effects from dynamic effects, and one also observes both effects on head and eye movements and also truly postural responses involving the limbs.

Static visual responses

In so-called civilized surroundings, such as an urban street, our visual world is largely made up of horizontal and vertical elements, and our expectations about their orientation mean that we can in principle

use our eyes to estimate head position. Many experiments have demonstrated that this tonic visual information is indeed used in making postural judgements and responses, and if subjects are seated on a tilting chair inside a dummy room which can itself be titled to various angles (Fig. 11.9), it is found that their sense of the upright direction generally lies somewhere between the true upright and the apparent upright of the room. However, it is not entirely obvious that information of this sort was very readily available in the more natural surroundings – jungles and so forth – in which this ability presumably evolved: perhaps it is entirely learnt.

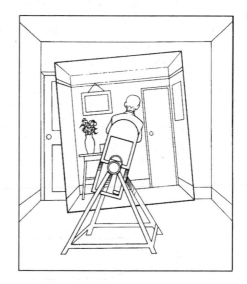

FIG. 11.9 Experiment with tilting room and tilting chair, to investigate relative visual and vestibular contribution to the sense of being upright. (Walsh, 1964, after Witkin, 1949)

Dynamic visual responses

We have already seen in Chapter 7 that one division of the visual system, the *visual proprioceptive system*, has neurones that are specialized in responding to movement of the retinal image across the retina. If a sufficient number of these cells fire off simultaneously – in other words, if most of the visual field is in motion – the brain assumes, logically enough, that the world is in fact stationary and that it is the eye that is moving. This sense of self-movement is a very powerful one, as anyone who has had the experience of sitting in a train at a station while a neighbouring train moves off will agree. However, misleading circumstances like these are most infrequent in nature, and by and large when most of the visual field moves it is indeed because the head has moved relative to the visual surroundings, providing information that supplements what is provided by the semicircular canals, and is used in the same way to generate postural and oculomotor responses. Experiments in which victims are required to stand in seemingly normal rooms whose walls are then suddenly moved can be made to stumble and fall, even though the ground has remained still. A visit to a 'surround' cinema can be instructive: look at your neighbours during the sickening turns of the switchback ride and you will see them swaying about in helpless unison.

Movement of the visual field also generates eye movements that are extremely similar to the dynamic vestibulo-ocular reflexes. If we seat someone in front of a rotating striped drum, close enough for it to fill a substantial part of his visual field, the result is a sawtooth-like movement of the eyes called *optokinetic nystagmus*, in which the eyes follow the moving stripes during the slow phase, and flick back again during the quick phase. One might think that this was merely the result of a conscious decision by the subject to track the stripes with his eyes but this is not so, as in fact if the subject tries very hard to keep his eyes still and ignore the movement, the nystagmus is nevertheless still observed, and indeed is in some ways more pronounced and more regular.

How does the eye tell us about head movement?

Now movement of the retinal image does not really tell us about head movement. Strictly, it can tell us only that an image of an object in the outside world has moved relative to the retina, and cannot say whether this was because the object itself moved, because the eye moved relative to the head, or because head and eye moved together. We have already seen that movements of large areas of the visual field are generally interpreted by the brain as being due to movement of oneself rather than of the world around us. But from the point of view of controlling posture, it is obviously very important to be able to disentangle the effects of movement of the head from those of movements of the eye, since it is the former that we really want to know about. How is this done? For a long time there were two rival theories. One, due to Sherrington, was that spindles in the eye muscles sent signals to the visual system telling it where the eye was in the orbit; this estimate of eye position relative to the head – call it E_H – could then in effect be subtracted from the estimate of eye position relative to visual space (E_S) provided by the visual system to generate an estimate of head

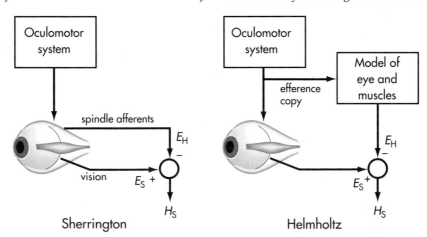

Sherrington   Helmholtz

FIG. 11.10 The sense of eye position. Left, Sherrington's scheme: proprioceptors in eye muscles provide information about the position of the eye in the head (E_H), and this is then compared with visual information concerning the position of the eye relative to the visual world (E_S) to give H_S, the position of the head in space. Right, in Helmholtz's scheme, a copy of the oculomotor commands is used to calculate, from knowledge of the behaviour of the eye on past occasions, the expected value of E_H: this is then combined with E_S as before, to give H_S.

position in space, H_S (Fig. 11.10). Helmholtz, however, argued that it was unnecessary to have receptors in the eye muscles to tell one the position of one's eyes. Since the eyes are never subject to external forces in the way that our limbs are, we can always deduce their position from the motor commands that we send to them; so Helmholtz suggested that a copy of the oculomotor commands – *efference copy* – was sent to the visual system to provide the required estimate of E_H. This theory, called the *outflow* theory in contradistinction to Sherrington's *inflow* theory, is supported by a number of pieces of experimental evidence. One of them is something you can do yourself: if you press on the side of your right eye with the left one shut, you will perceive an illusory movement of the outside world. This is exactly what would be expected from Helmholtz's model but is not easy to explain with the inflow theory, since the muscle spindles ought still to be providing the necessary information to cancel the signal produced by the movement of the retinal image. More convincingly, if the oculomotor commands are prevented from carrying out their usual effects on the eye muscles – for example, by some pathological condition affecting the oculomotor nerves or the eye muscles, or by artificial paralysis induced by local application of drugs like curare – then we would expect that every time the subject *tried* to make an eye movement, the E_H signal resulting from the efference copy would no longer be matched by the usual E_S signals from the retina, and the subject should therefore perceive an illusory movement of the visual world in the opposite direction; and this is precisely what is found. It seems therefore that efference copy is indeed the means by which the postural system can work out E_S, the position of the head in visual space, from the purely visual signal E_H.

Vestibular and visual interactions

We now have two quite different estimates of the position of the head in space, one provided by the vestibular apparatus, and one by the visual system. These two signals complement one another almost uncannily. The vestibular signal is extremely fast but not very accurate because the hair cells tend to suffer from low-frequency noise; the visual signals, on the other, are much slower (reaction times of the order of 150–200 msec) but potentially hugely accurate, limited only by the size of the retinal receptors. How are these two signals combined? And what happens if they conflict with one another?

Recordings from the vestibular nuclei show that most neurones here respond appropriately to optokinetic as well as vestibular stimulation, their response being roughly the sum of the two. In addition, under steady stimulation the optokinetic stimulus increases with a time-course that exactly complements the decline in the vestibular signal that is due to adaptation of the canals. We saw earlier, in the tilting room experiment, that in fact the brain seems to take something like the weighted mean of these two estimates of head position in arriving at a final answer. This in turn raises the interesting question of how one type of information is *calibrated* in terms of the other. How does the brain know that one particular rate of firing of certain fibres in the vestibular nerve is equivalent to such-and-such a rate of firing of a movement-sensitive neurone in the visual system?

The answer seems to be that this correlation of the two inputs is one that is *learnt* by the brain as the result of experience, and that in fact the signals from the vestibular system are continually being checked against, and calibrated by, the signals from the eye: a good example of *parametric feedback* of the kind described in Chapter 9. If the vestibulo-ocular reflex is not working properly, this will show up as slippage of the image across the retina when the head moves; this error signal is then used to make corrective adjustments in the vestibular response. Wearing spectacles, for instance, causes a change in the magnification of the retinal image which means that vestibulo-ocular reflexes that were previously just the right size to keep the image stationary despite head movement are now incorrectly matched. But within a very short period of time the reflexes are modified by parametric feedback so that they operate correctly. Even more dramatically, if a man wears prisms in front of his eyes that effectively reverse his visual field, so that an object moving from left to right appears to him to be moving from right to left, one finds that after a surprisingly short space of time – a matter of days – his vestibulo-ocular reflexes follow suit by reversing as well, even when measured in the dark.

A similar kind of long-term adaptation can be seen after unilateral damage to the vestibular apparatus. You may recall that vestibular fibres are tonically active but that central neurones in the vestibular nuclei are excited by afferents from one side and inhibited by those from the other, so that at rest in the normal subject the tonic activity cancels itself out. So unilateral damage leads to an imbalance in the vestibular signals coming from each side, for the tonic discharge from one side is now unopposed by that from the other. The result is a false sense of rotation (giddiness) combined with postural reactions, and spontaneous vestibular nystagmus. However, these effects gradually decline, and in a matter of weeks may have disappeared altogether. This seems to be because the visual system has informed the central vestibular pathways that the signals are false, resulting in some kind of tonic shift of activity that once again cancels out the continual signals from the unaffected side. That this is so may be demonstrated by subsequently cutting the vestibular nerve on the good side. Despite the fact that there is now no vestibular system at all the result is a nystagmus (*Bechterew* nystagmus) in the opposite direction to the first, presumably resulting from the central tonic activity that had been set up to correct the original imbalance; and this in turn gradually declines. This plasticity appears to be controlled by the cerebellum, the vestibular division of which (the flocculonodular lobe) is supplied with fibres both from the vestibular apparatus and from the visual system. This cerebellar mechanism is discussed more fully in Chapter 12, where it will be seen that it is a specific example of a general function of the cerebellum in learning motor responses to stimuli.

Conflicts between visual and vestibular information about head position and movement also tend to give rise to *motion sickness*. It is a matter of common experience that motion sickness is most likely to occur when our vestibular system tells us we're moving but the visual field appears stationary. In a car one may feel perfectly well as long as one is looking out of the window, when visual and vestibular estimates of head movement match, but feel sick when trying to read, when the visual field moves with the head and the two sources of information conflict with one another. One may also feel motion sickness under precisely the opposite conditions. Sitting near the cinema screen, watching something like *Moby Dick* with its storm-tossed seas and heaving decks, our eyes tell us we are moving up and down but our canals insist that we are stationary; the result is nausea. Removal of the vestibulocerebellum in dogs is said to eliminate motion sickness entirely, presumably because it is in this region that the correlation of the two kinds of input is made.

Incidentally, it seems also that the nausea sometimes associated with alcohol intoxication is also, in effect, a kind of motion sickness. One of the effects of alcohol is to alter the relative density of the cupula and endolymph in the canals, so that they are no longer exactly equal. This means that the cupula is influenced by gravity – becomes, in effect, an otolith – and is deflected by static head position as well as by angular velocity. Under these conditions one may see what is called a *positional* nystagmus, a nystagmus that occurs spontaneously when the head is held in different positions. It is a matter of common experience that one of the effects of overindulgence can be a sense of giddiness, particularly on changing head position, and if one goes to lie down there may often be a sensation of the bed turning head over heels.

NECK REFLEXES

So we need to know the position of the eye in the head before we can use vision to tell us about head position in space; but in exactly the same way we need to know the position of the head relative to the body (H_B) before we can use information about the position of the head in space (H_S) to tell us how our body is situated (B_S). And B_S is the variable that we need to know about to control posture since, as has been repeatedly emphasized, postural control is all about keeping the centre of gravity of the *body* in the right relationship to its supports. Whether the *head* is upright actually matters rather little.

This signal, H_B, comes from proprioceptors in the neck, mostly joint receptors around the vertebrae. Since H_B must be subtracted from H_S in order to produce B_S, we would expect the effects of bending the neck on its own to be as powerful as, and in the opposite sense to, the postural effects of changing the position of the head in space described earlier. This is found to be approximately true: the resultant responses are the *tonic neck reflexes* (Fig. 11.11). Thus

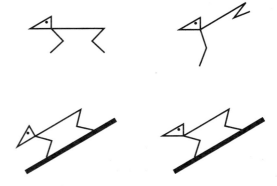

Fig. 11.11 Tonic neck reflex: if an animal is suspended with its head horizontal, dorsiflexion of the head (by tilting the back up) results in front-leg extension and rear-leg retraction (compare Fig. 11.7). Below, this means that if an animal has its body tilted downwards, then whatever the position of the head, there will still be a postural drive to right itself: if the head is horizontal, this is because the head is dorsiflexed; if there is no neck flexion, because the head is tilted downwards.

if an animal's vestibular system is destroyed, and its head moved about while the body is suspended horizontally, we find that tilting the head up – resulting in dorsiflexion of the neck – gives front-leg extension and back-leg retraction. This, as you will recall, was the vestibular effect of tilting the head down. Thus corresponding to the vestibular mnemonic 'head down, front legs extend' we have the neck reflex mnemonic 'dorsiflexion, front legs extend'. As in the case of the vestibular reflexes, moving the head in other directions produces exactly analogous limb responses.

The use of these reflexes in maintaining posture is clear. If an animal is standing facing down a slope, this time with its head in the normal horizontal position so that there is no vestibular stimulation, the result is exactly the same as if the head were pointing down. In fact, the animal will produce the same correct postural response *whatever* the position of the head. This consequence of the opposition of vestibular and neck reflexes is a very important one: if it were not so, then every time a cow tried to bend down to eat some grass, its front legs would extend, neatly frustrating its endeavours.

This is why, although the head is the single most important source of information about body position, nevertheless it can still move around freely without producing inappropriate postural responses. It is exactly analogous to the mechanism described earlier that permits us to move our eyes around without at the same time perceiving apparent shifts of the visual world.

POSTURE AS A WHOLE

Figure 11.12 is intended to summarize this chapter by bringing together the various sources of postural information and the way they interact in a hierarchical scheme that helps illustrate the parallels between the modes of operation of many of its parts. It is obvious that the scheme is highly redundant, in the sense that there are three separate channels from which B_S, body position in space, can be deduced. In fact, it is clear that one can manage without any one of them,

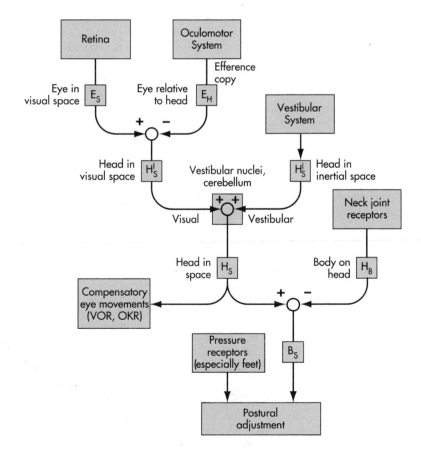

FIG. 11.12 Summary scheme of the sources of information used in the control of posture, and their interrelations.

or even two, without completely losing one's ability to make postural adjustments. When swimming underwater, for example, only our vestibular system can provide us with information about body position; and in fact, although patients with bilateral destruction of their vestibular apparatus can get about perfectly well in normal life by using the senses in their eyes and feet, it is precisely in circumstances like swimming underwater or running over a ploughed field that they may no longer be able to respond satisfactorily. But performance is always impaired by loss of one of the inputs. A simple sign of vestibular malfunction is simply to ask the subject to stand, and then to close their eyes. Most people sway around a little more as a result, especially if standing on something soft; with vestibular impairment, the additional instability is very marked.

Though one can get along without any one of these sources of information, a sufficiently strong stimulation of one of the inputs can cause disequilibrium despite the correct functioning of the other two. As already mentioned, we may be thrown to the ground by our own vestibular reflexes after a spin in a revolving chair, and misleading visual information may similarly make us fall over if we stand looking up at the clouds.

Finally, there is another source of information that is not sensory at all but the result of another kind of efference copy: feedforward rather than feedback. Many of our voluntary actions are themselves threats to equilibrium, as for example if we pick up a heavy object and then throw it, or even for that matter as we simply walk along. In these cases the threat can of course be anticipated, and postural compensations initiated even before the disequilibrium has been sensed by the afferent pathways shown in Figure 11.12. A striking example of this kind of learnt postural response is the transient jolt one feels on stepping on to an escalator that has been turned off and is therefore stationary, representing a temporary failure to suppress the normal, learnt postural reaction to the sudden movement of the feet that would occur if the escalator were actually working.

References

de Kleijn, A. (1921) Tonische Labyrinth- und Halsreflexe auf die Augen. *Pflügers Archiv* 186, 82–97.

Martin, J. P. (1967) *The Basal Ganglia and Posture*. Pitman, London.

Rademaker, G. G. J. (1935) *Réactions Labyrinthiques et Équilibre. L'ataxie Labyrinthique*. Masson, Paris.

Walsh, E. G. (1964) *Physiology of the Nervous System*. Longmans, London.

Witkin, H. A. (1949) Perception of body position and the position of the visual field. *Psychological Monographs* 302 (3), 1–46.

NOTES

A very intelligent account of posture, with many interesting examples (but long out of print), is Roberts, T. D. M. (1967) *The Neurophysiology of Postural Mechanisms* (Butterworths, London). Rothwell, J. C. (1993) *Control of Human Voluntary Movement* (Chapman and Hall, London) has a more up-to-date, but less full account. Sherrington, C. S. (1906) *The Integrative Action of the Nervous System*. (Yale University Press, New Haven, Conn) is a classic description of some basic responses, of some historical interest.

Page 220 Dynamic visual posture It is probably the main explanation for the postural instability associated with *heights:* if one is standing at ground level in a typical urban environment, most of one's visual field is filled with highly detailed visual texture, and the slightest head movement is likely to cause a brisk response from movement-detecting visual neurones. But on top of a high building, things are very different. Most of the field is now occupied by clouds and sky, of low contrast and low spatial frequency, so that movements of the head are no longer so likely to be noticed by the visual system; the consequence is an increased instability, a tendency to sway about. Worse still, if one looks up, one's visual field is likely to contain nothing but the clouds moving past, which therefore give the visual system the illusion that one is falling over: the resulting postural compensation may well result in one actually falling over in the opposite direction.

Page 222 Motion sickness The most comprehensive account is Reason, J. T. and Brand, J. J. (1975) *Motion Sickness* (Academic, London). Nausea can occur even with quite mild visual/vestibular mismatch, for instance on putting on an unfamiliar pair of spectacles, when the slight degree of magnification or minification they produce temporarily upsets the natural relation between head movement and retinal slip.

Page 222 Alcohol and the cupula It has been reported that the ingestion of heavy water may provide an instant antidote, by restoring cupular density, but it is obviously important to titrate accurately. See Money, K. E. and Myles, W. S. (1974) Heavy water nystagmus and effects of alcohol. *Nature* 247, 404–405.

NEUROLAB

 ## Postural stability

Page 216, 218, 223

A stick-creature with endearingly well-developed postural responses, on a terrain whose tilt can be modified by the control called Slope. You can use the check boxes to turn any one of the three sources mentioned on or off, and you can move the head. Look at positive supporting on its own, and the improvement that comes from having vestibular information as well. See for yourself the severe disadvantage of having no neck reflexes when you move your head, especially in the absence of the positive supporting reaction.

 ## Eye movements

Page 218, 220

This exhibit shows examples of various kinds of eye movements: its general operation has already been described, in Chapter 9, p. 198. Here, you may like to look at optokinetic and vestibular nystagmus. The duration of the stimulus for both of these is indicated by the red trace, with the eye movement in green. The vestibular stimulus is a period of rotation at constant velocity, followed by a sudden cessation. Per- and post-rotatory nystagmus are seen, the slow-phase velocity and the frequency of the nystagmus gradually declining as the canals adapt. With optokinetic stimulation at constant velocity, the slow phase accelerates quite rapidly (in humans) to a steady value, and stops almost instantly when the stimulus stops. You may also like to look at the demonstration of fixation movements, instructions for which are provided on-screen. The wandering is due to a large extent to low-frequency noise in the vestibulo-ocular reflex, interrupted by microsaccades when the eye moves too far from the target. Go back to the main screen and select Fixation, then start a sweep: the relationship between the slow noise (drift) and the microsaccades should be obvious.

Parametric feedback

Page 221

This exhibit shows the functioning of parametric feedback in the vestibulo-ocular reflex. Start by selecting the Dark button. The head is moving sinusoidally from side to side: its window shows the time-course, and the one on the right shows the resultant eye movement. As it is dark, there is no visual stimulation, and we are looking at the VOR on its own. At top right, head movement is shown together with gaze, the direction of the eye in space. In the dark, the gain (the ratio of output to input, in this case eye movement amplitude divided by head movement amplitude) is a little less than one, so that the gaze is not in fact stationary. Now select Visual assistance. Additional windows appear with the target movement (none) and the degree of retinal slip: because of the extra visual information, gaze is now held steady. Now select Visual suppression: this is equivalent to making the visual world move with the head, so that the VOR actually generates retinal slip instead of being useful. Very quickly, this retinal slip changes the VOR gain to zero, so that gaze moves with the head as it should. A more extreme perturbation is Reversing prisms, which invert the visual world from left to right. This introduces very large visual slip at first, which acts to drive the VOR gain so far down that it actually reverses: now when the head moves to the right, the eyes do too (as they now need to do). Finally, Magnifying lens and Minifying lens are milder stimuli, in which only a small degree of gain adjustment is needed to match the visual and vestibular signals: adaptation is complete relatively quickly. The learning mechanism can be turned on and off with the check box.

12 GLOBAL MOTOR CONTROL

Motor cortex 226
Cerebellum 231

Basal ganglia 238

We must now consider the levels of the motor system at which detailed information from the special senses first begins to be important: in ascending hierarchical order, they are the cerebral motor cortex, the cerebellum, and the basal ganglia.

MOTOR CORTEX

By the middle of the last century, there was an increasing interest in the interactions between electricity and living tissues, and particularly in the kinds of responses that could be obtained by electrical stimulation of the central nervous system. It turned out that there was a conveniently accessible region in the middle of the cerebral cortex where stimulation evoked reproducible movements of parts of the opposite side of the body; since no other area of the cortex generated movements on stimulation, this region was called the motor cortex. At about the same time, the English neurologist Hughlings Jackson had been studying the relation between paralysis of different parts of the body due to stroke, and the post-mortem location of the associated cerebral lesions. He was also interested in a special variety of epilepsy called Jacksonian epilepsy in which there are characteristic motor signs, such as spontaneous twitching, that start at one particular location – often an extremity such as a finger tip – and then move progressively and systematically, for example up the hand and arm, until they culminate in a more generalized convulsion. Putting these two types of observation together, he suggested that the progress of the epileptic signs over the body was the result of a 'march' of the region of pathological abnormality over the cortex itself. This is now known to be perfectly correct. An epileptic focus of overactivity in one cortical region tends to spread to the regions with

which it communicates, a fact of importance in trying to treat epilepsy by surgical means.

The orderly representation of parts of the body in the cortex was wholly confirmed when accurate motor maps were made by investigators such as Sherrington in the monkey, and later by Penfield and others in human patients in the course of operations to treat Jacksonian epilepsy. This area, the *primary motor area*, lies just in front of the central sulcus (Figure 12.1), and corresponds to Brodmann's cytoarchitectonic area 4. It thus lies alongside the primary somatosensory projection area (areas 3, 2, and 1), and indeed, shows a similar distribution of the representation of different parts of the body. Some regions of the body, such as the hands and mouth, have a disproportionately larger representation than others in this motor homunculus: a possible reason for this will be considered later. Next to area 4 lies another motor area 6, often called the *premotor* area, and in humans some five or six times larger than area 4 itself. There is also a quite separate secondary motor area (called MII, the first being MI; it is also known as the *supplementary* motor area or SMA: Figure 12.1) which, like the corresponding sensory area SII, is more bilaterally organized than the strictly contralateral MI.

At this point we need to break off in order to consider the neural structure of the cerebral cortex in general. In most mammals by far the largest part of the cortex is neocortex, a sheet made up of six layers of cells and fibres (Figure 12.2) and elaborately wrinkled into the complex pattern of sulci and gyri that enables a large surface area to be stuffed into a relatively small volume. The main output from the cortex comes from the large *pyramidal cells* of layer V, forming what are known as the projection efferents, that go to subcortical destinations. The dendrites of these pyramidal cells extend vertically as well as branching sideways, so that the cells are capable of being

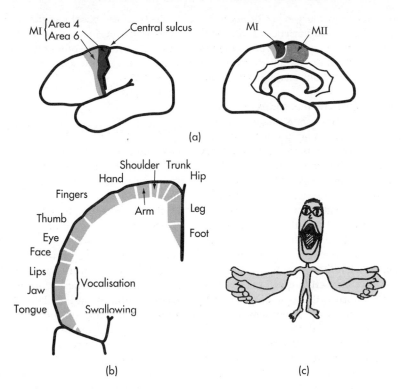

FIG. 12.1 **(a)** Lateral and medial views of human brain, showing the approximate positions of motor cortex, areas MI and MII. **(b)** Transverse section through MI, showing the distributions of areas devoted to different parts of the body. **(c)** Motor homunculus (compare the corresponding sensory homunculus, Figure 4.8). (Partly after Penfield and Rasmussen, 1950)

influenced by all layers of the cortex, within a radius of half a millimetre or so. Corresponding to the projection efferents, on the input side there are the specific projection afferents of subcortical origin (mostly in fact from the thalamus) that ramify into large terminal trees around layers III and IV.

However, in a sense the whole point of the cortex is to bring many diverse types of input and output into functional association, and to a large extent this is brought about by associational neurones having cell bodies in layer III of one cortical area, that send off axons terminating in vertical columns in some other

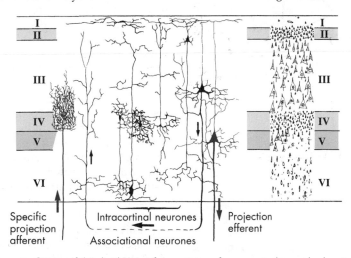

FIG. 12.2 Diagrammatic representation of the distribution of some types of neurone in the cerebral cortex, and their principal connections. On the left, afferent systems and on the right, efferent. Far right, the general histological appearance of the six layers.

area. In addition to these primary types of neurone, there is also a host of different varieties of interneurone that communicate from layer to layer as well as horizontally, many of which are inhibitory in nature and probably carry out functions analogous to lateral inhibition.

It is important to appreciate that cortex and thalamus work together very much as a single unit, and that the latter is not merely a relay for fibres on their way to the cortex but receives back from the cortex almost as many fibres as it sends there. Two thalamic nuclei are paired in this way with the cortical motor areas (Figure 12.3): they are the *ventrolateral nucleus*, which projects mostly to area 4 and receives fibres back from both area 4 and the somatosensory cortex; and the *ventroanterior nucleus*, which projects to area 6 and receives reciprocal connections from both area 4 and area 6. Unlike, for example, the ventroposterior nucleus, which sends spinal information to the somatosensory cortex, the ascending input to the motor nuclei of the thalamus is not sensory at all but comes partly from the basal ganglia and cerebellum and partly from the reticular formation; these regions also project to the more diffuse centromedial thalamic nuclei, which communicate more widely with both somatosensory and motor cortex, and other areas as well. These relationships are summarized in Figure 12.3. The output from the sensorimotor regions is diverse: some of course makes up the corticospinal tract, some can reach the cord indirectly via the red nucleus and the nucleus gigantocellularis of the reticular formation, but most

projects to the basal ganglia and – via relays in the pons and inferior olive – to the cerebellum. These indirect routes are sometimes lumped together under the heading of *extrapyramidal* pathways, those outputs that do not simply go straight down into the spinal cord.

Corticospinal concepts

Now area 4 is differentiated from all other areas of the cortex by having a number of particularly big cells in layer V, the giant *Betz cells*. Their size suggests that they might be the origin of the corticospinal tract, and for a long time the notion was current that the essence of the voluntary motor system was something like what is shown in Figure 12.4, with 'volition' triggering off in some way the Betz cells of area 4, which in turn synapsed directly with spinal motor neurones. The former were called the 'upper motor neurones' and the latter the 'lower motor neurones', with the implication that the effects of stimulating the motor cortex were entirely due to stimulation of the cortical tract. This is an unhelpful and misleading picture in a number of ways. In the first place, it is clear that the Betz cells are not the sole origin of the corticospinal tract: for one thing, the latter contains about a million fibres, whereas there are only some 30 000 Betz cells. It is not even true that the tract comes only from the motor cortex: in primates about 30 per cent comes from area 4, another 30 per cent from area 6, and the rest from more posterior areas, somatosensory and parietal. Nor is it true that the effects of cortical stimulation are even mainly due to activation of corticospinal fibres. If in the monkey one traces the motor map by electrical stimulation both before and then after completely severing the pyramidal tract, the distribution of responses is found to be essentially unchanged (though they may tend to be a little slower and require a larger current to be evoked). And finally, as we have already seen, even in the primates only some of the corticospinal fibres end directly on motor neurones, while in other species none do: cortical control is probably rather of spinal circuits than of individual muscle units. The corticospinal tract is not a particularly rapid conduction route: some 5% are unmyelinated in humans, and of the myelinated fibres, 90% of the fibres are quite small, with diameters around 1–4μm.

Lesions of the corticospinal tract give similar, but not identical, effects to lesions of the cortex itself: generally some hypotonia and weakness (paresis), but more specifically loss of skilled movements, particularly of extremities such as the fingers as in picking up a small object. Lesions of area 4 are in

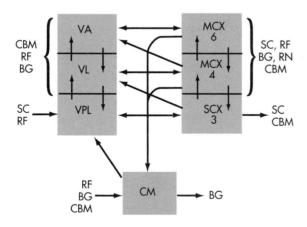

FIG. 12.3 Stylized representation of the main connections of motor cortex and thalamus. Cortical regions: MCX, motor; SCX, somatosensory. Thalamic nuclei: VA, ventroanterior; VL, ventrolateral; VPL, ventral posterolateral; CM, centromedian. Other regions: CBM, cerebellum; BG, basal ganglia; RF, reticular formation; SC, spinal cord; RN, red nucleus.

general rather more severe, resulting at first in a wholly flaccid paralysis, and typically in greater functional loss than pyramidal section by itself. There are certain difficulties of interpretation, however, both by reason of the marked species variation that is seen – a cat can still apparently run about after complete resection of its pyramids – and also because gradual (though variable) recovery is a feature of lesions of both cortex and pyramidal tract. In time, the immediate flaccidity resulting from a lesion in area 4 usually develops into a spasticity, presumably through some kind of release phenomenon. Lesions that are large enough to encroach on area 6 as well as 4 also tend to produce spasticity, which might be interpreted as suggesting that area 6 has some kind of tonic inhibitory action, a notion reinforced by observations of the effects of stimulating area 6 during voluntary or evoked movements. At all events, the classic clinical description is that an 'upper motor lesion' gives a spastic paralysis, without muscle wasting, while a 'lower motor lesion' produces a flaccid paralysis and degeneration of muscles.

Another associated early misconception was that the upper motor neurones coded for movements rather than for individual muscles, and that the translation from one to the other was a function of the manner in which the descending axons were distributed within the cord. It is certainly true that if extracellular electrodes are used to elicit movements by electrical stimulation of the motor cortex, then even at threshold one tends to observe not isolated twitches from separate muscles but the simultaneous and apparently co-ordinated contraction of several muscles at once. But it is now clear that this is essentially because the current from extracellular electrodes of this kind spreads out over a wide area of cortex, and that one cannot avoid stimulating large numbers of pyramidal cells and interneurones simultaneously, even at the threshold for overt movement. More recent work with intracellular electrodes indicates clearly that the effect of stimulating one pyramidal tract neurone is the excitation of only one muscle at a time, either directly (most obviously in humans) or via the specific facilitation (or sometimes inhibition) of one particular stretch reflex. There is also a systematic representation of muscles in the cortex, analogous to that found in somatosensory or visual cortex, with a grouping of neurones corresponding to synergistic muscles in columns; it is presumably for this reason that extracellular stimulation gives the appearance of co-ordinated activation of synergists. A reverse mapping of pyramidal cells making monosynaptic connections with individual motor neurones in the monkey shows them to be distributed typically over an area of some 10 mm in diameter.

Co-ordination of somatosensory input with motor output

One of the most interesting findings comes from using the same microelectrode for recording as well as stimulation. What is found is that pyramidal cells have very wide, multimodal receptive fields, from joint receptors and tendon organs as well as skin receptors, and with a small representation of spindle afferents as well. If one looks at the relationship between what any particular cell does when it is stimulated and what it actually responds to, it is striking that frequently the cutaneous receptive fields represent areas of skin that are normally brought into contact with one another when that particular muscle contracts (Figure 12.5), and are found to be most active during precision grip rather than power grip. This suggests rather strongly that the cortex is the site of the kinds of sensorimotor correlation that are obviously necessary whenever grasping or touching or some other *manipulation* is being performed.

That this is perhaps the most important single function of the motor cortex is suggested also by the relative sizes of different parts of the body in the motor map. In humans, only two areas of the body are used to any large extent for tasks of this kind that

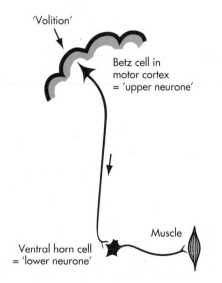

FIG. 12.4 Classic but misleading concept of 'upper' and 'lower' motor neurone.

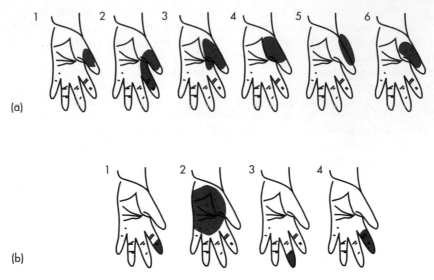

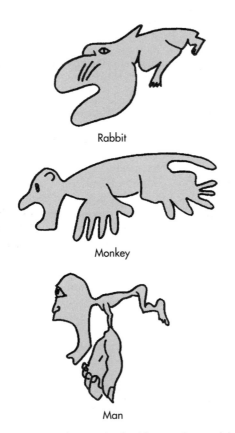

FIG. 12.5 Cutaneous sensory fields associated with pyramidal cells of monkey causing **(a)** thumb flexion, and **(b)** digital flexion on stimulation. The cutaneous fields correspond with areas that would be brought into contact by resultant movement. (After Rosen and Asanuma, 1972)

FIG. 12.6 Motor homunculi of rabbit, monkey and human, showing differences in the relative degree representation of different regions (highly schematic). Partly after Woolsey, 1958)

require accurate feedback from the skin, namely the hands and the mouth; and both of these together form by far the greatest proportion of the motor map. In the monkey, which makes more use of its feet for handling objects, they have almost as large a representation as the hands, and relatively much larger than in humans. In most four-footed animals it is only the mouth and lips that are used for grasping and exploration, and their representation is correspondingly enlarged (Figure 12.6); virtually the whole of the pig's motor cortex is said to be devoted to its snout! It is also perhaps significant that lesions in area 6 – which we saw to be predominantly inhibitory in effect – often produce uninhibited grasping of the kind frequently observed in very young children: any object touched against the palm results in immediate forceful seizure, with an unwillingness to let go. Destruction of the motor cortex also abolishes the tactile placing reaction described in Chapter 11.

One further function of the cortex, of a related kind, is probably the generation of the 'expected force' commands that were described in Chapter 10. We saw there that these commands need to be adjusted to match the load that is to be encountered, and that one source of information about load that seems to be used to do this comes from pressure receptors in the skin; tendon organs, which as we have seen also project to pyramidal cells, are another likely source of information about load (see Figure 10.14). Could the pyramidal tract fibres be the route by which force commands are sent to the spinal cord?

They certainly have the right kinds of information at their disposal to carry out such a function, and also appear to give the expected effects of facilitating stretch reflexes when stimulated. And if one records from the pyramidal tract of a conscious freely moving animal, and observes the circumstances under which pyramidal fibres actually fire during voluntary movements, one finds that whereas the correlation between pyramidal activity and muscle length or velocity is poor, there is a clear correlation between frequency of firing and the *force* that is being produced at any moment to generate the movement, suggesting very strongly that this tract does indeed provide force commands.

Finally, we have seen that the effect of lesions to motor cortex or pyramidal tract is not just a loss of the kinds of skilled movements that require close co-ordination between skin sensation and movement, but also a general weakness of the muscles, with a correspondingly increased sense of effort on the part of the patient. Sense of effort seems to be found in situations where the gain of stretch reflexes is insufficient, for example in the experiments of Figure 10.13 when the pressure receptors in the subject's thumb were blocked by local anaesthesia, and may well be associated with voluntary excitation of motor cortex neurones. Partial paralysis tends to result in an apparent increase in the heaviness of a weight being lifted.

If it is true that the main function of the motor cortex is a relatively simple co-ordination between skin and other spinal afferents and the gain of stretch reflexes, one might well wonder why this function has to be carried out in the cortex and not in the cord itself, where the inputs and outputs actually are. Why bother to go all the way up to the top of the head? There are probably two reasons why the spinal cord is essentially unsuited to the task. The first is that most spinal reflexes seem to be organized in a segmental manner. But the feedback from skin receptors resulting from contraction of a particular muscle will not always return to the cord via the dorsal roots of the same segment; in the cortex, however, information from different segments is brought into much closer approximation, and the large amount of convergence and divergence – in the monkey, each pyramidal cell receives some 60 000 synapses – means that connections from different inputs can presumably be attached more easily to their appropriate muscles, rather as subscribers' lines converge on a telephone exchange.

The second point is that it is difficult to see how appropriate connections could ever be set up in the cord in the first place: how can an incoming sensory fibre from the skin know which of the hundreds of thousands of ventral horn cells are the ones to which it is supposed to make contact? It seems much more likely that such connections are established through *experience,* by frequent association of stimulation of a particular afferent with contraction of a particular muscle. This implies a richness and flexibility of connections, an ability to form functional contacts as the result of experience, that the cortex seems specifically adapted to perform, through memory-like mechanisms of association, discussed in Chapter 13. Lesions in the supplementary motor area seem to cause a specific detriment in internally generated movements made from purely motor memory, though the animal can still learn the same movements in response to external signals.

Finally, it should not be forgotten that if it is convenient for the control of movement to have cutaneous information readily available in areas 1, 2 and 3 right next door to the motor cortex, it is equally important in analysing cutaneous sensations to have information immediately on hand about what movements are being executed. It was emphasized in Chapter 4 that such common sensations as softness, resilience, roughness, stickiness, and the like rely on knowledge of what forces are being applied to the surface in question by the motor system, knowledge that is easily supplied by pyramidal tract neurones through the rich interconnections between the two cortical areas. In human patients, electrical stimulation of the motor cortex produces sensory effects not very different from those resulting from stimulation of the somatosensory cortex: numbness, tingling, and a sense of movement which may or may not be accompanied by actual movement; if it is, the subject feels that he has been 'made' to carry out the action by the experimenter rather than 'wanting' to make it.

CEREBELLUM

The cerebellum and basal ganglia are, very broadly speaking, at a higher hierarchical level in the motor system than the cortex, in the sense that when they go wrong they tend to produce disorders of function, sometimes of a subtle kind, rather than discrete paralysis or weakness. We have already seen that anatomically they are considerably further from the final output, in that they send no fibres directly into the spinal cord. They are also older structures than neocortex, prominent in all vertebrates; in birds and reptiles the motor cortex or its equivalent does not appear to exist, so that one is forced to conclude that

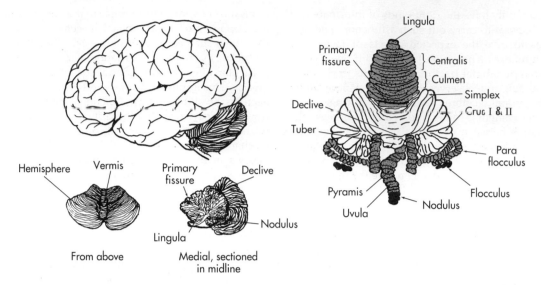

Hemisphere   Vermis   Primary fissure   Declive

Nodulus

Lingula

From above

Medial, sectioned in midline

Lingula

Primary fissure

Centralis

Culmen

Declive

Simplex

Tuber

Crus I & II

Para flocculus

Pyramis

Flocculus

Uvula

Nodulus

FIG. 12.7 Gross structure of the cerebellum. Left, viewed from various directions, and in sagittal section. Right, 'unrolled', showing the main anatomical divisions. Functionally, it may be divided into vestibulocerebellum (black), spinocerebellum (colour) and neo-cerebellum (unshaded), though the divisions are not as clearcut as this diagram implies.

the cortex has developed more for *refining* actions than for generating them in the first place.

The cerebellum seems to have grown out of the brainstem as an adjunct to the vestibular system but this oldest part of it, the *archicerebellum* or vestibular cerebellum, is now dwarfed by two newer areas: the *palaeocerebellum* associated with the spinal cord, and hence also sometimes called the spinocerebellum, and the large and central *neocerebellum* or corticocerebellum, whose development has been in step with that of the cerebral cortex from which most of its input is derived (Figure 12.7). The cortex of the cerebellum has a very regular and beautiful neuronal structure quite unlike the chaos seen practically everywhere else in the central nervous system, which has led to it being called 'the neuronal machine', and has provoked more speculation than anywhere else – particularly from mathematicians and computer scientists – about how its circuits might work.

Cerebellar neurones and their connections

The most conspicuous type of cell in the cerebellar cortex is the Purkinje cell, which has a huge dendritic tree that is confined to a plane perpendicular to the surface and roughly anteroposterior (Figure 12.8); the cells are lined up in soldierly rows over the whole of the cortex, with their dendritic trees thus stacked like a pack of playing cards. There are about 15 million of

them, and each has a dendritic surface area equivalent to two average-sized front doors. They form the sole output of the cerebellar cortex, for their fibres run downwards to the deep nuclei that lie in the core of the whole structure. In primates there are four of these nuclei on each side (fastigial, emboliform, globose and dentate); in other species the second and third of these are fused into one, called the interpositus. The projection from the cerebellar cortex on to

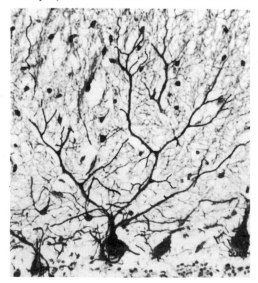

FIG. 12.8 Cerebellar cortex, stained by the Golgi silver method, to show a large part of the dendritic tree of a single Purkinje cell.

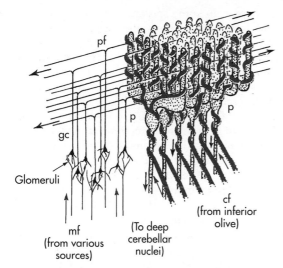

FIG. 12.9 Diagrammatic representation of the connections between mossy afferents (mf) (bottom left), granule cells (gc) and parallel fibres (pf) (left), Purkinje cells (P) and climbing fibres (cf).

these nuclei is a systematic one: medial areas project to the fastigial region, lateral ones to the dentate, and the intervening region to the interpositus. A curious feature of the Purkinje cell is that although it is the only output from the cortex, it is entirely inhibitory (the transmitter is GABA) on the deep nuclei. Finally, the deep nuclei themselves project to various other motor structures: the fastigial primarily to the vestibular nuclei, interpositus to the red nucleus, and dentate to the thalamus (mainly ventrolateral) and hence to the cerebral cortex; all probably also send fibres to the reticular formation of the brainstem. Thus there are several routes by which the cerebellum can influence the spinal cord.

Afferent information reaches the Purkinje cells by two quite distinct pathways (Figure 12.9). In the first place, each Purkinje cell receives a unique single fibre that climbs up its efferent axon and then branches to clamber all over its dendrites like ivy on a tree, forming synaptic contacts that are very strongly excitatory. These *climbing fibres* come from the *inferior olive* in the brainstem, which receives its input in turn mostly from the cerebral cortex but also from the spinal cord and to some extent from the special senses (as, for example, from the visual system, in the case of the vestibulocerebellum); as well as these contacts with Purkinje cells, they also excite the deep nuclei to which the Purkinje cells project. Such specificity of synaptic contact with a single cell is rather a rarity in the central nervous system, where wide divergence and convergence seem to be the general rule, and experimentally it is found that a single shock to a

climbing fibre never fails to fire the associated Purkinje cell, sometimes repetitively.

The other type of afferent system is utterly different. Here, the incoming fibres enter the lower layers of the cerebellar cortex and branch to form large terminal structures (giving them their name of *mossy fibres*) that synapse in glomeruli with a number of dendrites from granule cells in the cortex. These in turn send ascending axons to the surface, where they bifurcate and send two thin axons (called *parallel fibres*) in opposite directions, perpendicularly piercing the planes of the stacked Purkinje cells, to whose dendritic trees they form side connections, like telephone wires on a telephone pole (Figures 12.9, 12.10). In this way, and in complete contrast to the highly specific climbing fibres, each parallel fibre can contact a large number of Purkinje cells; conversely, each Purkinje cell receives nearly half a million contacts from parallel fibres. Mossy fibres carry information from a very wide range of sources: directly, from vestibular and spinal afferents, notably from muscle spindles, and visual, auditory and spinal afferents also indirectly through the *precerebellar* nuclei in the reticular formation (*lateral reticular nucleus, the nucleus reticularis tegmentum pontis and the paramedian reticular nucleus*), and finally from the cortex via relays in the pons. The receptive fields of Purkinje cells are very large indeed – sometimes extending over a whole limb – and are remarkably multimodal. This arrangement of parallel fibres and flat Purkinje cells is an efficient way of providing the largest possible number of output channels with access to the largest number of input sources, within the smallest possible space.

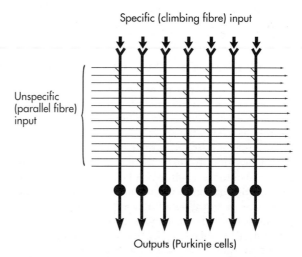

FIG. 12.10 Highly schematic diagram of cerebellar inputs and output, equivalent to Fig. 12.9.

Thus the basic structure is essentially simple: one system of inputs – the climbing fibres – which is extraordinarily precise, and a second system – the mossy fibres – which is equally extraordinarily diffuse and non-specific (Figure 12.10). It is slightly complicated by the existence – as everywhere else in the central nervous system – of various types of interneurone that mostly appear to provide lateral inhibition, sharpening up any spatial patterns of excitation that may be present. These include basket cells, excited by parallel fibres and inhibiting a parasagittal row of Purkinje cells, and Golgi cells, also excited by parallel fibres but inhibiting granule cells instead and thus acting at the input rather than at the output (Figure 12. 11).

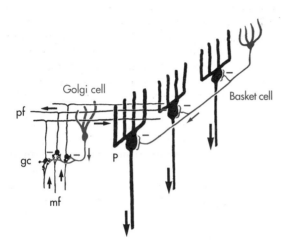

FIG. 12.11 Inhibitory interneurones in cerebellar cortex. Left, a Golgi cell inhibiting a cluster of granule cells (gc); right, a basket cell inhibiting a row of Purkinje cells (P). pf, parallel fibres; mf, mossy fibres.

Disorders of the cerebellum

Although our knowledge of the neuronal structure of the cerebellum is quite precise, our knowledge of its function is less secure, and until recently was almost entirely limited to the effects of cerebellar lesions and other kinds of damage, which are often quite specific and revealing (*Clinical Neurology*, Ch. 9). Damage to the vestibulocerebellum leads to difficulties of postural co-ordination that are similar to what is found with damage to the vestibular apparatus with which it is associated. There may be difficulty in standing upright, a tendency to dizziness, and sometimes a staggering gait when walking. It is very likely that this area acts as the centre of co-ordination for the various postural mechanisms described in the previ-

ous chapter. In some species, as was noted earlier, visual information enters the vestibulocerebellum through the climbing fibres, and vestibular fibres via the mossies; it seems probable that it is here that the comparison and integration of postural information from these two sources takes place. As mentioned earlier, cerebellar ablation in dogs leads not only to abolition of the effects of prism reversal on vestibular reflexes but also to freedom from motion sickness: these will be considered in more detail below.

Difficulties of gait – *ataxia* – are also found after damage to other cerebellar areas but the effects are then found to be more generalized and not just postural: a lack of co-ordination of all kinds of movement *(asynergia)*, generally in association with a loss of muscle tone *(hypotonia)*. It is worth considering some specific examples of these defects in more detail, since they reveal a good deal about the nature of cerebellar disability. Many can be explained in terms of the patient's motor system taking too long to respond to sensory information, of added delay round a feedback loop. Thus *dysmetria* or overshoot may be seen: when the patient reaches out to touch something, his hand goes too far, presumably because the command to stop the movement is sent out too late. A consequence of this is *intention tremor*, in which the overshoot is subsequently corrected by a movement in the opposite direction which then itself overshoots, resulting in a new correction, and so on – the result being an oscillation or tremor around the desired position. The tremor is not seen at rest but only when the patient is aiming to achieve a particular limb position. This slowness to react to changed circumstances is seen also in *rebound*: if, for example, the patient is asked to flex his arm against a force which is then suddenly removed, whereas in the normal patient the resultant inward movement of the hand is quickly checked, in the cerebellar patient it is not, and may strike his body with considerable violence. A related defect is *adiadochokinesis*: the patient is unable to make rapid alternating movements, as for example rapid oscillatory rotation of his wrist between pronation and supination; he cannot apparently issue the command to reverse a movement sufficiently soon after having sent the command to start it (Figure 12.12). In the same way, he may show *scanning speech*: whereas a normal person does not have to think about the sequence of mouth and tongue actions that he makes while speaking, the cerebellar patient seems unable to generate the series of commands sufficiently rapidly, and appears to have to think about the formation of each separate phoneme, like someone trying to speak an obscure foreign language for the first time.

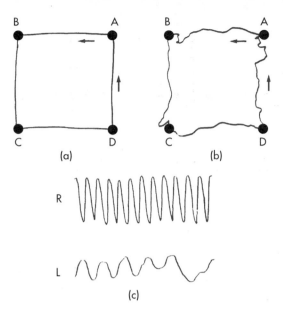

FIG. 12.12 Illustrations of some signs of cerebellar damage. Above, the (normal) subject was instructed to draw a pencil line linking the dots ABCD in the order shown; **(a)** is with normal vision, **(b)** looking in a mirror. Dysmetria, intention tremor and decomposition of movement, of a kind similar to the signs of cerebellar damage, are obvious. Below, adiadochokinesis: records from a patient with damage to his left cerebellum, who can make rapid alterations of pronation and supination with his right arm (R) but not with his left (L). The duration of the trace is 5 seconds. (Holmes, 1922)

Altogether, in fact, the patient has to bring much more conscious control into his movements and it is the time required to think that slows things up. A normal person can walk along, pick things up and so on without thinking much beyond merely willing the final outcome but a cerebellar patient has to plan and think about the details not just of what to do but how to do it. This is perhaps most clearly demonstrated in another dysfunction called *decomposition of movement*: complex movements that require the temporal co-ordination of several different muscles are simplified by being broken down into their components, being executed in effect by one muscle group at a time. Normal people can see for themselves what it is like to be in this condition by the simple expedient of getting drunk: alcohol seems to have a particularly noticeable effect on the cerebellum, and in such circumstances one does indeed sense the need to think consciously about putting one foot in front of the other in order to walk, and one's conversation may begin to approximate to scanning speech.

The difficulty that cerebellar patients have is essentially in using stored programs to carry out

Box 12.1 Classic signs of cerebellar impairments

Ataxia

Hypotonia

Asynergia: *dysmetria*
                  intention tremor
                  decomposition of movement
                  adiadochokinesis
                  scanning speech

Rebound

In general, impairment of execution rather than of initiation; more conscious intervention required in actions previously performed automatically.

motor sequences that are usually automatic: their actions are performed as if they were learning them for the first time. In fact, the execution of any new task by a normal subject is strikingly similar to what is seen in cerebellar patients all the time. A simple experiment you can do yourself is to try drawing whilst looking at what you are doing not directly but in a mirror. If you attempt to move your pencil smartly towards a particular point on the page, you will see both dysmetria and intention tremor; more complex manoeuvres are only achieved by decomposition of movement and all the time one is painfully aware of the need for continual thought about the details of the movements one is making (Figure 12.12). With enough practice, of course, one would in time learn to execute mirror-drawing without these defects, and without the need for continual conscious intervention. Presumably some part of the brain is then carrying out automatically, perhaps by means of some kind of internal model, as in Figure 9.7, what previously had to be thought about. It seems increasingly probable that the cerebellum is the part of the brain that carries out this kind of motor learning; that it acts, in a sense, as the body's autopilot.

Theories of cerebellar action

What has always captured the imagination of neurophysiologists is the way the cerebellum seems so beautifully regular, a sort of neural crystal. In particular, the contrast between the tight, one-to-one coupling of climbing fibres and Purkinje cells, and the grid-like arrangement of the connections with the myriad parallel fibres has suggested that whereas the

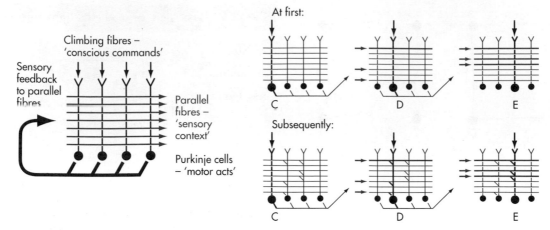

FIG. 12.13 A model of how the cerebellum may learn sequences of motor actions. Left, highly simplified diagram of cerebellar inputs and outputs (see Figure 12.10) showing feedback from motor actions to the parallel fibres. Right, the hypothetical sequence of events before and after learning to play a piano scale C, D, E, . . . (for explanation, see text).

former are in a sense hard-wired, the parallel fibre synapses might be of variable strength: programmable in a way that would account for the cerebellum's ability to learn. A plausible rule for such programming is for synaptic strengthening to occur if there is a coincidence of presynaptic and postsynaptic activity: if, in other words, a particular parallel fibre fires at the same time as the Purkinje cell. On this hypothesis, originally put forward by the late David Marr, it is possible to provide a ready explanation for the kinds of defects associated with cerebellar damage, as well as for more recent and precise observations. He suggested that the cerebellum stores and executes specific sequences of actions by means of a gradual process in which the sequences are first generated consciously while the subject is attempting to master the task, but as the result of repetition are gradually taken over by the cerebellum itself. A crucial idea here is that every movement takes place in a sensory *context*, some of which will be due to feedback from the last movement that has been made. If we have a device that can learn to form an association between the feedback generated by one movement, and the initiation of the next, then we can use it to generate each fragment of a movement automatically from its predecessor. In its final form the theory is a complex one, requiring complex mathematics to be fully appreciated, but a simplified example may help to convey Marr's basic argument.

Consider how we might learn to play a scale on the piano. To simplify things, let us begin by supposing that there is one Purkinje cell that corresponds to each of the fingers playing 'C, D, E, F' (Figure 12.13), and that when the cell fires, it causes that finger to

play the corresponding note. (The fact that the Purkinje output is inhibitory need not be an embarrassment: if we inhibit an inhibitory cell, the result is excitation, and neuronal circuits within the CNS can work equally well whether we consider either an increase or a decrease in firing rate to represent a 'positive' signal: one need only think of the hyperpolarization of retinal receptors in response to light.) Now we have seen that the Purkinje cells are powerfully and specifically excited by their climbing fibres, and that one important source of these fibres, via the inferior olive, is the cerebral cortex. What is suggested is that during the initial learning phase, the Purkinje cells are driven by these climbing fibres – activated by some kind of volitional process – in the correct sequence C,D,E,F; under these circumstances the cerebellum is doing nothing more elaborate than simply relaying this sequence of commands to some lower level.

But consider what meanwhile is happening to the parallel fibres: with their diffuse activation from every kind of sensory input, the pattern of their firing embodies the sensory context in which the action is taking place. Every time we carry out a motor act, it necessarily results in a kind of echo that comes back to us through our senses. When we play a note on the piano, we get feedback not only from proprioceptors, the muscle spindles, tendon organs and joint receptors but also from endings in the skin, not to mention the visual stimulus of seeing the finger move and the note go down, and the auditory stimulus of hearing the result. Each note that is played consequently generates a particular pattern of sensory feedback that will be quite specific to that particular action and to no other. This pattern will be reflected in the pattern of activity of the parallel fibres, which we saw to convey information of the most diverse kinds to the dendrites of the Purkinje cells. Thus when we play the note D, having just played C, the Purkinje cell corresponding to D is activated by its climbing fibre during a sensory context that is quite specific to the state of having just played C, and is quite literally present at its dendritic branches in the form of a particular and specific pattern of parallel fibre activity. And if we now recollect our original supposition that the condition for their synapses getting stronger is that the parallel fibre should often fire at the same time as the Purkinje cell, then we have a system that will learn to recognize the context associated with a particular action, and eventually respond to it automatically by generating the action itself. For if we play the sequence C–D over and over again, each time we do it the parallel fibres that are activated by the sensory feedback from C will fire at the same time as Purkinje cell D, so that their synaptic contacts with the latter will gradually get stronger and stronger. Eventually they will get so strong that they can fire D off even in the absence of a volitional command from the climbing fibre: D will then be produced spontaneously simply as the natural result of having played C, with no conscious intervention. In the same way, E will come to follow automatically from D, F from E, and G from F; and in the end all the subject needs to do is to initiate the sequence, and it will follow automatically – and more rapidly.

Such a model explains the phenomenon of adiadochokinesis particularly simply. If we imagine just two Purkinje cells, one for supination and one for pronation, then what we are doing when we learn to make the rapid alternation of hand position is to connect the two cells up reciprocally so that the context produced by one eventually comes to fire the other, resulting in almost automatic oscillation; those familiar with electronics will recognize that we have in effect built an astable multivibrator out of our cerebellar components. That these alternating movements have to be learnt in the first place is clear if you try and execute them with some less familiar part of the body: most people – unless they've been practising – suffer from adiadochokinesis of the toes, as you can easily verify for yourself.

Finally, it is perhaps worth mentioning that Marr's model has already found a potentially useful application in the field of industrial robots: machines have been built that incorporate similar circuits and are equipped with sensors from the work area, and will learn to perform complex sequences of operations by first being driven 'consciously' (by a human operator, in fact) and then gradually recognizing the patterns of sensory input that are to act as triggers for particular items of motor output.

With slight modifications, the same model can also form the basis of the other two types of motor learning discussed in Chapter 9, namely the storage of ballistic programs, and the prediction of expected results from copies of motor commands, by means of a stored model of the behaviour of the body. In the first case, we need only assume that a part of the mossy fibre input comes from other motor areas at a lower hierarchical level, rather than from sensory receptors (as indeed is the case, particularly in the neocerebellum). Then instead of relying on actual feedback from the results of any particular item of a motor sequence, the command for one such item can trigger the next, producing ballistic sequences of motor acts that do not have to wait for actual feedback from results. Under these circumstances, the climbing fibre input (whose function in Marr's model is in effect to say to the Purkinje cells 'now learn this!') could be used to provide parametric feedback in order to improve ballistic performance through experience.

For example, we have already seen that in the vestibulocerebellum there is evidence that visual information enters through climbing fibres and vestibular through the mossy fibres. In Marr's model, this would imply that visual information would not only drive postural responses such as eye movements directly, but also strengthen those vestibular connections to Purkinje cells that were appropriate, in the sense that they were in close correspondence with the visual signal. Such a mechanism could explain very nicely the way in which visual information appears to be capable of continually calibrating the vestibular input in such situations as the prism-induced reversal of vestibulo-ocular reflexes mentioned earlier. The synapses of those vestibular parallel fibres whose activity was in agreement with visual climbing fibre input would strengthen, and those in disagreement would weaken (Figure 12.14).

And lastly, if we imagine the parallel fibres to convey copies of motor commands, and the climbing fibres to be activated by actual sensory feedback from the results of those commands, then we have a system in which Purkinje cell output will, as a result of experience, come to provide an estimate of the result of motor commands of the kind required in internal feedback systems like that of Figure 9.7. Marr's model is thus a very versatile one, capable of embodying almost any kind of motor learning by defining its inputs and outputs in different ways. Many would say, in fact, that it explains almost too

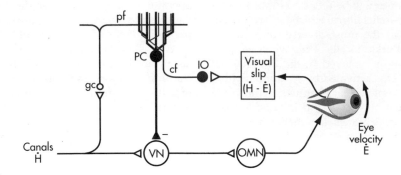

FIG. 12.14 Postulated role of the flocculonodular lobe (FNL) of the cerebellum in adaptation of the VOR. At bottom, head velocity signals from the semicircular canals drive the oculomotor nuclei (OMN) via the vestibular nuclei (VN). In addition to this direct route, canal fibres also project to cerebellar cortex, where they impinge on Purkinje cells (PC) as parallel fibres (pf). Since the FNL Purkinje cells inhibit the VN pathway, this provides a route by which the gain of the VOR can be altered. Climbing fibres (cf) to the FNL come from the dorsal cap of the inferior olive (IO) and are driven by visual slip; since this is an error signal (it represents the difference between eye and head velocity) it is ideally suited to alter the strength of the connections between parallel fibres and Purkinje cells, and thus alter VOR gain to improve performance. However, experiments show that the learning in VOR adaptation is not confined to the cerebellum.

much, and is consequently difficult to test; and it has to be admitted that elegant and powerful though it is, there is as yet little direct neurophysiological evidence to support it. Its value at present is perhaps essentially explanatory, in that it helps to tie together in a coherent way both the observed effects of cerebellar dysfunction and what is known of cerebellar microanatomy and function. There are several details of it which certainly require correction in the light of subsequent work. For instance, while it is true that NMDA synapses showing the expected strengthening in response to coincidence of afferent and efferent activity are indeed found in the cerebellum, they are on granule cells rather than on the Purkinje cells where they ought to be. Synaptic plasticity of the connections from parallel fibres to Purkinje cells can be demonstrated, but it is a weakening rather than strengthening (long-term depression rather than long-term potentiation). This in itself is not fatal, for shortly after Marr's work was published it was pointed out that the model would in some respects work better with just such a modification. Much more seriously, in the case of modification of the vestibulo-ocular reflex, it is now clear that while some learning changes occur in the cerebellum, the most important ones occur in the *brainstem,* though they are certainly cerebellum-dependent. A picture is beginning to emerge of a cerebellum that learns but also *teaches:* it learns to predict errors before they actually occur, and these errors – whether real or virtual – are then used to modify the behaviour of the more primitive circuits in the brainstem.

BASAL GANGLIA

Unfortunately the functions of the basal ganglia are as uncertain in detail as their structure is complex. A prominent component of the basal ganglia is the *corpus striatum* lying in the mesencephalon at the level of the thalamus; in higher animals it has suffered the fate that frequently falls to older structures in the brain – as we saw in the case of the archicerebellum – in that it has been elbowed out of the way by newer structures that have consequently distorted it into an even more tortuous shape than is altogether necessary (Figure 12.15). Thus what was originally a relatively compact mass of cells has been disrupted by the arrival of the internal capsule – like a motorway through a village – with the result that it is now an elongated structure that twists its way round the newer ascending fibres. The stripes seen in cross-section, that give it its name, divide it into a number of different regions: of these, the most important distinction is between the older part, the palaeostriatum or *globus pallidus* which lies on the inside, and the outer *putamen,* which is continuous with the long arc of the caudate nucleus, the two together forming the *neostriatum* or simply 'striatum'. There are other nuclei which conventionally are also considered part of the basal ganglia, though not everyone agrees as to what should or should not be included. They include the *subthalamus* lying below the thalamus, and the *substantia nigra* (so called because certain of its cells are darkly pigmented with melanin). Some authors also include the red nucleus.

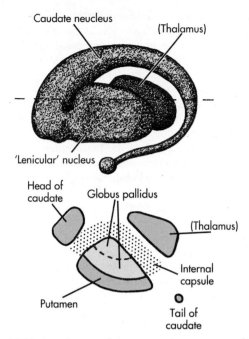

FIG. 12.15 Lateral view of the principal components of the basal ganglia, together with the thalamus; right, a horizontal section at level of the dotted line, showing in addition the fibres of the internal capsule pushing their way through. (Partly after Netter, 1962; copyright CIBA Pharmaceutical Company)

The connections between these structures are very complex and their functional significance largely a matter for speculation. The important flow of information seems to be a projection from the cerebral cortex to the putamen and caudate nucleus, thence to the internal and external layers of the globus pallidus and substantia nigra pars reticulata (SNPR), both of which then project to VA and VL of the thalamus, and thus back to the cortex again (mostly to the supplementary motor area, but also to motor and premotor areas), forming two large feedback loops (Figure 12.16). In addition, there is a second output route from SNPR to the superior colliculus, through which head and eye movements can be controlled. More is known about the transmitters here than in most parts of the brain: keen transmitter spotters will be glad to know that the striatopallidal and striatonigral projections are GABinergic, and that the efferent cells of the striatum receive glutamate-secreting fibres from the cerebral cortex, and serotonin fibres from the raphe nucleus, dopaminergic fibres from the substantia nigra and inhibitory cholinergic fibres from neighbouring interneurones. The subthalamus has connections to and from the globus pallidus, and the substantia nigra receives an input from the putamen while sending fibres back to both parts of the corpus striatum (Figure 12.16). Other connections are difficult to establish, though it is likely that there are indirect connections from the older areas of the brain such as the limbic system (which is concerned with motivation and emotion), possibly via the *nucleus accumbens*, and at least in fish one may demonstrate a functional projection from the olfactory system which, as we have seen, is one of the oldest senses and one that is particularly associated with limbic functions. A suggestive recent finding is that within the striatum here appear to be two distinct populations of cells, one forming relatively dense clusters (*'striosomes'*) and the other forming a looser background (*'matrix'*). The input to the striosomes appears to be predominantly from motivational areas of the limbic system, while that to the matrix is mostly from cerebral cortex.

As with the cerebellum, such meagre information as we have about the functions of the basal ganglia is almost entirely derived from clinical observations of

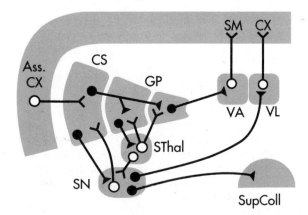

FIG. 12.16 Schematized representation of the principal connections of the basal ganglia. NS, neostriatum; GP, globus pallidus; SN, substantia nigra; SThal, subthalamus; Ass CX and SM CX, cerebral cortex, associational and somatomotor; VA, VL, ventroanterior, ventrolateral thalamic nuclei. Inhibitory cells and endings in black.

the effects of damage in humans. The best known of these disorders is *Parkinsonism* or paralysis agitans, associated especially with damage to the pathways linking the substantia nigra and the putamen (*Clinical Neurology*, Ch. 9). The main feature of classic Parkinsonism is a general poverty of movement *(akinesia)*. Expressive movements, such as the normal mobility of the face, may be absent, giving the patient a lifeless and apathetic appearance, and there may be a loss of associated movements, movements that normally occur in conjunction with a particular primary activity but are not strictly necessary (such as swinging the arms when walking). The patient may blink less often than a normal subject; there is often a shuffling gait, and he may be very slow in walking about. None of these things are defects of the peripheral motor apparatus, for under the right circumstances, especially under strong emotional stimulation, quite normal movements may be made. Thus a Parkinson patient may be shuffling his way across the road when a car comes: he then runs briskly to the other side, only to continue his slow shuffle along the pavement. The difficulty, in other words, is not in the *execution* of the movement but in its *initiation*. A patient may find it very difficult to start to walk but some martial music or even a few lines drawn on the ground to act as a visual stimulus may be sufficient to get the movement going. Equally, once started it may be difficult to stop: *perseveration* of movement. It is clear that these are difficulties at a very high level of the motor system, and it is significant that Parkinsonian patients often show emotional disorders of a related kind: a more general apathy and immobility of mind as well as body. Other common features of Parkinsonism are a general rigidity and slowness (bradykinesia), vague postural difficulties, and a tremor that is the exact opposite of the intention tremor of cerebellar damage, being present only at rest, and disappearing as soon as some voluntary action is attempted.

If Parkinsonism is essentially a state of poverty of movement, other disorders of the basal ganglia, by contrast, result in the spontaneous production of *unwanted* movements. Lesions of the subthalamus in particular give rise to *ballismus* in which the patient may throw his limbs about in a violent manner. In other regions, damage may give rise to less energetic spontaneous movements called *chorea* ('dancing'), for example continual shaking or twitching, or to slow writhing movements known as *athetosis*. Some of these symptoms get worse as the patient tries to reach a particular goal. There may also be an exaggeration of associated movements. With the exception of the ballismus that can be produced in

monkeys as well as humans by damage to the subthalamus, these effects are not clearly associated with lesions of specific areas of the basal ganglia, and indeed it has not proved possible to simulate them very closely in experimental animals. Consequently, treatment of these disorders is generally of a rather rough-and-ready kind: it is sometimes found, for example, that a Parkinson patient's rigidity and tremor may be alleviated by actually making further lesions in other parts of the basal ganglia. Another treatment for Parkinsonism that is often helpful and has the appearance of being more scientific is to treat the patient with DOPA, a precursor of dopamine, the transmitter in the projection from substantia nigra to putamen; it is possible that it is some defect in the production of transmitter here that gives rise to the condition in the first place.

At all events, it is certainly not yet possible to use the existence of these clinical disorders to deduce the detailed functioning of the basal ganglia; and single-unit recording is only just beginning to make a contribution to our understanding of what they do. To suggest, as some of the older accounts do, that because damage to a certain area gives rise to tremor or to sudden violent movements, the function of that area is to reduce tremor or smooth movements out in some way, is only slightly less absurd than the analogy presented in Chapter 1, of removing a circuit

---

Box 12.2 Classic signs of basal ganglia impairments

Hyperkinetic:

Ballismus (subthalamus)

Chorea (corpus striatum)

Athetosis (corpus striatum)

Hypokinetic: Parkinsonism (nigrostriatal)

Rigidity

Bradykinesia

Tremor at rest

Akinesia:
> *loss of associated movements*
> *loss of expressive movements*
> *difficulty of initiation*
> *bradykinesia*

In general, difficulties are at a higher level: of initiation rather than of execution. In the right circumstances, movements may be performed relatively normally.

board from a hi-fi and deducing that its function was to inhibit whistling. As yet, recording from basal ganglia has – apart from a specific role in the control of eye movements – produced only equivocal findings. In the case of the putamen, it is not even at all clear that the neurones are motor and not sensory (if that distinction has meaning at this level): most are best described as responding to a stimulus if it has some behavioural significance for the animal.

But one can deduce a great deal about the hierarchical level at which the basal ganglia operate. In all these cases, whether there is loss of voluntary initiation of movements that can be evoked involuntarily or the intrusion of unwanted movements that are, in

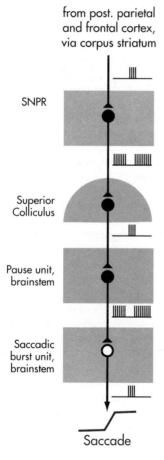

from post. parietal and frontal cortex, via corpus striatum

SNPR

Superior Colliculus

Pause unit, brainstem

Saccadic burst unit, brainstem

Saccade

FIG. 12.17 Cascade through basal ganglia causing the initiation of saccades. Saccadic burst units in the brainstem drive oculomotor neurones; they are tonically inhibited by pause units, which stop firing to permit a saccade. The pause units are in turn inhibited by burst units in the superior colliculus, under visual control, but these too are held tonically in check by inhibitory pause units in substantia nigra pars reticulata (SNPR); these in turn appear to be gated by higher areas, including parietal and frontal cortex. Inhibitory neurones black, excitatory white.

their way, quite well executed (or even elegant, as in athetosis), it is clear that we are at a very high level in the motor system. Lesions of the cerebellum give rise to defects of execution but not of initiation, and lesions of the cortex lead to even 'lower' defects like weakness or frank paralysis. But damage to the basal ganglia clearly interferes with the level at which movements are *strategically planned and initiated*: we saw in Chapter 7 that recent experiments have provided direct evidence for precisely such a role for SNPR in the control of eye movements (Figure 12.17). So if we had to represent, in general terms, what the relative hierarchical positions of these three higher levels were, we would put the basal ganglia at the top, responsible for the initiation and perhaps the large-scale or strategic planning of movements, particularly in cases where the movement is not simply an automatic response to an external stimulus; the cerebellum underneath, automatically translating these commands into sequences of unitary actions, with reference to feedback from the periphery; and at the bottom the primary motor cortex, where commands concerning the desired positions of the limbs and so forth may be converted into yet more detailed instructions governing the forces required from moment to moment in order to achieve these results.

One might well ask what, if anything, lies above the basal ganglia in such a scheme. The problem here is partly one of terminology. In the general representation of the brain presented at the beginning of Chapter 9, it was emphasized that there is in effect a gradual series of neuronal levels that convert sensory information into motor movements. When we are considering areas near the centre of such a scheme, at the highest hierarchical levels, the distinction between 'sensory' and 'motor' becomes a somewhat arbitrary one. (Of course, one might cut through this problem at one stroke by introducing a 'ghost in the machine' which is both conscious of incoming sensory information and also capable of willing volitional movements: by definition, any structure upstream of such an entity is sensory, and downstream, motor. The question of whether such a notion is necessary in understanding human behaviour is postponed until Chapter 14.)

Meanwhile, all one can usefully say is that it is simply a matter of convention that the inputs that provide the drive for motor acts are normally reckoned not to be part of the motor system. There are in fact two distinct types of input that must be considered; first of all the sensory information about the environment without which one clearly cannot make decisions about how to plan one's motor acts, even on a large scale; and secondly, the neural mechanisms that decide what is to be done, that choose between all the various possible courses of action that are open to the brain at any particular moment. The first type of input, that of high-level integrated sensory information about the environment, forms the subject of the next chapter; the second type, which is what motivates the motor system, and requires information not just about the outside world but also about one's internal environment as well, one's state of need, forms the subject of Chapter 14.

References

Holmes, G. (1922) Clinical symptoms of cerebellar disease and their interpretation (Croonian Lectures). *Lancet* 203, 59–65, 11–115.

Netter, F. H. (1962) *Nervous System: The CIBA Collection of Medical Illustrations.* CIBA, Basle.

Penfield, W. and Rasmussen, T. (1950) *The Cerebral Cortex of Man: a Clinical Study of Localization of Function.* Macmillan, New York.

Rosen, I. and Asanuma, H. (1972) Peripheral afferent inputs to the forelimb area of the monkey motor cortex: input–output relations. *Experimental Brain Research* 14, 257–273.

Woolsey, C. N. (1958) Organization of somatic sensory and motor areas of the cerebral cortex. In *Biological and Biochemical Bases of Behaviour*, ed. H. F. Harlow and C. N. Woolsey. University of Wisconsin Press, Wisconsin.

NOTES

Page 226 Higher motor areas Some excellent general accounts: Evarts, E. V., Wise, S. P. and Bousfield, D. (1985) *The Motor System in Neurobiology* (Elsevier, Amsterdam); Rothwell, J. C. (1993) *Control of Human Voluntary Movement* (Chapman and Hall, London); Brooks, V. B. (1988) *The Neural Basis of Motor Control* (Oxford University Press, Oxford).

Page 228 Motor cortex Useful accounts include: Passingham, R. (1993) *The Frontal Lobes and Voluntary Reaction* (Oxford University Press, Oxford); Phillips, C. G. and Porter, R. (1977) *Corticospinal Neurones: Their Role in Movement* (Academic, London); Porter, R. and Lemon, R. (1993) *Cortico-spinal Function and Voluntary Movement* (Oxford University Press, Oxford); Schmitt, F. O., Worden, F. G., Adelman, G. and Dennis, S. G. (1981) *The Organization of the Cerebral Cortex* (MIT Press, Massachusetts).

Page 231 Cerebellum Two comprehensive accounts: Ito, M. (1984) *The Cerebellum and Neural Control* (Raven, New York); Palay, S. L. and Chan-Palay, V. (1974) *Cerebellar Cortex* (Springer, Berlin).

Page 234 Effects of cerebellar damage Someone is sure to tell you that the cerebellum can't be that important since just the other day a body turned up in the dissecting room where the cerebellum had been totally absent from birth, yet the man had made his living as a steeplejack (or ballet dancer or pole-vaulter or something similar). Professor Mitchell Glickstein has traced the origin of this extraordinarily resilient urban myth in Glickstein, M. (1994) Cerebellar agenesis. *Brain* 117, 1209–1212.

Page 236 Marr's theory Marr, D. (1969) A theory of cerebellar cortex. *Journal of Physiology* 202, 437–507.

Page 238 Cerebellum as motor learner And perhaps not just motor: some believe that it may play a part in purely cognitive functions, but this is somewhat controversial. See Leiner, H. C., Leiner, A. L. and Dow, R. S. (1993) Cognitive and language functions of the cerebellum. *Trends in Neuroscience* 16, 444–454, with its lively commentaries and discussion afterwards.

Page 238 Cerebellar predictive models? There is an excellent recent discussion of this possibility in Miall, R. C., Weir, D. J., Wolpert, D. M. and Stein, J. F. (1993) Is the cerebellum a Smith predictor? *Journal of Motor Behaviour* 25, 203–216.

Page 238 Depression and not potentiation See Albus, J. S. (1971) A theory of cerebellar function. *Mathematical Biosciences* 10, 25–61.

Page 239 Striosomes See Graybiel, A. M. (1990) Neurotransmitters and neuromodulators in the basal ganglia. *Trends in Neuroscience* 13, 244–253.

Page 240 James Parkinson It is worth reading Parkinson, J. (1817) *An Essay on the Shaking Palsy* (Whittingham and Rowland, London) partly as an admirable example of clear clinical description, and partly to see how excellent observation and plausible deductions can lead to an utterly false conclusion, in this case that the cause was *'some slow morbid change in the structure of the medulla, or its investing membranes, or theca, occasioned by simple inflammation, or rheumatic or scrophulous affection'.*

Page 240 The need for external cues A description of such a patient from that unusually thoughtful and wise analysis of what is really happening in Parkinsonism, Sacks, O. (1982) *Awakenings* (Pan, London): *'Once a first step was taken – and walking could be inaugurated by a little push from behind, a verbal command from the examiner, or a visual command in the form of a stick, a piece of paper, or something definite to step over on the floor – Miss D. would teeter forward in tiny rapid steps. ... In remarkable contrast was her excellent ability to climb stairs stably and steadily, each stair providing a stimulus to a step; having reached the top of the stairs, however, Miss D. would again find herself "frozen" and* unable to proceed. She often remarked that "if the world consisted entirely of stairs" she would have no difficulty in getting around whatever.'

Page 240 Single unit recording See for instance Brotchie, P., Iansek, R. and Horne, M. K. (1991) Motor functions of the monkey globus pallidus. I. Neuronal discharge and parameters of movement. *Brain* 114, 1667-1684.

NEUROLAB

Cortical regions

Page 226

A simple map of functional cortical areas, for self-testing. Click on one of the radio buttons designating an area of cortex, and the name and Brodmann number will appear in the box at right. Alternatively, click on the pull-down button at the right of the box to display the whole list, and click on an item: the corresponding radio button will be selected.

Anatomical pathways

Page 228

A database of nuclei and other areas in the CNS, and the tracts and pathways that join them, that you can use for reference or for self-testing. The two upper windows list sources and destinations, the lower one has the names of tracts that join them. If you click on the name of a tract, its origin(s) and destination(s) appear in the upper windows. To restore the full lists, click on Show all. If you click on a source in one of the upper windows, the destination window lists the major areas to which it projects, and the corresponding tracts are listed below. Similarly, clicking on a destination shows the sources and their linking tracts. Double-clicking on a destination takes you one stage further on, by treating it as a source and showing you *its* destinations; similarly, double-clicking on a source takes you one stage further back.

Cerebellar dysmetria

Page 235

This exhibit shows how upsetting the normal relationship between movement and visual feedback results in phenomena very similar to those of cerebellar damage, including dysmetria, decomposition of movement and intention tremor. Click on the centre spot, then – holding the mouse button down – move as quickly and accurately as possible to each of the other three spots in turn. This demonstration relies on your not being *too* skilled in using the mouse; if you are, use your other hand, or – even more spectacularly – turn the mouse through 180° so its cable is towards you and your movements are reversed.

Cerebellar learning

Page 237

A very simple implementation of Marr's model of cerebellar sequence learning. The screen shows a row of (dark blue) Purkinje cells, A – E. Clicking on their corresponding buttons activates them, and also causes sensory feedback whose spatial patterning is characteristic of each response: see this for yourself by clicking on each of the buttons in turn. Now, in Learn mode (check box at bottom) press the buttons in a particular sequence at a steady pace, and repeat this training a few times. You will see that sensory feedback in parallel fibres from one button coincides with firing of the next Purkinje cell. Then select Execute, and press the first button of the sequence only: the model should then perform the rest of the sequence. Explore the limitations of its learning capability. The Forget button resets the synapses to their original (ineffective) state.

Parametric feedback

Page 237

This exhibit shows the functioning of parametric feedback in the vestibulo-ocular reflex: it has already been described in Chapter 11 (p.225).

PART

4

HIGHER FUNCTIONS

13 RECOGNITION AND MEMORY: CEREBRAL CORTEX

Prefrontal cortex 248
Parietal cortex 251

Temporal lobe 258

The processes covered by this chapter – unlike those discussed in previous ones – are those that we humans are best at, and to which we owe any temporary biological success that we have managed to achieve. Many animals are more agile and better co-ordinated than we are, can hear better or see better, and practically all of them have more sensitive noses. Our special virtue is that we are quite good at *storing* and *processing* such sensory information as gets through to us, so that we use it better in making effective responses to our environment. There is no very sharp distinction between us and other creatures in this respect. Nor are these functions particularly mysterious or magical: they are, after all, performed even better by some computers. It is simply that the parts of the brain that carry out these functions in a rudimentary way in other species have in us been very greatly expanded and developed. If we compare the cerebral hemispheres of a series of animals from different evolutionary stages, what is striking is not just the expansion in the absolute mass of neural tissue by the time one reaches humans (Fig. 13.1) but also the changes in the relative proportions of the cortex devoted to different functions. Very little of a rat's cortex is not either primary motor or a projection area for one of the senses; in humans, by contrast, most of the human cortex neither responds in an obvious way to simple sensory stimulation nor produces movements when electrically activated: they are what are sometimes called silent areas.

Now these are precisely the properties we would expect from neural levels somewhere in the middle of the model of the brain that was first discussed in Chapter 9 and is shown again in Figure 13.2: because each neurone at any level is only activated by a particular pattern of activity in the preceding layer, as we penetrate deeper into the sensory side we find

that individual neurones become fussier and fussier about what they respond to, until eventually the chance of our finding out, in an experiment of finite duration, what they *do* actually do becomes extremely

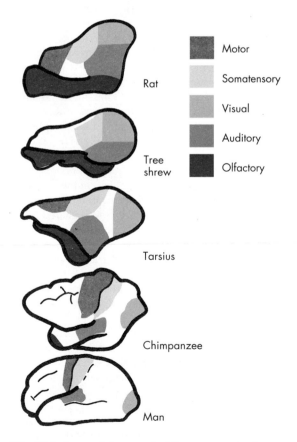

FIG. 13.1 Series of brains of different species, showing increase in extent of 'silent', associational cortex (unshaded) in the course of evolution. (After Stanley Cobb, in Penfield, 1967)

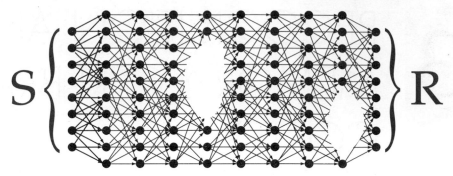

FIG. 13.2 Representation of the brain as a series of neuronal levels (as in Fig. 9.1) showing the differing effects of a lesion at a high hierarchical level (centre), and one nearer the periphery.

small; and on the output side, unless we happen to stimulate them in a pattern that makes some kind of neural sense, nothing will happen at all. Equally, because these areas integrate or associate information from diverse sources which cut across the conventional divisions of sensory modality (for which reason the corresponding cortical areas are also known as *association areas*), lesions in them are unlikely to have the same kind of circumscribed effects that are found, for example, in damage to the primary visual or motor cortex (Fig. 13.2): we are at a high hierarchical level, in the sense discussed in Chapter 9. Nor, at this level, is there likely to remain much topological orderliness of the kind found at more peripheral levels. This situation is not unlike what happens in a telephone exchange: at the periphery – the region where the incoming cables arrive – there is a systematic relationship between a subscriber's number and the position of his particular connection, but the selector switches in the heart of the exchange that set up the circuits and form, in effect, associations between different subscribers are shared by all of them and used to set up different circuits on different occasions. The capacity of an exchange – the number of associations it can make at any one time – is thus simply proportional to the quantity of this common switching equipment it contains. Might the neural elements of associational cortex also be in some sense shared in this way?

Such a notion, of associational cortex being uncommitted to any particular task but providing a reserve of computing power that can be applied to whatever job is on hand, was originally suggested by the experiments of Karl Lashley described on p. 15. Lashley's 'law of mass action' – that the effect of lesions in associational cortex depends more on how large they are than on their exact location – is now less in favour. Recording from units in associational areas shows in many cases that their 'silence' is the

result of unnatural or boring stimuli; with adequate sensory patterning they can often be made to respond, in a way that may be complex and highly time-dependent but does not alter radically from one experiment to the next. And it is clear from clinical observations in particular that discrete lesions in associational cortex can sometimes lead to fairly circumscribed functional defects, rather than something like a generalized loss of 'intelligence'. What is true, as we shall see, is that these functional defects may be of the wide-ranging and subtle kind that is characteristic of damage at a high hierarchical level – for instance the loss of the ability to speak French, while spoken English is unimpaired – and also that there is very little reproducibility from subject to subject, in the sense that a lesion in a particular place in one person may have a completely different effect in another person. The idea of an uncommitted pool of 'brain power' is almost certainly wrong; the neurones are specialized in their function, but at a high level in the hierarchy: it is this that gives lesions in associational cortex their subtle and unpredictable quality.

In primates there are essentially three distinct regions of associational cortex (Fig. 13.3): they are the *frontal lobe* (strictly, prefrontal), occupying the entire region anterior to the motor cortex; the *parietal lobe*, bounded by somatosensory, visual and auditory cortex; and the *temporal lobe*, bounded above by visual and auditory cortex, and occupying the rest of the inferior portion of the cerebral cortex – the thumb of the cerebral boxing glove.

PREFRONTAL CORTEX

The prefrontal lobes form the largest single division of the cortex in humans, with a diverse output that

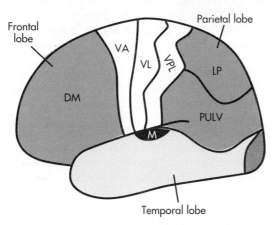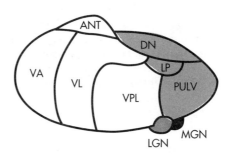

FIG. 13.3 Schematic lateral views of cerebral cortex and thalamus, showing corresponding regions of each. DM, dorsomedial; LP, lateroposterior; PULV, pulvinar; VA, VL, VPL, ventroanterior, -lateral, and -posterolateral; MGN, LGN, medial and lateral geniculate nuclei; ANT, anterior. VA also projects diffusely to the frontal lobe. (After Carpenter, 1976)

extends to the hypothalamus as well as to the striatum, subthalamus and midbrain. It receives afferents from the correspondingly large *dorsomedial nucleus* of the thalamus (Fig. 13.3: it is not just sensory projection areas that have afferent fibres relayed through the thalamus). This nucleus in turn receives fibres not only back from the frontal lobe, but also from the hypothalamus and other parts of the limbic system, an area predominantly associated with such functions as emotion and motivation, to be discussed in Chapter 14. These are very old parts of the brain indeed, found practically unchanged throughout the animal kingdom, and it is striking that their cortical projection is to the very newest part of that new area,

the cerebral cortex. Man is in fact distinguished most from primates by the absolute and relative size of his frontal lobes; until a century or so ago it was assumed that they must therefore be the seat of the very highest functions – intelligence, morality, religion, etc. – those that were thought to differentiate Man most clearly from the apes.

The case of Phineas Gage in 1848 came as a rude shock. He was an American mining engineer, who was one day tamping down dynamite with an iron bar (one cannot help wondering about his intelligence *before* his accident). The consequence can be imagined (Fig. 13.4). Astonishingly, when one considers contemporary standards of medical care, he

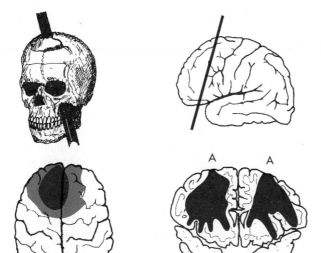

FIG. 13.4 Prefrontal damage. Left, Phineas Gage's skull, with crowbar; horizontal section below indicates the subsequent area of destruction (black) and probable neural damage (shaded). (After Cobb, 1946) Right, deliberate frontal leucotomy, showing (above) the approximate plane of the cut, and below, cross-section of an actual cut of this kind, performed by means of a spatula inserted through skull openings at the points marked A on each side. (After Freeman and Watts, 1948)

survived, and made a precarious living for some years by exhibiting himself in public, together with the bar. Post-mortem examination showed that most of the frontal cortex had been destroyed; what was extraordinary was how little effect this seemed to have on him: far from turning into an ape or losing his powers of reason, he seemed to suffer little more than a slight change in personality. His doctor described him as *'fitful, irreverent, indulging at times in the grossest profanity (which was not previously his custom), manifesting but little deference for his fellows, impatient of restraint or advice when it conflicts with his desires, at times pertinaciously obstinate, yet capricious and vacillating'* – what nowadays we would call perfectly normal. Indeed, his friends said that in some ways he was actually happier – more carefree and less inhibited – after the accident than before.

As a result of this dramatic demonstration, controlled experiments were performed on animals, with the same conclusion: that lesions in the frontal lobes seem generally to reduce anxiety – monkeys worry less when they make mistakes in learning tasks – and inevitably the idea developed that such a procedure might even be of benefit to depressive patients or anxious schizophrenics. This operation, *frontal leucotomy* or lobotomy (Fig. 13.4), began to be practised around 1935 and remained popular until the introduction of pharmacological agents doing much the same thing in a more reversible manner, in the early 1960s. There is no doubt that the operation gave a great deal of relief: not only alleviation of tension and anxiety but better adjustment to work, and increased weight and energy. A difficulty was that the changes in personality might go too far, developing into euphoria, tactlessness, a lackadaisical approach to life, and a lack of social inhibitions such as those that discourage urination in the fireplace. One circumstance where these side effects seemed worth putting up with was in the treatment of intractable pain, not easily dealt with by other measures. The result in this case was not so much loss of the objective knowledge of the pain – not, in other words, analgesia – but rather a loss of the *'affekt'* of the pain, its unpleasant or emotional quality. Thus when asked what the pain was like, a patient might reply 'Oh doctor, it's absolutely appalling, unbearable', yet would be smiling as he said it and not – apparently – really feeling it despite being able to sense it.

What is perhaps most notable about the effects of frontal lesions is how little defect of ordinary intelligence occurs, with one exception: there are almost always difficulties in carrying out two programs of activity simultaneously. Thus a patient may be asked to recite the letters of the alphabet 'A,B,C,D', and then be interrupted and asked to add together 13 and 15: '28'. If then told to carry on the response may be '29,30,31,…': the original task is forgotten. Similarly, there may be an inability to organize actions in proper temporal sequence; this may become apparent when trying to prepare a meal, where one has of course to plan well ahead, bearing in mind the different times that different things take to cook, so that everything is ready simultaneously. These effects can be demonstrated in monkeys by means of the *delayed reaction test*. Here a monkey sits behind a glass partition in a cage, in front of which are two boxes, one of them containing a reward such as a banana. The doors of the boxes are first opened to show what is in them, then closed again; after an interval of perhaps 10 minutes the partition is raised, allowing the monkey to go and open the correct box and receive his reward. Normal animals can do this very well: frontal animals cannot, unless they spend the waiting period doing nothing except sitting and concentrating single-mindedly on the correct door. Recordings from neurones in prefrontal areas during delayed response trials confirm the idea that these areas are in some sense to do with *waiting to do something*, with activity in many units starting up on receipt of the command, then firing in a sustained way until the response is finally made.

These miscellaneous observations concerning the prefrontal areas can be unified quite satisfactorily once it is appreciated that each involves a defect in the ability to *store a program of action*, for deferred rather than immediate use. Anxiety is of course a side effect of the sense that something has to be done in the future, and lack of anxiety may sometimes merely indicate a lack of forethought: worry, if rational, is a thoroughly good thing. Thus it was anxiety that presumably made our ancestors save some of their seed harvest to plant for next year, despite their immediate needs, and it is perhaps not going too far to suggest that the enhancement of useful anxiety of this kind is indeed what separates us most from the other primates. Finally, it may also be that the unpleasantness of pain, particularly when it results from terminal illnesses (it is this type of pain that frontal leucotomy seems best at alleviating), is at least in part due to the anxiety it causes us by reminding us of our impending death: the painfulness of an injury depends very much on the significance that we attach to it (see Chapter 4). By stripping pain of its meaning for the future, we also relieve its emotional threat.

PARIETAL CORTEX

The parietal lobe consists of an anterior part, the purely somatosensory strip already considered in Chapter 4 (p. 77), and the associational *posterior parietal lobe* (Brodmann areas 5, 7, 39 and 40) which is what we are concerned with here. It occupies a central position in the cerebral hemisphere (Fig. 13.3), and one might therefore expect it to be concerned with the co-ordination of information from the visual, auditory, somatosensory and motor areas which surround them; and by and large this seems to be true. There are massive fibre bundles connecting these neighbouring cortical regions with the parietal region, and it also receives a projection from the pulvinar and lateral posterior nuclei of the thalamus. The pulvinar in turn receives sensory information from visual areas 18 and 19, and from the colliculi and lateral and medial geniculate bodies; in addition it receives the usual reciprocal fibres from the parietal cortex itself. The lateral posterior nucleus obtains its input partly from the pulvinar and partly from the (somatosensory) ventral posterolateral thalamic nucleus (Fig. 13.3). Efferents from parietal cortex go to the premotor and supplementary motor areas, to the frontal eye fields, to basal ganglia (and hence to colliculus) and indirectly to the cerebellum. As might be expected from such a diversity of input, neurones in parietal cortex show complex responses to stimulation of many modalities, that are greatly influenced by context and attention. For instance, many are visually driven, with receptive fields that can be mapped out; but unlike visual cells in visual cortex itself, they may or may not fire when a stimulus appears within the field, depending on whether or not the stimulus is sufficiently interesting to evoke a subsequent motor response such as an eye movement. For this reason, this area is better regarded as sensorimotor rather than purely sensory (if indeed such a distinction has much meaning).

A great deal of what we know of the parietal cortex comes from the effects of damage to it; there are very many kinds of defects that can arise from such damage. They are not well localized, and some are associated with lesions in other associational areas as well, notably the upper parts of the temporal lobe. In this respect it is better to think of parietal and temporal neocortex as a single functional unit. These clinical disorders fall essentially into three groups:

1. *agnosia* – disorders of high-level sensory analysis;
2. *apraxia* – disorders of high-level motor co-ordination and appropriateness;
3. *aphasia* – disorders in communicating and using symbols.

Agnosia

One kind of agnosia has already been mentioned in Chapter 4: lesions of parietal cortex near the somatosensory region may give *tactile agnosia*. Here there is no appreciable peripheral disorder – the subject has normal sensitivity to touch or temperature, and his acuity as measured by the two-point discrimination test may be unimpaired – but what is lacking is the ability to use this sensory data properly in order to recognize and respond to objects that are sensed by the skin. Such a patient may not recognize a matchbox when he is given one to hold, but can do so if he is allowed to see it; such difficulties in feeling the shape of an object in the hand are sometimes called *astereognosia*. (The -*gnosia* root, incidentally, means 'knowledge': 'astereognosia' means 'no-shape-knowledge'. A little Greek helps make some sense of the forbidding clinical jargon for parietal lobe defects.) A comparable defect of vision is called *visual agnosia*. Again, simple tests of visual performance reveal no abnormality – acuity, colour vision and sensitivity may all be normal – but the subject cannot always *appreciate* what he sees, and recognition of objects and places may be difficult. One highly intelligent patient described by Oliver Sacks, when asked to identify a flower, described it as 'a convoluted red form, with a linear green

Name	Area of difficulty
Astereognosia	*Tactile recognition*
Visual agnosia	*Visual recognition*
Auditory agnosia	*Auditory recognition*
Spatial agnosia	*Orientation, drawing, maps, etc.*
Anosognosia	*Appreciation of body topography*
Prosopagnosia	*Recognition of faces*
Motor apraxia	*Execution of skilled sequences*
Constructional apraxia	*Assembling components into a whole*
Ideational apraxia	*Formulation of plans of action*

Box 13.1 Examples of specific agnosias and apraxias

attachment' but only recognized it as a rose when allowed to smell it. As in all agnosias, it is generally the most difficult tasks that are most affected, and in this case a difficulty in recognizing people's faces may be the first sign that something is wrong.

A related but distinct defect is *spatial agnosia*: the subject has difficulty in appreciating the spatial relationships between objects, tends to get disorientated more easily or may have difficulty in trying to draw a map or sketch a complicated object like a bicycle (Fig. 13.5). Very commonly the defect is unilateral, as a result of one-sided brain damage, and the disability is then confined to half of the visual field, which may often show lack of use or neglect. There is in fact increasing neurophysiological evidence that cells in parietal cortex may be specifically involved in the representation of visual and somatosensory space, and in dealing with the transformations and reorientations that are necessary every time we make a movement.

A curious feature of many of these high-level defects is that the subject may often be strikingly unaware that anything much is wrong, and resent suggestions to the contrary; the defective field is simply ignored – much as we ignore our own blind spot – and it may require specially designed neurological tests to reveal the disorder. One particularly bizarre example of this is when the agnosia takes the specific form of defects in the perception of one's own body image *(anosognosia)*. Such a subject may emphatically deny that a particular part of his body such as a leg

actually exists, and disown it when it is forcibly brought to his attention. This is not merely a conscious fabrication on the part of the patient: he may be completely consistent in his attitude to the limb, not drying it after a bath, not bothering to dress it, tending to bump it against door-frames, and the like. Nor can one talk about any lack of intelligence in the normal sense: rather the lack of a certain kind of synthesis between somatosensory and visual inputs.

Apraxia

Apraxia implies clumsiness, but of a kind that is much more specific for particular tasks than the more general impairment associated with lesions of the cerebellum or motor cortex. It may be especially noticeable when the subject had previously been extremely skilled at using a particular tool or carrying out a highly trained sequence of actions, as in the case of a fish-filleter whose biparietal lesion led her to forget how to do it: although she 'knew in her mind' how to set about filleting a fish, she was unable actually to execute the manoeuvres that she wanted, and was sent home by the foreman for 'mutilating fish'. Sometimes a patient cannot produce specific actions on command – for example, gestures such as beckoning or saluting – but can do so spontaneously in appropriate circumstances, illustrating the high hierarchical level of the deficit. A more specific variety of apraxia is *constructional apraxia*, a sort of motor version of spatial agnosia: though the patient may

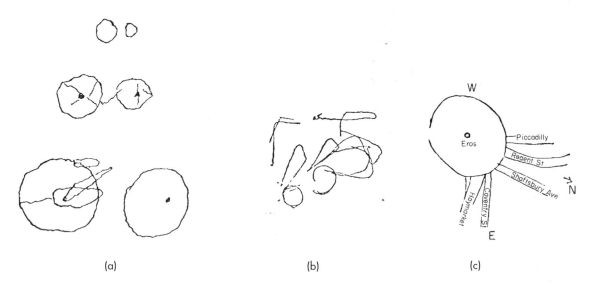

(a)   (b)   (c)

FIG. 13.5 (a) Attempts at drawing a bicycle: left parietal lesion. (b) Another attempt: biparietal vascular lesion. (c) An attempt at a map of Piccadilly Circus, showing neglect of top and left: right parietal lesions. (Critchley, 1971)

seem to perceive spatial relationships quite readily, he may for example find it difficult to put building blocks together to make a particular shape or construct a simple jigsaw puzzle.

Aphasia

There are many different ways in which aphasia may be manifested: a useful classification is into *sensory aphasia, motor aphasia* (these being in effect agnosia and apraxia in the particular field of language and communication), and *central aphasia*. (Strictly speaking, disorders of these kinds should be called *dysphasias* since there is not usually complete loss of function; but aphasia is nevertheless the term commonly in use.)

It is helpful to think of the processing of language by the brain in the same hierarchical terms as the generation of other kinds of movement (Fig. 13.6). Raw sense information enters through the eyes or ears, and is analysed by successive levels to the point at which letters, words, and larger syntactic units are recognized. At the highest level, *meaning* comes about by association of these symbols with other kinds of sensory information to form concepts; these in turn may result in speech or writing by an exactly converse process of elaboration down the motor side, ending up with the firing of motor neurones in appropriate patterns to form phonemes or fragments of writing or typing. Defects at the most peripheral levels – simple blindness or paralysis of the writing

Box 13.2 Examples of specific aphasias	
Name	**Area of difficulty**
Anarthria	*Articulation*
Aphonia	*Speaking*
Dyslexia	*Reading*
Dysgraphia	*Writing*
Broca's (expressive) aphasia	*Expression of communication*
Wernicke's (sensory) aphasia	*Understanding communication*
Conduction aphasia	*Repeating*
Nominal aphasia	*Recalling names*
Global aphasia	*All aspects of communication*
Amusia	*Music*
Acalculia	*Arithmetic*

arm – will prevent certain kinds of communication, but do not count as aphasia because the effects are unspecific.

In *sensory aphasia*, the patient's sense of hearing, for example, may be perfectly normal, and the sounds of speech are heard, but they make no sense:

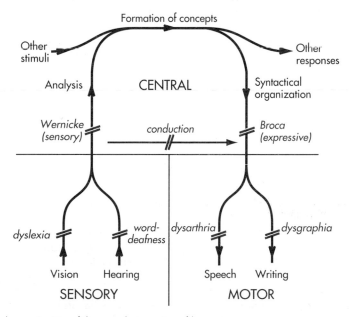

FIG. 13.6 The hierarchical organization of the neural processing of language.

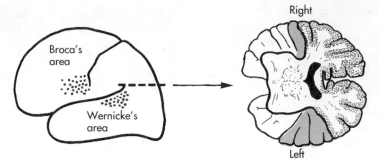

FIG. 13.7 Left, lateral view of left hemisphere, showing approximate location of Broca's and Wernicke's areas. Right, section along the dotted line above showing relative enlargement of the left planum temporale (approximating to Wernicke's area, colour) in comparison with the right. (After Geschwind and Levitsky, 1968; copyright AAAS)

he may complain that everything sounds like a foreign language. This is what is meant by *word deafness*, and may indirectly lead to speech defects as well, since the patient can no longer monitor effectively the words he is producing. A similar disability specifically affecting reading is word blindness or *alexia* (dyslexia in milder forms). These sensory aphasias are generally associated with a relatively localized region that borders on both visual and auditory cortex, called Wernicke's area (Fig. 13.7).

In *motor aphasia* the subject can show by his actions that he understands what is said to him or what he reads, but has difficulty in initiating such communications himself. Thus one may find *agraphia*, an inability to write, and apart from the actual absence of speech (*expressive* or Broca's aphasia) there may be less severe disabilities such as stuttering, and other more generalized defects of articulation (*dysarthria*). That this is not simply a peripheral motor defect is shown by the fact that emotional expression is sometimes unaffected – swearing may continue unabated – and stutterers often find that under sufficient duress, when they are not thinking consciously about what they are saying, the disability may suddenly vanish. Lesions specifically affecting speech and articulation are associated with another cortical area, *Broca's area* (Fig. 13.7), which is close to the tongue and mouth regions of the motor cortex, and is not actually in the parietal lobe at all but in the posterior frontal lobe. Damage here can frequently result from stroke due to a vascular accident.

Central aphasia

This term covers a number of miscellaneous conditions in which the defect is not primarily either sensory or motor but involves the mental mechanisms for forming concepts, for understanding symbols, and making sentences. A patient may be shown a common object such as a knife and be unable to name it (*anomia*). Yet he can use it, and by employing a paraphrase – 'what you use to cut with' – he may show that he can designate it in speech. Nor is the defect simply motor, since he can repeat the word 'knife' when told to do so; what seem to be at fault are the normal central *connections* that ought to link the sight of the object to the utterance of its name. Sometimes such a patient may use the wrong word for something without realizing it: given a pair of scissors he promptly describes them as a nail-file, and on being corrected may say 'No, of course it's not a nail-file, it's a nail-file'. He may produce speech sounds that are correctly executed and sound grammatical but actually make no sense; one such patient, for instance, shown a bunch of keys, came out with: 'Indication of measurement or intimating the cost of apparatus in various forms'. Such a response, often with much repetition of meaningless phrases, is described technically as *jargon*: in many cases it appears to be related to a sensory aphasia (Wernicke aphasia) that interferes with normal feedback of what is spoken.

All these defects may be quite specific for only one category of symbolization: thus in bilingual patients, only one of the languages may be affected, and morse aphasia or aphasia of sign language in deaf and dumb patients have also been described. An interesting case of specificity of this kind occurred in the composer Maurice Ravel, who was affected by aphasia in later life yet, though unable to speak or write, could still sing and play and compose music. Other specialized aphasias of the central kind that have been described include *acalculia*, an inability to perform arithmetical operations, and *amusia*, an inability to appreciate music. Conversely, individuals are not infrequently found with extraordinary development of these same faculties – the *idiots savants* or calculating prodigies, infant musicians, and those

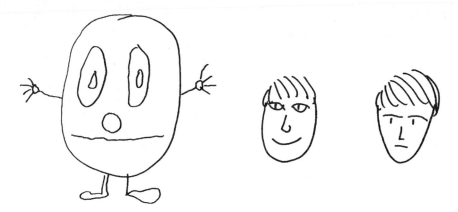

FIG. 13.8 Left, young child's drawing of a person; middle, untrained adult's, showing incorrect proportions, especially in the position of the eyes, compared with reality (right): the eyes are half-way down the head.

remarkable people who seem to find it no trouble at all to learn 20 or 30 different languages: but these are not normally reckoned to be disorders.

It is important to appreciate that normal people suffer from all types of aphasia on occasion. Not everyone can guarantee to complete *The Times* crossword puzzle; we all sometimes stutter or stumble over words; we are often at a loss for the name that goes with a face we know well or for something that a moment ago was 'on the tip of our tongue'; and all of us are guilty from time to time of generating jargon, especially in social situations where we are compelled to speak but have nothing to say. In people of limited education, one may observe a tendency for remarks to be repeated endlessly with only slight variations, or for a small number of concise adjectives to be applied indiscriminately; at a more exalted level we find 'ongoing situations', 'meaningful scenarios' and so forth. Equally, we all suffer at times from more or less severe attacks of spatial agnosia: few normal people are really very proficient at, say, drawing a map of the town where they live, and untrained drawings of the human face reveal obvious distortions of the proportions between the various parts that amount to a kind of disorder of body-image perception (Fig. 13.8). All this suggests that the parietal lobes are a fruitful area for human improvement, that might well become better developed in the course of future evolution. We'd all like to be able to speak several languages, to be 'good with our hands', to have a good ear for music, to be able to recollect everyone we meet, and be quick at doing mental arithmetic; but it seems that our cerebral cortex is just not up to doing all these things well at once. What we mean by 'intelligence' is perhaps no more than a relative freedom from the more obvious kinds of aphasia.

Finally, a rather curious kind of aphasia called conduction aphasia results in a specific inability to repeat what has just been heard, although speech may, in other respects, be relatively normal. It is thought to be associated with damage to fibres that link Wernicke's area to Broca's (the arcuate fasciculus).

Left–right asymmetry in the brain

One important point of interest in connection with the aphasias is that they show a functional asymmetry between the left and right halves of the brain. Although the agnosias can on the whole be found with lesions of either hemisphere, aphasia is nearly always associated with lesions of the left hemisphere (that governs the right side of the body), at least in right-handed people. This asymmetry is reflected in the relative anatomical size of certain parts of the cerebral cortex on the two sides, notably in Wernicke's area (Fig. 13.7). In living subjects this cerebral *dominance* (the dominant hemisphere being the one associated with aphasia) may be demonstrated by injecting a substance such as sodium amytal into the carotid artery on one side or the other, while the subject is carrying out some such task as reciting the letters of the alphabet. If the injection is on the dominant side, the recitation is interrupted for a short time and then continues; on the non-dominant side, very little is observed or felt by the subject. The various types of brain scan described in Chapter 1 (p. 14) enable both dominance and other aspects of cerebral localization to be shown in a dramatic manner (Fig. 13.9), with graphic pictures of the changing patterns of activity associated with different types of mental process.

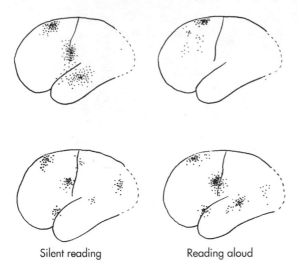

Silent reading   Reading aloud

FIG. 13.9 Regional blood flow in the cerebral cortex of a conscious human subject, revealed by a radioactive marker, under the various conditions shown. (After Lassen *et al.*, 1978)

In most people with left-hemisphere dominance, one finds that not only is the right hand used preferentially for writing and other skilled tasks but often the subject is right-legged and right-eyed as well: one may discover this by observing which foot is used to kick a ball or which eye looks through a peep-hole. Other, more unconscious actions may be revealing: thus the right leg may be crossed over the left when sitting; or if asked to fold his arms, the right arm may be placed on the left. But in the 7 percent or so of the population who have right-hemisphere dominance, most (but not all) are found to be left-handed. Some statistics relating to this correlation between dominance and handedness are shown in Figure 13.10. It is clear that although there is a strong correlation between the two, it is not an absolute one; one factor that tends to distort such figures is that there are considerable social pressures from school and family for 'natural' left-handers to learn to use their right hands in preference, producing an artificial shift of the distribution towards right-handedness, shown by the horizontal arrows. It is likely in fact that in the absence of such pressures the number of left-handers in the population would be rather more than the 10 percent or so usually reported, though this percentage has remained essentially unchanged throughout recorded history. It also appears from these statistics that there are essentially two distinct ways in which left-handedness can come about. The first is what might be called 'normal' left-handedness, and is probably genetically determined and essentially independent of dominance. The second type may be

the result of slight brain damage to the left hemisphere early in development, which causes both speech and handedness to shift to the other hemisphere, as indicated by the downward diagonal arrow in the figure; of these, some are again converted to apparent right-handedness by social pressures. Left-handers in this category may often show vague disabilities of speech such as stuttering or mild forms of apraxia or agnosia, a fact that has given left-handers as a whole – including the 50 percent of left-handers who are in every way perfectly normal – a bad name: literally so, when one considers the etymology of words like 'dextrous' and 'sinister', not to mention 'right'!

One interesting consequence of the lateralization of speech occurs in patients who have undergone surgical section of the fibres of the corpus callosum (see Fig. 1.5), an operation sometimes performed when there is an epileptic focus on one side of the cortex, in an attempt to prevent its spread to the mirror-image position on the other side by the mechanisms described earlier. What is most surprising in such cases is the apparent lack of ill effects, despite the severance of a massive fibre bundle containing more than 200 million fibres (a fact that prompted the facetious suggestion that the function of the corpus callosum is to allow the spread of

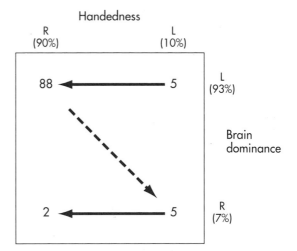

FIG. 13.10 Incidence of right- and left-handedness and brain dominance, expressed as percentages of the whole population. The horizontal arrows indicate the social pressures tending to turn natural left-handers into apparent right-handers; the dashed arrow indicates the likely effect of early damage to the left hemisphere. The data are derived from observations of the incidence of aphasia after unilateral brain lesions in right- and left-handers (Zangwill, 1967) and are therefore necessarily somewhat approximate.

epilepsy across the brain). However, although in the course of everyday life the patient may not perceive that much is amiss, more careful testing in the laboratory reveals an extremely interesting state of affairs: each half of the brain now appears to act independently, receiving information from the opposite half of the visual field, and controlling the opposite half of the body but only the left hemisphere is able to speak and thus tell you what it is thinking. Each half can perform matching tasks, so long as input and output are both on the same side – an object in the left visual field can be chosen by the left hand to match a picture shown on the left, but not by the right hand – but tests involving a *comparison* of left and right cannot be done. The non-dominant side is not entirely aphasic, for it can understand speech and also read: the left hand will pick up a cup to correspond with the word 'cup' presented in the left visual field, but the patient will be unable to name the object he has just selected because the specific function of speech is wholly localized in the other hemisphere. In general, the non-dominant hemisphere has great difficulty with things like selecting from a list of alternatives the word needed to complete the sentence 'The cat sat on the. . .', indicating that it suffers from central as well as motor aphasia. Some communication appears

to be possible between the hemispheres, but of a sub-conscious, emotional kind rather than of 'facts'. Thus a patient whose non-dominant hemisphere is allowed to see a pornographic picture may blush or giggle, and when asked what was there, may indicate the awareness of the emotion without being able to describe exactly what was seen. Some functions – for example, spatiovisual tasks like drawing, and probably musical appreciation as well – appear to be performed better by the non-dominant hemisphere (Fig. 13.11), and when asked to choose one of a set of drawings to go with another drawing, although the dominant side may select according to similarity of function, the non-dominant side uses similarity of appearance. Findings of this sort have led to a certain amount of semi-mystical speculation about the possibility of a fundamental split in the human psyche between the rational and factual left hemisphere and the intuitive and artistic right, and the importance of not allowing one hemisphere to develop at the expense of the other.

Finally, one may sometimes observe in such split-brain patients the effects of evident struggles between the two sides about what should be done, one hand perhaps trying to tie up the patient's shoelaces while the other unties them. Such observations raise rather

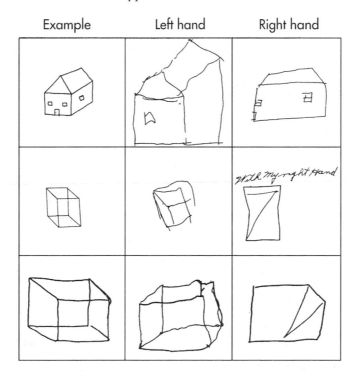

| Example | Left hand | Right hand |

FIG. 13.11 Right- and left-handed attempts by a split-brain patient to copy the series of drawings on the left; the superiority of the left hand in dealing with the implied three-dimensional relationships is evident, although the right hand is slightly better at carrying out the drawing movements. (Gazzaniga, 1967; copyright Scientific American Inc.)

difficult problems concerning the nature of consciousness and its relation to the brain: do we here have two minds in one body? The one thing we cannot do, of course, is to ask the patient what *he* thinks is going on: only the dominant hemisphere will reply.

TEMPORAL LOBE

There is no very clear distinction between temporal and parietal cortex, and we have already seen that some of the areas mentioned in the preceding section – Wernicke's area, for one – lie partly in the temporal lobe. There is, however, a specific type of disability associated with damage to the temporal cerebral hemispheres, *amnesia*, which is quite different in kind from anything seen with damage to frontal or parietal cortex. It is now recognized that these and other classic 'temporal lobe' disabilities are probably more related to structures forming part of the *limbic system,* lying within the temporal cortex itself. To make clear the distinction between these two quite different areas that are sometimes lumped together as 'temporal lobe', it is necessary to begin by outlining the structure and development of those deeper and older structures that form the limbic system, and which on account of their close association with the olfactory sense, discussed in Chapter 8, are sometimes classed together as the *rhinencephalon* or 'nose-brain'.

We have noted several times before that older structures of the brain tend to get elbowed out of the way by newer ones, and thus often become twisted into complex and at first sight incomprehensible shapes; this is markedly true of the limbic system. It consists of nuclei (notably the *amygdala, septal nuclei, mammillary body* and *hypothalamus*) and areas of cortex (in particular the *hippocampal gyrus, cingulate gyrus,* and *entorhinal, periamygdaloid* and *prepyriform cortex,* the latter two having particularly important olfactory connections), all joined together by fibre tracts (for instance the *fornix, medial forebrain bundle,* and projections from the mammillary body to *anterior thalamus,* and from there in turn to the cingulate gyrus); some of these are shown schematically in Figure 13.12.

Originally, it seems that the two main areas of limbic cortex, hippocampal and cingulate, formed almost the entire cortical surface of the brain, lying side by side immediately over the relatively compact group of their associated nuclei. But in the course of time, this simple three-layered *archicortex* was infiltrated by the newer six-layered *neocortex* which, by expanding almost explosively in the region separating the two areas, swelled into the modern balloonlike cerebral hemispheres, leaving the now dwarfed limbic cortex out on a limb (hence the name) round the edge (Fig. 13.13), and tucked away out of sight. Meanwhile, the massive fibre tracts required to link all this bulk of new cortex to the thalamus and other subcortical structures have forced their way between the older nuclei, cutting them off from one another and making their communicating nerve fibres wind their way right round the outside in circuitous fashion. At the same time, the amygdala, originally a structure on the wall of the hemisphere,

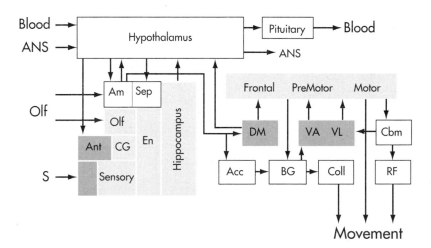

FIG. 13.12 Highly schematic and simplified representation of the principal areas of the limbic system and their connections to other structures. Cortical areas: Olf, olfactory: periamygdaloid, prepyriform; CG, cingulate; En, entorhinal; Thalamic nuclei: Ant, anterior; DM, dorsomedial VA, ventroanterior; VL, ventrolateral; Other regions: AM, amygdala; SEP, septum; Acc, nucleus accumbens; BG, basal ganglia; Coll, colliculi; RF, reticular formation; ANS, autonomic nervous system.

became – like the corpus striatum – submerged beneath the incoming tide of neocortex, and ended up as an additional subcortical nucleus.

All this makes the neuroanatomy of the limbic system look a great deal more complex than it really is, and a schematic representation of the functional connections, as in Figure 13.12, is in many ways more helpful than trying to reproduce in one's mind all the three-dimensional muddle of its actual form. Most of the limbic system appears to be concerned with such functions as emotion and motivation, with the neural control of the body's internal environment, and to some extent with olfaction; these aspects will be dealt with in the next chapter. The cortical regions, and especially the hippocampus, seem on the other hand to be more concerned with learning and memory, and will be discussed here.

As we have seen, the *hippocampus* lies along the bottom edge of the temporal neocortex, and it is perhaps not too fanciful to think of it as a kind of cortical gutter, with sensory information being increasingly analysed and refined as it trickles from neuronal level to neuronal level down from sensory projection areas, through the complex associational networks of parietal and temporal cortex, and finally draining into the hippocampus itself. Certainly in the more posterior region of the temporal neocortex, which borders on visual areas, the logical progression already noted in the visual cortex by which cells are found first with simple concentric fields, and then with more and more specificity in terms of such parameters as line orientation, colour movement, or width, appears here to be continued; in Chapter 7 (p. 154) we saw that cells have been found in the temporal cortex which respond to quite specific objects – faces, hands and so on – with significant behavioural implications.

In humans, electrical stimulation in this region has been undertaken occasionally as a preliminary to the surgical treatment of epileptic foci. What has sometimes been reported is that stimulation at particular sites gives rise not to the discrete flashes and spots of light characteristic of electrical stimulation of the human visual cortex but rather to complex and repeatable hallucinations of an unusually realistic kind, sometimes apparently not static but moving in 'real time' (for example, of a tune played by an orchestra, to which the patient could beat time), and often producing an experience which is a synthesis of many sensory modalities at once. In one case a patient described a sense of it being Sunday morning, a bright summer day, the car being washed, children shouting, and so on. Such experiments have naturally been rare, and there must be some doubt as to how they should be interpreted: necessarily, they have not been carried out on normal people, and one can never be quite sure that the effect of electrical stimulation is not merely to evoke an epileptic discharge of some kind. Nevertheless, it does seem probable from electrical recording in animals that some kind of progressively more detailed analysis of sensory information, and its integration across sensory modalities, does occur on its way down to the archicortex that runs round the bottom edge of the

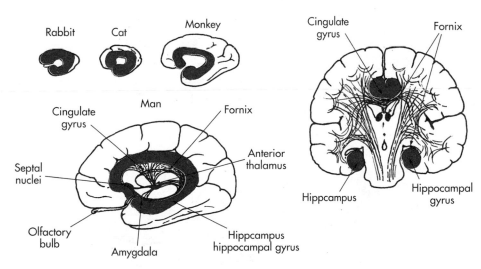

FIG. 13.13 The eclipse of the limbic cortex. Left, approximate area of limbic cortex (shaded) in rabbit, cat, monkey and human, showing the relative growth of neocortex and consequent relegation of limbic structures to medial and central regions. (Partly after Ochs, 1965) Right, transverse section of human brain, showing limbic cortex (shaded) and fornix, in relation to the massive fibre bundles serving the neocortex.

temporal cortex, and that this analysis – unlike what is seen in the parietal lobe – is of *recognition* rather than *localization*.

A cross-section through this gutter – its seahorse-like shape giving rise to the name 'hippocampus' – reveals a surprisingly regular neuronal structure, almost as machine-like as the cerebellum (Fig. 13.14). Archicortex differs from neocortex in having only three layers instead of six; there is only one layer of pyramidal cells, with fibres running predominantly transversely above and below them, and making afferent synaptic contact with the pyramidal cell dendrites. There appears to be a regular sequential arrangement, with each pyramidal cell in the entorhinal cortex projecting to a long row of pyramidal cells in the dentate gyrus, each of these in turn projecting to a row of cells in the CA3 region of the hippocampal gyrus, and finally these cells in turn projecting to the pyramidal cells of the CA1 region. Branches of the CA3 cells form the large fibre bundle called the *fornix*, which projects to the mammillary bodies and septal nuclei and in humans contains more fibres than either the pyramidal tracts or optic nerves. The CA1 cells project to the neighbouring *subiculum* and thence, amongst other areas, to the anterior and central regions of the thalamus, by which route they may ultimately influence the basal ganglia and neocortical areas. Apart from receiving fibres from temporal neocortex, the entorhinal region has projections also from the neighbouring olfactory areas, prepyriform and periamygdaloid cortex, and septum. Thus the entire structure can be represented in the highly schematic form shown in Figure 13.15, a strongly hierarchical arrangement well adapted to integrating together information from neocortex and from the olfactory system, recognizing specific patterns of activity, and producing both motivational responses through the motor system and emotional responses via the limbic nuclei. The question of what its output actually does must wait until the next chapter; what we are concerned with here is how the output is derived from its input.

That the hippocampus does indeed form in a sense the final output from the sensory analysers of the neocortex is clear from electrical recordings from its pyramidal cells. Ninety-five percent of the pyramidal cells of area CA3 have been described as totally multimodal, responding to almost any combination of sensory modalities, and they are also described as being 'novelty-conscious'; that is, that they tend to show *habituation* to a stimulus if it is repeatedly presented, and respond more readily to things that are new; this in itself represents a kind of memory process. The main reason for believing that the limbic cortex is concerned with memory functions comes from the effects of lesions, and in particular with a somewhat rash operation that has sometimes been performed with a view to alleviating certain types of epilepsy, in which parts of one or both temporal lobes have been excised. The first operation of this kind, carried out by the American surgeon W. B. Scoville, consisted of the removal of the tips of the temporal lobes on both sides. This had the disastrous result that although the patient's memory for events

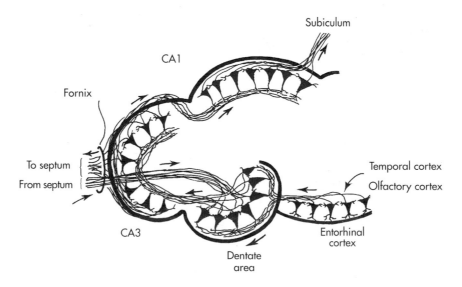

FIG. 13.14 Simplified transverse section of the hippocampus, showing the main neuronal connections.

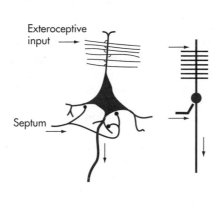 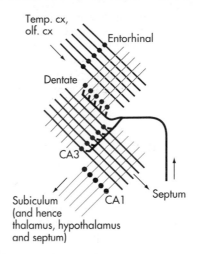

FIG. 13.15 Left, schematic representation of single hippocampal pyramidal cell from CA3, showing different regions of termination of septal and 'exteroceptive' afferents. (MacLean, 1975) Right, stylized representation of neural circuitry of the hippocampus.

that had occurred *before* the operation was good, he was in effect unable to remember for more than 10 minutes or so anything that had happened *after* it, a condition known as *anterograde amnesia* (Fig. 13.16). Subsequent work in animals has confirmed that it is damage to the hippocampal region that is responsible for this defect, and that it only happens when the lesion is bilateral, in which case the deficit is quite unspecific as to the nature of the material to be learnt: it can be recalled for some 5–10 minutes, but after that time, unless the subject can in some way rehearse it in his mind – as for example when trying not to forget a telephone number in the interval between looking it up in the book and dialling it – it is lost for good. Significantly, purely *motor* skills are unaffected: previously learnt ones are not lost, and new ones (like learning to type or to ride a bicycle) may be acquired: motor skills are learnt elsewhere, presumably either in cerebellum or neocortex. Unilateral lesions do not have the same dramatic effect, although some difficulty has been reported in learning verbal material if the lesion is on the dominant side.

The commonest type of anterograde amnesia is seen as a result of chronic alcoholism, and is called the *Korsakov syndrome* (*Clinical Neurology*, Ch. 20). It is thought to be the result not so much of the effects of the alcohol itself as of the malnutrition that goes with it, in particular of thiamine deficiency. After death, one may see degenerative changes to various areas on the limbic system, notably the mammillary bodies and anterior thalamus, both of which lie on the output from the hippocampus; however, one cannot of course be sure whether or not other regions, such as the hippocampus itself, may be functionally deranged even though their gross visual appearance may be normal. Again, long-term storage of memories is impaired and things cannot be remembered for more than a few minutes without conscious rehearsal. The victim consequently often seems to be stuck in a past era: if asked who the Prime Minister is, he might reply 'Harold Macmillan', and asked to describe the latest fashions for men, would talk about winkle-pickers and drainpipe trousers. As with the agnosias associated with parietal cortex, the patient

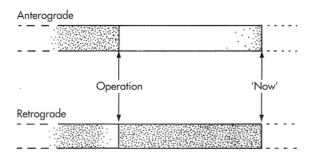

FIG. 13.16 Two kinds of amnesia. Above, anterograde amnesia: shaded areas represent the stretches of past experience that can be recalled (in this case only very recent events or those before the operation). Below, in retrograde amnesia there is a loss of recall of occurrences just before the operation or other precipitating event.

is often strikingly unaware that anything is wrong, and if confronted with facts that don't fit in to his private time-warp, may start to *confabulate,* making up elaborate fantasies to explain the discrepancies; he may also become paranoid and aggrieved, believing that there is some kind of global conspiracy directed against him.

The neural mechanism of memory

It is one thing to find a particular region of the brain that appears to be concerned with a particular function, but quite another to deduce exactly how the neurones of that region actually perform that function. In the case of memory, there is an additional complication in that there is not just one type of memory but at least three, apparently associated with different regions of the brain. In the first place, we have the kind of *sensory* memory which is implied by the ability of higher order sensory cells – for example, in the visual cortex – to develop for themselves a selectivity to those particular patterns of input that actually occur in the environment (see below). Secondly, we have the ability of the *motor* system to learn, through practice, to produce ballistic sequences of actions, using sensory feedback to modify the responses if they do not lead to success. And finally we have the kind of *central* memory that seems to be lost in the Korsakov syndrome or after bilateral hippocampal damage: the ability to put together analysed information from different sources, attach some kind of significance to it, and then store it so that it can be recalled at will. Can we hope to find any common mechanism for each of these types of memory, performed by different areas of the brain?

Certainly the first and third of these varieties are not conceptually very different: one can imagine a continuum of types of learning between, say, learning to associate patches of light on the retina into lines and edges, learning to associate these geometrical fragments into letters of the alphabet, and learning to recite a poem composed of the same letters. In each case, the key operation is one of forming *associations* between those elements of the stimulus that tend to recur together. If retinal units tend to fire in rows, we learn to recognize lines; if lines quite often lie in a certain relation to one another, we learn to recognize an 'E'; and after we have seen a particular configuration of such letters a few times, we have learnt 'Mary had a little lamb'. And as was emphasized in Chapter 1, sensory analysis and coding

necessarily imply a degree of plasticity in the connections from one level to the next – imply in fact a kind of memory – if the brain is not to be of astronomical size. Furthermore, in the case of Marr's plausible model of motor learning by the cerebellum examined in the previous chapter, it is the associations formed between sensory feedback patterns and ensuing fragments of action that ultimately result in the learning of motor sequences. Thus all learning by the brain amounts, in the end, to the formation of physical connections between neurones in such a way as to mirror the associations that exist in the real world between the stimuli that those same neurones code for. Memory is the process that models the world within our heads.

Consider for example the classic example of the Pavlov dog, trained by frequent association of sound and food to salivate when a bell is rung (Fig. 13.17). What can we deduce about what must be going on in his brain? Here there are, in simplest terms, two stimuli or inputs (S_1, sight of food; S_2, sound of bell), and one output or response (R, salivation). In the end, since either input will produce the output, there must be at least one chain of neurones forming a functional pathway from S_1 to R, and another from S_2 to R. Before the period of training, the second pathway either does not exist or perhaps exists in the structural sense but is functionally incapable of initiating salivation. It follows that learning the association between S_2 and R is brought about either by growth of new neuronal connections or by the activation of pre-existing ones. The only questions that remain are, firstly, *"What are the conditions under which such growth or activation occurs?* and secondly, *'What is the neuronal mechanism of these processes?'*

Now there is one further point that may be deduced about the Pavlov dog's brain when it has finally learnt to make its conditioned response. There must be at least one neurone – the one that actually innervates the salivary gland, if none other – that is common to both pathways, and where they first come together; this is the cell X shown schematically in Figure 13.17, and in the simplest case of all might have exactly one synapse (A) driven ultimately by S_1, and one (B) driven by S_2. Let us for the moment consider only the second and more likely of the two possibilities mentioned earlier, namely that both synapses are structurally in existence before the training period but that the synapse B is in some kind of inactive, dormant state; we assume that synapse A on the other hand is always capable of firing X and hence producing salivation. What we observe is that after sufficient pairings of food with bell, the bell alone eventually produces salivation. Translating this

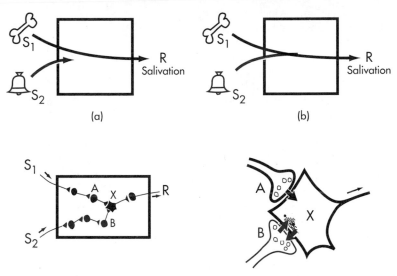

FIG. 13.17 Memory and neuronal connections. Above, schematic representation of functional pathways before **(a)** and after **(b)** Pavlovian conditioning of salivation (R) to the sound of a bell (S_2) by frequent pairing of bell and food (S_1). Below, simplified representation of the functional chains of neurones that must exist after conditioning : X (shown in more detail on right) is the first neurone common to both paths. It has an afferent A that is driven by S_1 and an afferent B, driven by S_2, whose effectiveness has increased because of frequent joint activity of X and B.

into what is happening in the region of X, this means that the more often A (and hence X) fires at the same time as B, the stronger becomes the connection from B to X, until in the end B is able to fire X all by itself: the bell produces salivation.

Note that it is the *associated* firing of B and X that is necessary to strengthen the synaptic connection: mere overactivity of B alone (if for example the unfortunate dog were to be subjected to continual bell-ringing except at meal-times) is not a sufficient condition. In other words, it is the conjunction of presynaptic and postsynaptic activity that is postulated to cause synaptic strengthening: *fire together, wire together*. That this must be so was deduced – as we shall see, with extraordinary prescience – more than 50 years ago by D. O. Hebb, and synapses with these properties are called *Hebbian synapses*. You may recall that exactly the same hypothesis was used in Marr's model of cerebellar learning (Chapter 12): once again, it is the paired association of Purkinje cell firing with parallel fibre activity that results in strengthening of the connection from one to the other. In terms of Figure 13.17, A is the climbing fibre, B is the parallel fibre, and X the Purkinje cell itself.

It may of course be objected that the notion that the connection from B to X already exists structurally before the period of training is an implausible one, even granted the amount of convergence and divergence of pathways that occurs in the brain, and the bringing together of diverse sources of information

in such regions as the hippocampus. However, the model will still work without that assumption, if we imagine that paired firing of B and X results in some way in growth of B towards X and eventual functional contact (or alternatively, in growth of dendrites of X towards B).

Until a few years ago, Hebbian synapses were a purely theoretical construct; then suddenly an entirely novel kind of synaptic mechanism was discovered – the NMDA receptor – that exactly embodied what had been predicted so long ago. The principle of its operation is simple, and it is perhaps surprising that it had not been proposed earlier: whereas other ionic channels known at that time were either voltage- or ligand-gated, the NMDA receptor is *both*. The condition for it to open is first that the postsynaptic cell is depolarized, and second the presence of the transmitter glutamate. If both conditions are met, calcium enters the postsynaptic cell, where it appears to turn on cellular machinery for the manufacture of more glutamate receptors: not NMDA ones but conventional KQ ones that require only the presence of glutamate to produce depolarization (Fig. 13.18). Once there are enough of them, the synapse will be strong enough to fire the postsynaptic cell on its own.

There is a peculiarity of the dendrites of neurones in those regions of the brain that are particularly associated with learning of one sort or another – the pyramidal and stellate cells of neocortex and of hippocampus, and the Purkinje cells of the cerebellum – which supports the idea of local postsynaptic change. Certain classes of afferent in each case terminate not directly on the soma or dendrite surface but rather on a sort of bud sticking out from it (the dendritic spine, Fig. 3.14), which contains a prominent Golgi apparatus, implying a specifically localized production of protein, presumably of new KQ receptors; on visual cortical cells, the number of spines on visual cortical cells is greatly reduced by visual deprivation. It is of course essential that synaptic strengthening should be strictly limited to only the one particular synapse and not over the whole cell. At many sites there is also evidence for presynaptic changes, an increase in the amount of transmitter released being triggered by NO diffusing from the postsynaptic cell, generated as response to the entry of calcium through NMDA receptors.

Finally, it is clear that whereas a stimulus that one remembers for a lifetime may only be present for less than a second, growth or strengthening of synapses must take some time to implement. There must therefore be a period of consolidation during which the event to be remembered is actually converted into some kind of semi-permanent structural change. There is in fact good evidence that there are really two distinct memory stores in the brain: a *long-term memory* (LTM) which takes the form of the kind of synaptic changes that we have been considering, and a *short-term memory* (STM; there is evidence that it has a number of separate components) which retains information temporarily to cover the period – probably of the order of 20 minutes or so – during which consolidation takes place. It appears that STM is much more vulnerable than LTM, suggesting that the short-term store is a dynamic one, perhaps consisting of impulses continually circulating round looped chains of neurones. Sudden shocks of any kind – a blow on the head or the passage of a large electrical current across the skull, as in electroconvulsive therapy – are sufficient to disrupt STM, and cause a characteristic type of amnesia called *retrograde amnesia* in which the ability to recall events that occurred

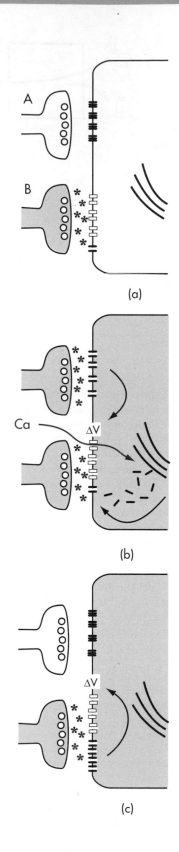

(a)

(b)

(c)

FIG. 13.18 NMDA synapses and learning. **(a)** Synapse A and B both release glutamate, but B has NMDA receptors under it, (white) whereas A has only KQ receptors (black). Before training, B alone is ineffectual because of the lack of KQ receptors, and the postsynaptic cell does not fire. **(b)** If A is active as well, causing postsynaptic depolarization, the NMDA channels now open in response to the transmitter from B, allowing calcium to enter. This calcium then improves the effectiveness of B, either (as here) by increasing the number of KQ receptors or possibly through presynaptic mechanisms. As a result **(c)**, B is now effective on its own.

either after the shock or long before it is unimpaired, but a period of some 20 minutes or so before the shock remains more or less blank (Fig. 13.16). It seems as though memories need to be stored for a certain time in STM in order to make, as it were, a sufficient impression on the permanent memory trace, as suggested by the two-tank analogy of Figure 13.19, and that violent disruption of the brain's activity through electroconvulsive therapy or some other shock simply empties the STM of its contents. *Anterograde amnesia*, characteristic of hippocampal damage and the Korsakov syndrome, is in a sense exactly the opposite: it is as if the flow from the upper to the lower tank, from STM to LTM, had been permanently disconnected, leaving the patient with a functional STM but fossilized LTM. Finally, the leak in the STM tank in Figure 13.19 is a reminder that not everything in STM – perhaps fortunately – finds its way into permanent memory, and there is little conscious control, if any, over what is or is not permanently stored. Some unconscious control certainly does occur, since experiences with a strong emotional significance are almost always transferred to LTM. (A striking instance of this, for those of my own generation at least, is that nearly everyone remembers with unusual vividness exactly what they were doing when, in 1963, they heard the news that President Kennedy had been assassinated.)

One complicating factor is that things may have been stored perfectly well in LTM, but cannot be recalled because the mechanism for *retrieval* is not working properly – this is particularly obvious in the case of unpleasant experiences and psychiatric help may be required in order to bring such repressed memories to consciousness. In other cases, forgetting may be the result of learning new material. Since retrieval is essentially by association, memories that are linked together by too many associations may become irretrievably entangled. Unique and strange events are easy to recollect; boring things like telephone numbers are much more difficult, because of the vast number of pre-existing associations in our minds between each of the digits, the result of having remembered many other numbers in the past. Commonly advertised methods for improving one's memory generally work by translating each digit into a unique and vivid mental image: thus if 7 is 'elephant', 3 'cigar' and 4 'bicycle', the number 734 could be recalled by picturing an elephant smoking a cigar and riding a bicycle. The snag is of course obvious: after a while, there will be such a tangled knot of connections between elephants, bicycles and cigars and so forth as a result of learning one's friends' telephone numbers that new numbers will be just as difficult to remember as ever.

Sensory learning: recognition

Recognition implies classification. A classification based on only one criterion is trivial to implement: it is easy, for example, to build a machine that will sort peas out according to size before stuffing them into appropriate tins. The problems start when there are a large number of attributes to be taken into account before a stimulus can be assigned to one or another category, and when it is the relation between them that is the crucial factor, rather than exact correspondence

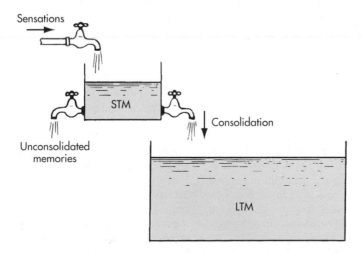

FIG. 13.19 The two-tank analogy of short-term and long-term memory (STM and LTM).

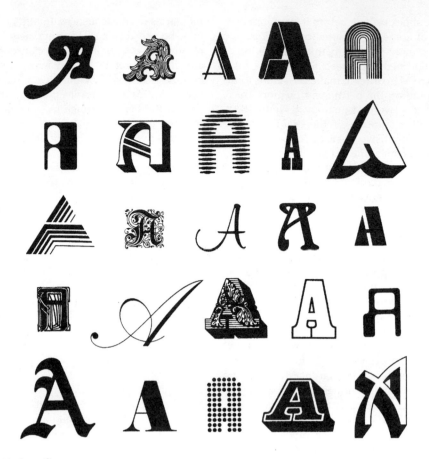

FIG. 13.20   What is A-ness?

with some kind of template. If the objects to be recognized are highly stereotyped, like £10 notes, it is not difficult to make a device that looks for a match between a stored 'ideal' bank note in the machine's memory, and the actual specimen that is presented. But how, for instance, do we recognize sets of objects as different as the A's in Figure 13.20 as actually belonging in the same category? It is hard to define an 'ideal' letter A or say what essentially is the A-ness that all the examples in Figure 13.20 have in common. And we recognize a rose not because it is identical to some archetypal rose but because some aspects of it are similar to other specimens that we have seen, and although in other respects – perhaps its size or its colour – it may be different, we know these aspects are irrelevant and can be ignored. Thus there are two components to recognition: one is to do with associating together those attributes of a stimulus which define what it is; the other is the *filtering out* of aspects of the stimulus that are irrelevant.

The filtering out part of it is something we have already met when considering the functions of adap-

tation, more particularly in the eye. We saw that one of the functions of dark adaptation is to enable us to perceive the intrinsic albedo of an object despite the fact that on different occasions it may be brightly or dimly illuminated. It is often forgotten that it is the *object* that has to be recognized and not the stimulus. Objects in the real world are seen at different times under lighting of different intensities and colours, and from different distances and directions. The stimulus, in other words, is partly a function of what the object is, and partly a function of quite accidental and arbitrary factors that are nothing to do with the object at all. A particular retinal image of a cube under particular conditions is as much a coded version of the cube, that has to be deciphered, as are the four letters CUBE: in many ways the latter presents an easier task! So the job of the visual system (and indeed, any sensory system) is to separate off those aspects of an object's image which are its *essential* attributes in the sense of defining its essence, and those which are merely *accidental* and the result of temporary circumstances (Fig. 13.21). Thus in the

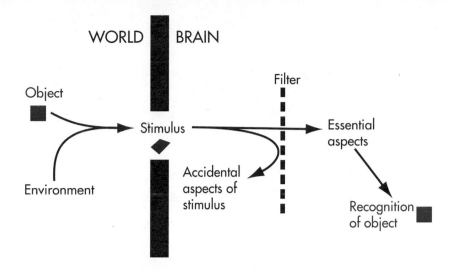

FIG. 13.21 A stimulus is a coded version of the object that causes it, some aspects of it being due to the object itself, and some to accidental factors. It has to be decoded by the brain filtering out the accidental properties to leave behind those that are essential to the object itself.

case of luminance and illuminance, it is the albedo of an object which is essential, and not how brightly it is illuminated: adaptation here filters out the accidental part to leave behind something that is essential.

It is not hard to extend this idea – of filtering out accidental properties to leave behind what is most characteristic of an object – to much higher levels of perception. When we look at a coin on a table, it looks circular even though its retinal image is in fact an ellipse. We recognize that all the different elliptical images that it forms as we change our viewing angle represent the same essence, and we are filtering out the accidental aspects of the stimulus that depend on us and not on the coin. Or again, when we perceive that Figure 13.20 is composed entirely of A's, we are filtering out the accident of the way in which they happen to have been designed. At a higher level, we recognize that *arbre, baum* and *tree* are all essentially the same by disregarding the accident of what language they happen to have been expressed in. The same principle operates at the very highest levels of thought: in chess, rather than laboriously calculating all the possible consequences of a given move, a good player will perceive that a given position is essentially the same as some other one with which he is familiar, even though many of the accidental details are different.

The second principle, that of *association,* can be explained quite readily in terms of the mechanism described in the previous section, in which neurones form functional connections between themselves when their activities are correlated. We recognize a figure '3' because it has certain topological features that are found in association together: a single continuous line with a cusp in the middle to the left and a couple of bulges to the right. If we imagine individual neurones that respond to each of these features, we can see in general terms how, with sufficient repetition, they would tend to strengthen their mutual connections and form a functional cluster corresponding to the existence of 3s in the outside world. To take a more specific example, it is not difficult to imagine how a cortical line detector might be 'built' in this way. Imagine that the projection of thalamic units to cortical neurones is initially rather random, with a good deal of convergence and divergence (Fig. 13.22). At first the receptive fields of these 'naive' cortical units will be chaotic and disorganized. Let us suppose also that the synaptic connections from thalamus to cortex have the property that when the cortical unit fires it strengthens those synapses that are active at the same time, and weakens those that are not. On looking at a straight line, although no line detectors as such will yet exist, it is clear that some cortical units will fire and others not. Of the afferents going to the cells that fire, the ones corresponding to retinal units lying on the line will be strengthened, while the others will weaken. In time, when a sufficient number of straight lines of the same orientation have been experienced, it is clear that the inputs from the line will have been reinforced, and the other, irrelevant ones will have ceased to function: the receptive field of the cortical unit will

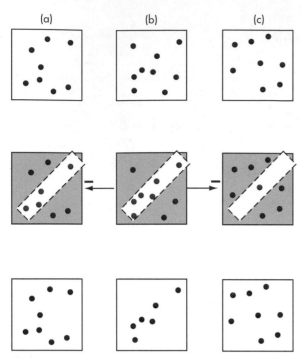

FIG. 13.22 Hypothetical mechanism by which the specificity of central visual neurones might grow from experience. Top row, receptive fields of three 'naive' neurones, indicated by dots. Middle row, on stimulation with a slit of light at a particular orientation, only **(b)** fires: its active afferent fibres grow stronger, while the others decay. Bottom row, after a sufficient number of presentations of this type, **(b)**'s receptive field is closely matched to the slit, and **(a)** and **(c)** are still available to learn some other stimulus.

then be that of an ordinary line detector. (Such a model can be extended to cover the generation of inhibitory surrounds as well but it must be said that recent work has indicated that the true mechanism, though not understood in full, is not quite as simple as the one presented here.)

It is not difficult to extend such a notion to yet higher stages of cortical processing, and imagine units that could learn in exactly the same way to respond to the more complex sets of essential features that make up things like teacups and human faces. It is certain that some such mechanism of learned connections must exist, for we know that young kittens brought up in a visual environment consisting entirely of lines having a single orientation are found on subsequent testing to have cortical units that respond only to lines of that same orientation. Once such a set of features have been associated together in this way, the detector may not mind very much if some of its inputs are missing on a particular occasion: so long as it fires more actively than any of its neighbours in response to a particular object, then it will in effect form a hypothesis about what is present, and the subject may then think he sees features of the object that he expects but which are not in fact there (Fig. 13.23).

Lateral inhibition is an important component of models of this kind. During the learning process it will ensure that only the cells that are most stimulated by a particular pattern will be activated enough to

increase the strength of their afferent synapses (Fig. 13.22). And subsequently it will help to sharpen up the discrimination between stimuli that differ only slightly by enhancing any differences in the patterns of neural activity that they evoke. Lateral

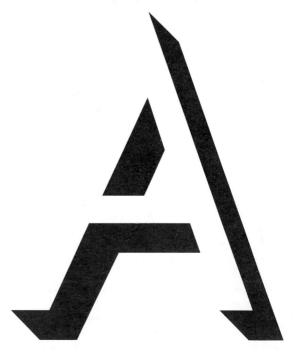

FIG. 13.23 Phantom contours.

inhibition of this kind is not strictly spatial, of the kind introduced in Chapter 4, but operates rather along what might be called an abstract sensory dimension. For example, the mutual inhibition between red- and green-sensitive channels in the retina that generates colour-opponent responses can be thought of as lateral inhibition along a wavelength axis, that sharpens up colour discriminations. In the same way, lateral inhibition between line detectors in the visual cortex acts along a dimension of orientation, improving angle discrimination. A consequence of this is that if two lines are presented at once, forming an angle, the effect of the lateral inhibition is to exaggerate the difference in their orientation, and thus make the angle seem larger. Many well-known optical illusions (Fig. 13.24) can be explained by angle expansion of this kind.

The most abstract example of all is perhaps in the olfactory bulb. We saw in Chapter 8 that olfactory receptors are very unspecific as to the chemical stimuli they respond to: to take a simplified example, while one receptor might respond to substances A, B, C and D, its neighbour might respond to A, B, C and E. But the effect of lateral inhibition between second-order neurones within the olfactory bulb (Fig. 13.26) will be to eliminate the overlap between the two 'receptive fields' and thus considerably sharpen up their modality specificity to particular stimuli. Here we have lateral inhibition that is in effect operating in a multidimensional stimulus space.

The final goal of recognition is not, of course, simply the identification of individual objects but of attaching *meaning* to them. This implies, in effect, associating them not only with each other but with

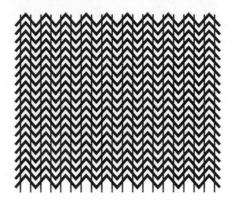

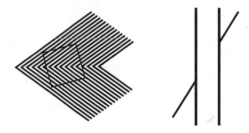

FIG. 13.24 Some illusions caused by lateral inhibition amongst orientation detectors; in each case, the apparent orientation of a line is twisted away from a neighbouring line of different orientation. Above, the thin lines are in fact parallel (the Zöllner illusion); below left, the figure is actually a square; right, the two thinner lines are in fact aligned, though the expansion of the angle they make with the vertical lines makes it look as though they would not meet if extended (the Poggendorf illusion).

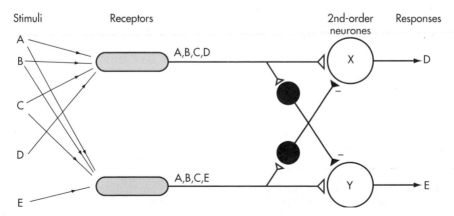

FIG. 13.25 Lateral inhibition as a means of increasing modality specificity. Left, two idealized olfactory receptors, each responding to its own list of substances (A, B . . .E) but with considerable similarity of response. The effect of mutual inhibition at the level of the second-order neurones (right) is to increase the specificity of the response by eliminating responses that are common to the two receptors: neurone X will respond only to D and neurone Y only to E.

words, actions, and above all with emotional states and with the satisfaction of physiological needs. The only way to make sense of what the brain does is to take a firmly pragmatic line, to insist all the time on asking what *use* things are. Our senses are not, after all, merely there to provide some sort of in-flight entertainment for the soul: they have evolved because they help us to survive. They are required by the motor system both in the planning and execution of actions, and also by the *motivational* systems that decide what action to take: whether an object is nice or nasty, whether it is something to eat or something that will eat us. It is not difficult to see how this can be done, by an extension of the mechanism for forming associations by means of synaptic strengthening, and this is what the next chapter is about.

References

Carpenter, M.B. (1976) *Human Neuroanatomy*. Williams and Wilkins, Baltimore.

Cobb, S. (1946) *Borderlands of Psychiatry*. Harvard University Press, Harvard, Mass.

Critchley, M. (1971) *The Parietal Lobes*. Hafner, London.

Edwards, B. (1979) *Drawing on the Right Side of the Brain*. Collins, Glasgow.

Freeman, W. and Watts, J. W. (1948) TheThalamic Projection to the Frontal Lobes. *Research Publications of the Association for Nervous and Mental Diseases* 27, 200–209.

Gazzaniga, M. S. (1967) The Split Brain in Man. *Scientific American* August

Geschwind, N. and Levitsky, W. (1968) Human Brain: Left–Right Asymmetries in Temporal Speech Region. *Science* 161, 186–187.

Lassen, N. A., Ingvar, D. H. and Skinhøj, E. (1978) Brain Function and Blood Flow. *Scientific American* October, 50–59.

MacLean, P. D. (1975) An ongoing analysis of hippocampal inputs and outputs: microelectrode and neuroanatomical findings in squirrel monkeys. In *The Hippocampus*, ed. R. L. Isaacson and K. H. Pribram. Plenum, New York.

Ochs, S. (1965) *Elements of Neurophysiology*. Wiley, New York.

Penfield, W. (1967) *The Excitable Cortex in Conscious Man*. Liverpool University Press, Liverpool.

Zangwill, O. L. (1967) Speech and the Minor Hemisphere. *Acta Neurologica Belgica* 67, 1013–1020.

NOTES

Page 248 Prefrontal cortex Two excellent and comprehensive accounts are Fuster, J. M. (1989) *The Prefrontal Cortex* (Raven Press, New York), and Levin, H. S., Eisenberg, H. W. and Benton, A. L. (1991) *Frontal Lobe Function and Dysfunction* (Oxford University Press, New York).

Page 251 Parietal areas Good general accounts may be found in Beaumont, J. G. (1983) *Introduction to Neuropsychology* (Blackwell, Oxford), Critchley, M. (1971) *The Parietal Lobes* (Hafner, London), Stein, J. F. (1991) Space and the parietal association areas, in *Brain and Space*, ed. J. Paillard (Oxford University Press, Oxford), and Walsh, K. W. (1978) *Neuropsychology, a Clinical Approach* (Churchill Livingstone, Edinburgh).

Page 251 Symptomatology Neurological anecdote has now – deservedly – achieved the status of a recognized literary genre, and sometimes reached the stage as well; some of the best are Critchley, M. (1979) *The Divine Banquet of the Brain* (Raven, New York); Klawans, H. L. (1989) *Toscanini's Fumble* (Bodley Head, London); Klawans, H. L. (1990) *Newton's Madness* (Bodley Head, London); Sacks, O. (1985) *The Man who Mistook his Wife for a Hat* (Duckworth, London).

Page 252 The representation of space See de Renzi, E. (1982) *Disorders of Space Exploration and Cognition* (Wiley, Chichester); de Renzi, E. (1988) Visuo-spatial agnosias, in *Physiological Aspects of Neuro-ophthalmology, ed.* C. Kennard and F. C. Rose (Chapman and Hall, London).

Page 252 Denial of body parts As in the following Monty Python-like dialogue:

> *Doctor:* Is this your hand?
> *Patient:* Not mine, doctor.
> *Doctor:* Yes it is. Look at that ring: whose is it?
> *Patient:* That's my ring. You've got my ring, doctor!

Sandifer, P.H. (1946) Anosognosia and disorders of the body scheme. *Brain* 69, 122–137.

Page 253 Aphasia Brain, L. (1975) *Speech Disorders* (Butterworth, London) is a classic account; see also Rose, F. C., Whurr, R. and Wyke, M. A. (eds) (1988) *Aphasia* (Whurr Publishers, London).

Page 254 Aphasia after a stroke A classic example is that of Dr Samuel Johnson, who has left a vivid account of what it is like to experience such a stroke. Johnson was a stutterer before this episode, and was notoriously clumsy: it is possible that he may in fact have suffered some slight brain damage in early life: *'I went to bed, and in a short time waked and sat up. I felt a confusion and indistinctness in my head that lasted, I suppose, about half a minute. I was alarmed, and prayed God, that however he might afflict my body, he would spare my understanding. This prayer, that I might try the integrity of my faculties, I made in Latin verse. The lines were not very good, but I knew them not to be very good: I made them easily, and concluded myself to be unimpaired in my faculties…. Soon after I perceived that I had suffered a paralytick stroke, and that my speech was taken from me. Though God stopped my speech, he left me my hand. My* *first note was necessarily to my servant, who came in talking, and could not immediately understand why he should read what I put into his hands. In penning this note I had some difficulty; my hand, I knew not how nor why, made wrong letters. My physicians are very friendly, and give me great hopes; I have so far recovered my vocal powers as to repeat the Lord's Prayer with no very imperfect articulation.'*

A number of features of this account are interesting: the aphasia was clearly predominantly expressive, with a little disturbance of writing, but no disorder either of the ability to comprehend speech or to formulate it in the mind – even in Latin verse! – and certainly no evidence of any general impairment of intelligent thought.

Page 255 Prodigies See for example Treffert, D. A. (1989) *Extraordinary People: an Explanation of the Savant Syndrome* (Bantam, London). There are also some good examples in Sacks, O. (1985) *The Man who Mistook his Wife for a Hat* (Duckworth, London).

Page 256 Dominance and handedness There is a good discussion in Morgan, M. J. and McManus, I. C. (1988) The relationship between brainedness and handedness, in *Aphasia*, ed. F. C. Rose, R. Whurr and M. A. Wyke (Whurr Publishers, London).

Page 257 Abilities of the non-dominant side A full account is Springer, S. P. and Deutsch, G. (1993) *Left Brain, Right Brain* (W.H. Freeman, San Francisco). With special exercises to encourage the right hemisphere, one can learn to draw better (it works – I've tried it): see Edwards, B. (1979) *Drawing on the Right Side of the Brain* (Collins, Glasgow).

Page 262 Anterograde amnesia A moving account of such a case (*The Lost Mariner*) can be found in Sacks, O. (1985) *The Man who Mistook his Wife for a Hat* (Duckworth, London).

Page 262 Memory A well-written popular account is Baddeley, A. (1983) *Your Memory: a User's Guide* (Penguin, Harmondsworth); Dudai, Y. (1989) *The Neurobiology of Memory* (Oxford University Press, Oxford) is more physiological.

Page 262 Memory and development Some accounts of neuronal memory mechanisms, particularly in relation to development: Abeles, M. (1991) *Corticonics: Neural Circuits of the Cerebral Cortex* (Cambridge University Press, Cambridge); Byrne, J. H. and Berry, W. O. (1989) *Neural Models of Plasticity* (Academic, New York); Gaze, R. M. (1970) *The Formation of Nerve Connections* (Academic, London); Hopkins, W. G. and Brown, M. C. (1984) *Development of Nerve Cells and Their Connections* (Cambridge University Press, Cambridge); Lund, R. D. (1978) *Development and Plasticity of the Brain* (Oxford University Press, Oxford).

Page 263 Hebb The postulate was most clearly stated in Hebb, D. O. (1949) *Organization of Behaviour* (Wiley, London): *'When an axon of cell A is near enough to excite a cell B and repeatedly or persistently takes part in firing it, some growth process or metabolic change takes place in one or both cells such that A's efficiency, as one of the cells firing B, is increased.'*

Page 265 Memory methods The technique of bizarre association is of very great antiquity, used, for instance, by the great Roman orators. In its original form it involved the mental placing of things to be remembered into a fixed sequence of locations in a real or imagined building: hence the expression 'in the first place ... in the second place....'. See the extraordinarily stimulating Yates, F. A. (1969) *The Art of Memory* (Penguin, Harmondsworth) and also Rossi, P. (1990) Creativity and the art of memory, in *Creativity in the Arts and Science*, ed. W. R. Shea and A. Spadafora (Science History Publications, Canton, Mass).

Page 266 Nature of perception See for example Kaufman, L. (1979) *Perception* (Oxford University Press, Oxford). Some of the most thoughtful and penetrating insights in this area have been voiced by the distinguished art historian E. H. Gombrich, who frequently shows a much better understanding of perceptual mechanisms than many neurophysiologists: see for instance Gombrich, E. H. (1982) *The Image and the Eye* (Phaidon, London).

Page 269 Angle expansion See Carpenter, R. H. S. and Blakemore, C. B. (1973) Interactions between orientations in human vision. *Experimental Brain Research* 18, 287–303. An excellent and comprehensive source of visual illusions in general is Robinson, J. O. (1972) *The Psychology of Visual Illusion* (Hutchinson, London).

NEUROLAB

 ## Cortical regions

Page 248

A simple map of functional cortical areas, for self-testing. Click on one of the radio buttons designating an area of cortex, and the name and Brodmann number will appear in the box at right. Alternatively, click on the pull-down button at the right of the box to display the whole list, and click on an item: the corresponding radio button will be selected.

Pavlovian conditioning

Page 263

An exhibit demonstrating classic Pavlovian conditioning. Two buttons (bone and bell) represent respectively the unconditional and conditional stimuli, UCS and CS; the response is indicated by the horizontal thermometer at the right. Click on the UCS, and observe the time-course of the response, and the existence of temporal summation. Wait for the response to die away, and then click on the CS: nothing happens, as the animal has not yet been conditioned. Now train it by pairing the UCS with the CS a number of times. The thermometer at the bottom shows the resultant strength of the synaptic connection from the CS to the response, which is subject to spontaneous decline (the rate depends on the Decay rate slider). Now test by giving the CS alone: a response should now be evoked, but if you go on testing without reinforcement from the UCS, you will see the synaptic strength decline quite rapidly. Experiment with various regimes of training and testing. Note that the model is a simple one and does not incorporate some of the more complex features of conditioning known to psychologists.

Neural network

Page 265

The elementary part of this exhibit has already been described, on p. 198. If you click on Learning, you are given a neural net that is smaller in size, but does have the capability of learning. Its task is to work out whether the number of activated check boxes on the left is even or odd, as indicated by the activity of the two output neurones on the right: red indicates excitation, blue inhibition. Each neurone in the middle layer receives a synapse from each of the three input neurones, and contributes to both the output neurones: initially, or after pressing Forget, the strengths of these synapses are set to small random values. Press Forget, and then start to teach the network the difference between 0 and 1 by repeatedly clicking to turn a particular check box on and off. You will see that quite soon the 'Odd' output neurone will turn red when the box is checked, and blue otherwise, and vice-versa for the 'Even' neurone. How it works is that those synapses that contributed to a correct response gradually get stronger, while the others get weaker. Try then to teach it to respond correctly to a different check box on its own: you will find it takes longer to learn it, because to some extent you have to

overcome the previous learning; when you return to test the original task, you may find that it has forgotten it. It is even more difficult then to teach it that 2 is even. With some patience, and several hundred trials, you may succeed it getting it to respond correctly to all possible combinations of checks. The best teaching strategy is to train it with examples of all the possible combinations rather than concentrating on one particular case at a time – as in real life. After it has been trained, observe what input patterns each middle layer responds to: they tend to be rather haphazard combinations, as in many parts of the brain.

Line learning

Page 267

This exhibit shows how a set of cortical units, initially connected rather randomly to retinal afferents, can learn to convert themselves into a set of line detectors for different orientations. The five units are shown at the top, each with a window indicating the position of their retinal afferents, the colour showing the strength of the connection; underneath a thermometer shows the degree of its excitation, and the button indicates that it has reached threshold for activation. When a line is presented (click on Give stimulus), the activity in each unit rises at a rate proportional to the amount of input it receives from the retinal afferents; the first to reach threshold then fires, inhibiting the other through lateral inhibition. When an afferent fibre fires at the same time as the unit itself, its connection is strengthened: the others to the same unit are weakened. Select an orientation with the slider, and present it a few times: one of the units will reach threshold first, and you will see the strength of its connections alter as a consequence. Train it with the same orientation a few times, then change to a different orientation and train again. See if you can make every unit respond to a different orientation. You should find this happening even if you just present orientations once each at random, without particularly attempting to train them. Click on Forget to reset the connections to their original values.

Olfactory recognition

Page 269

This exhibit shows how lateral inhibition between units which are intrinsically rather unspecific can lead to enhanced specificity: it shows lateral inhibition in an abstract multidimensional space (in this case, amongst different odorants). It has already been described in Chapter 8: see p. 184.

MOTIVATION AND BEHAVIOUR

Motivation 273
Emotion 275
The hypothalamus 278

Sleep and cortical arousal 283
A last look at the brain 286

The concept of the hierarchical structure of the brain and of its organization in an ascending series of levels was introduced in Chapter 9. This chapter is concerned with the very highest levels of all, those that determine *what* to do rather than how to do it. Actually, there is no very logical distinction between 'what' and 'how' in this sense: the task of deciding what to do amounts in the end to deciding *how* to stay alive or, at worst, how to immortalize one's genetic instructions. Thus the sensory inputs of this highest level come – somewhat paradoxically – not just from the special senses that tell us about the outside world but also from those interoceptive senses that are usually considered so 'low' as to be beneath our conscious notice: information, that is, about the physiological well-being of the body, the state of the milieu intérieur, and our distance from that final condition that awaits us all.

MOTIVATION

Why, in fact, do we ever bother to do anything at all? Teleologically, the answer is obvious: even if an animal is at rest, it is using up energy which it must replenish or perish. Unless it is completely sessile, relying on food that happens to pass by, this means that it must deliberately expend some of its energy on a sort of gamble in the hope of getting more back as a result, like a business investing part of its profits in the expectation of greater future returns. Whether or not to undertake the risk of such an investment is both the most important and the most difficult decision an animal has to make, and the whole of the recent expansion of the brain can be thought of as an attempt to reduce the risks involved by making *predictions* about the likely outcomes of alternative courses of action on the basis of the closest possible analysis of more and more information about the outside world, and past experience of the relationship between actions and results, stored not just in our brains but in our books.

Motivational maps

But the decision process need not be as complicated as this. In a simple creature like an amoeba this fundamental mechanism of *motivation* is easy to appreciate: its decisions take the form of tropisms in response to gradients of chemical stimulation in its environment. On the one hand, attractive stimuli like food set up a positive gradient down which the animal moves; while on the other hand, poisons or other threatening conditions create a negative gradient, and the animal moves away (Fig. 14.1). One can think of the amoeba's environment as a sort of motivational potential field, the amoeba itself acting like a little charged particle that moves about in response to local gradients, the path it traces out being a direct function of its environment.

Higher animals produce more complex behaviour but the fundamental mechanism is essentially the same. The added complexity comes about for two reasons. First of all, there are many more types of desirable and undesirable stimuli to which they may react, and many of them – perhaps most – are *learnt:* these are the secondary motivators (like money) that through experience become associated with other more self-evidently desirable goals (Chapter 8). Consequently each individual has its own classification of stimuli into desirable and undesirable categories, unique because it is the result of that individual's own personal experience. Secondly, the relative desirability of different attractants and repellents is constantly changing in response to the

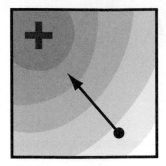 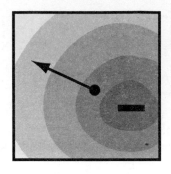

FIG. 14.1 Positive and negative motivational gradients.

organism's *needs;* thus changing patterns of need give rise to changing patterns of action even though the environment itself is the same, in a way that may seem to an outsider to be unpredictable. Thus Cambridge for me consists of a large number of separate gradient or contour maps, each corresponding to a different need: one for food, with high points at all the food shops and restaurants, one for money, centred on my bank, one for newspapers, for tobacco, and so on. Which one is operative at any particular moment depends on my need at that

moment, rather like those electrical maps sometimes seen at tourist resorts with bulbs that light up when you press one of a set of buttons marked 'parking', 'pubs', 'post offices', and so on.

In other words, the central mechanism of the motivational system of the brain can be thought of as a sort of Yellow Pages connecting particular gratifications to particular parts of one's internal representation of the outside world: like the tourist map, it translates information about need into the kind of tropistic data that can be turned by the higher

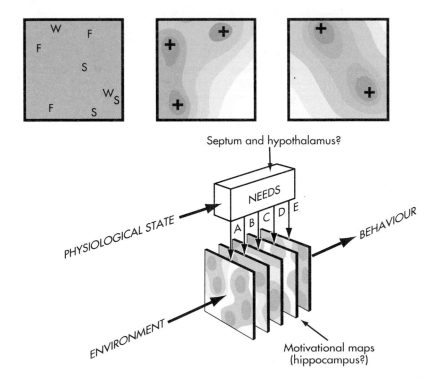

FIG. 14.2 Motivational maps. Above, **(a)** a neutral environmental map showing the location of food (F), water (W) and shade (S); and the corresponding motivational maps when the animal is hungry **(b)** or thirsty **(c)**. Below, hypothetical model of mechanism for computing directed behaviour from needs sensed by monitoring the body's physiological state. A, B, C, etc. are separate needs, as for example hunger, thirst, etc., and each has its own stored motivational map that is activated in appropriate circumstances.

levels of the motor system into actual patterns of activity (Fig. 14.2). It seems very likely that these Yellow Pages or motivational maps are embodied in the *hippocampus.* Hippocampal neurones have been found in the rat that respond specifically when the animal is at a particular point in its environment, for example within a maze that the rat has learnt (Fig. 14.3); their involvement in certain kinds of learning was discussed in the previous chapter. Equally, it is the *hypothalamus,* as the centre to which autonomic afferents project, and which itself monitors such physiological states of the blood as glucose concentration, temperature and osmolarity, as well as levels of circulating hormones, that defines one's state of need. It is also in the hypothalamus that primary consummatory responses such as eating and drinking may be triggered off by electrical stimulation.

Perhaps it is difficult for us to accept the notion that our own richly complex lives, with the apparent wealth of choices open to us, and our sense of liberty to choose among them, could possibly be determined by so simple a mechanism. But as Herbert Simon (1981) has said, human behaviour is really rather simple, but because most people live in very complex physical, man-made and social environments, their actual behaviour *appears* extremely complicated; thus the path traced out by an ant moving over rough ground may be very complex in appearance, even though its behaviour is simply directed at getting back to its nest. In fact, by averaging over large numbers of individuals, it is not difficult to measure quite

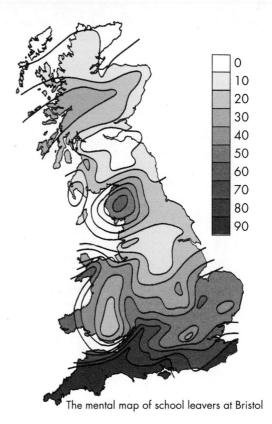

The mental map of school leavers at Bristol

FIG. 14.4 A human motivational map: preference contours defining relative desirabilities of different parts of Britain (the question the subjects were asked was simply 'Where would you like to be?'). (Gould, who lived in Bristol, and White, 1974)

directly the same kinds of tropistic gradients for us humans that work so well in describing what an amoeba does. If you take a group of people and ask them the very simple question 'Where in Britain would you like to be?', it is possible to obtain contour maps of average preferences (Fig. 14.4) which presumably, if the individuals had the means to do it, would be translated into actual migratory behaviour not very different in essence from our amoeba moving blindly down its tropistic gradient.

EMOTION

Apart from motivational tropism, another way in which behaviour is controlled is by switching on patterns of activity that are not directed at particular goals in the way that the tropisms are, but are rather in some sense preparatory or generally useful as an adjunct to the actual directed behaviour. This is what is meant in the widest sense by *emotional behaviour;*

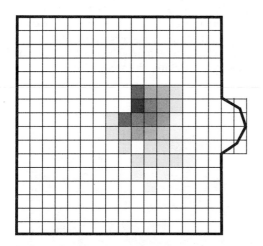

FIG. 14.3 Hippocampal mapping: plan view of an enclosure in which a rat with an electrode implanted in the hippocampus was free to move around. The shading represents the average firing frequency of a hippocampal unit in each of the squares, showing that the unit appears to code for a particular area within the enclosure. (Data from Wiener *et al.,* 1989)

the emotions that we may *feel* at the same time are the sensory side effects of this undirected behaviour (Fig. 14.5). There are as many types of emotional behaviour as there are types of motivational goal. Salivation, for example, is in this sense an emotional response accompanying the directed behaviour of getting food and eating it; and penile erection is an obvious preparatory response to another kind of goal. One may also include such internal responses as the release of hormones in this general category, as for example the surge of LH that triggers ovulation in response to copulation in some species, or the release of adrenaline associated with the need for sudden exertion. As Man has a richer set of possible needs and goals, including abstract or even spiritual ones, so his types of emotional behaviour and emotional sensations seem more varied and complex. But there are two basic emotional patterns found throughout the animal kingdom, and which are perfectly evident in Man as well, associated with tropisms of any kind: these are *arousal* and *conservation*.

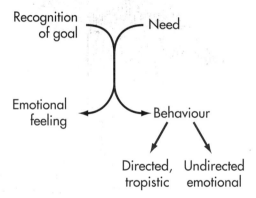

FIG. 14.5

Two basic emotional states

Arousal signifies the emotional state associated with a steep tropistic gradient, which may be either towards a desirable goal or away from a source of threat (Fig. 14.1): the state often described by physiologists as 'fight, fright or flight', that results in an increase in the general activity of the sympathetic system, and the release of adrenaline. The consequent bodily responses are all of more or less obvious use in preparing the body for the expenditure of the energy used to achieve the goal: blood flow through the muscles is increased, the heart rate is raised, glucose is released into the blood, the bronchioles and pupils dilate, the electrical activity of the brain increases, reaction times get quicker, and there is an

associated feeling of general excitement. All of this of course involves a certain expenditure of energy, and would be a drain on the body's resources if kept up for a long time: but much is now at stake, and the gamble is one worth taking.

Conservation or withdrawal is in a sense the opposite of arousal. In a situation like that shown in Figure 14.6, when every possible action is unpleasant – like standing in the middle of a minefield! – the sensible response is to conserve one's resources, and do nothing at all in the hope that the difficulties will go away of their own accord. The result is inactivity and stupor, a loss of muscle tone, sleep or even hibernation; if the situation is a sudden one, there may be abrupt immobility or freezing – the animal thus incidentally making itself inconspicuous and feigning death (a common response to oncoming motorcars but not a particularly helpful one). By all these means the rate of energy expenditure is greatly reduced, enabling the animal to ride out what may be only a temporary state of siege. The associated feelings are of apathy, tiredness and weakness: because of the reduction in muscle tone, one may actually feel heavier, pressed to the ground – the origin of the word 'depression'. Loss of muscle tone in the face produces a characteristic sagging of the lower jaw and of the corners of the mouth, and bowed head. In mild forms, the conservation state occurs only too commonly when a person feels that nothing is worth doing and circumstances are against him, giving rise to reactive depression. The more acute form of conservation is fortunately only rarely seen in civilized societies, except in response to cataclysmic disasters. The woman in Figure 14.7 has just emerged from shelter after an earthquake that has destroyed most of the town in which she lived. The objective signs of conservation are obvious: the stooped posture, the hand

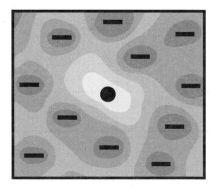

FIG. 14.6 The kind of motivational map for which the only appropriate response is conservation.

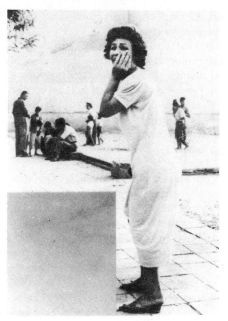

FIG. 14.7 Features of acute conservation. (Engel and Schmale, 1972)

lifted to the face to support the dropped jaw, the immobile staring eyes. In such circumstances one may find a general state of apathy and inactivity that continues for a long time and is not conducive to survival. A curious feature of such chronic depression, though one that is readily understandable in terms of motivational maps, is that in times of severe and particular stress, as in war, the incidence of this kind of emotional state actually decreases. The particular case of sleep as a form of conservation is considered in a separate section below.

Neither of these two kinds of emotional state is often seen in its pure form. Real objects tend to be both attractive and repellent: a hunting animal's prey may be both desirable as food and also dangerous, and in many species even the sexual act is a risky undertaking for the male. It can in fact be illuminating to think of emotions in terms of a continuum of types distributed around the two axes of arousal and conservation (Fig. 14.8), emphasizing the ambivalent nature of such states as rage and fear, the knife-edge between attack and retreat. Food does not usually have quite this effect on humans – dining is rarely a frightening experience in modern society – but rage can easily be elicited in situations of frustration, when the positive and negative aspects of a possible goal are nicely balanced. The generality of these two states can also be seen in human sexual behaviour, where sexual aggression shades off imperceptibly into sadism, and where affection may be expressed by licking and biting and other responses more appropriate to a food drive.

Of course any such scheme is oversimplistic; for one thing, it ignores the important part that memory, especially the kind of anticipatory memory discussed in the previous chapter in connection with the frontal lobes, may play in introducing an extra temporal dimension into our emotions: such emotional states as hope, worry, confidence and regret clearly involve an element of this kind. But it may help us to remember that there is nothing particularly recherché or high-falutin' about human emotional responses, and that there is no reason to suppose that they are produced by fundamentally different mechanisms from those generating the remarkably similar patterns of behaviour seen in animals.

Neural mechanisms

In short, keeping alive is a matter of monitoring the milieu intérieur and making homeostatic adjustments to it, adjustments that are partly neural and autonomic and partly hormonal: *internal* responses to *internal* stimuli. But this process is made much more effective by reacting to *external* stimuli as well, and by generating *external* responses. The development of the brain has permitted more and more sophisticated analysis of external stimuli, and greater and greater elaboration of patterns of external response, so that most of its bulk is concerned either with sensory analysis or motor co-ordination. But in the end, the

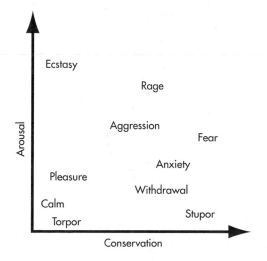

FIG. 14.8 Mixed emotional state as a result of stimuli that are partly attractive and partly repellent.

only part of it that really matters is the region where the four fundamental kinds of inputs and outputs actually come together. That region is the *hypothalamus:* though scarcely larger than a peanut, it determines all we do.

THE HYPOTHALAMUS

The hypothalamus lies on either side of the third ventricle, immediately above the pituitary (hypophysis) and below the thalamus, and consists of several fairly distinct subdivisions (Fig. 14.9). What is special about the hypothalamus is its uniquely intimate relationship with the blood and viscera. On the output side this comes about through its direct control of the pituitary and autonomic efferents; and on the input side through autonomic afferents, and also because many of its cells are themselves receptors that

respond to important parameters of the milieu intérieur, and to circulating hormones. At the same time, it has massive connections with the limbic system that provide it with processed information about external stimuli, and enable it to produce external responses in the form of overt behaviour. Its importance, in other words, lies in the fact that it is an *interface* between the blood and the brain, a region where internal stimuli and responses are co-ordinated with external ones (Fig. 14.10). It is both *need detector* and *response generator.*

Its hormonal output, the pituitary, is controlled by two distinct mechanisms. The axons of neurones in the supraoptic and paraventricular nuclei pass right down into the pituitary stalk to terminate in the posterior lobe (neurohypophysis). Here they release their transmitters, not at synaptic junctions but directly into the bloodstream; thus these neurones are acting directly as endocrine cells, and their transmitters are actually hormones. Neurones of the supraoptic region predominantly release *antidiuretic*

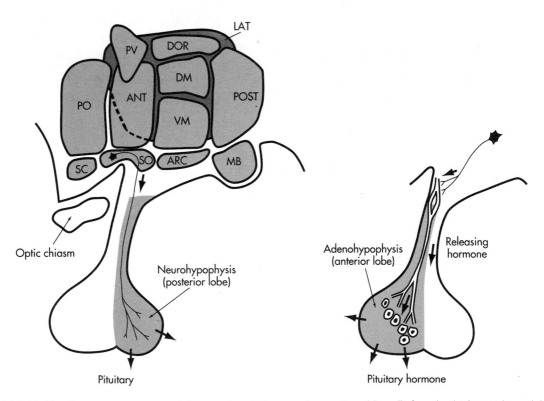

FIG. 14.9 Highly schematic representation of the main hypothalamic nuclei, as viewed laterally from the third ventricle, and their relationship to the pituitary. ANT, anterior; ARC, arcuate; DM, dorsomedial; DOR, dorsal; LAT, lateral; MB, mammillary body; PO, preoptic; POST, posterior; PV, paraventricular; SC, suprachiasmatic; SO, supraoptic; VM, ventromedial. Left, showing innervation of posterior lobe by hypothalamic fibres releasing pituitary hormones at their terminals; right, showing releasing hormones from hypothalamic neurones being carried by a portal system to the anterior lobe, where they control the release of pituitary hormones from pituitary endocrine cells.

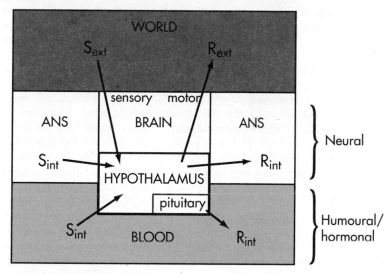

FIG. 14.10 The hypothalamus as an interface between blood and brain linking internal and external stimuli (S_{ext}, S_{int}) to internal and external responses (R_{ext}, R_{int}).

hormone (ADH), those of the paraventricular region mostly *oxytocin*. Both these hormones are nonapeptides of very similar structure, but their effects are very different. ADH helps control the osmolarity of the blood by stimulating the retention of water in the kidney; in large doses it may also increase blood pressure through arteriolar constriction (hence its alternative name of vasopressin), but this is probably not a very important physiological mechanism. Oxytocin stimulates the smooth muscle of the uterus in labour, and also causes milk ejection during lactation; in both cases the stimulus to its release is essentially neural, predominantly from mechanoreceptors in the regions concerned.

The other route by which the hypothalamus controls the secretion of hormones from the pituitary is quite different. Axons from other hypothalamic neurones terminate in a region on the ventral surface (the median eminence) where a system of fenestrated capillaries carries arterial blood down to the anterior pituitary through a portal system. The substances released from their terminals (*releasing* or *inhibiting hormones*) enter this portal system and are transported to the anterior pituitary where they each either stimulate or inhibit the release of some corresponding pituitary hormone. Thus the release of the pituitary hormone prolactin, which stimulates the secretion of milk and has other functions related to pregnancy, is stimulated by prolactin-releasing hormone (PRH) and inhibited by prolactin-inhibiting hormone (PIH) from medial regions of the hypothalamus. Other hypothalamic hormones have their

corresponding pituitary ones: apart from PIH (which is known to be dopamine) they are all small peptides. It is probably most helpful to consider them in a functional context, by examining a number of specific instances of homeostatic systems in which hormonal and neural signals are integrated by the hypothalamus to produce external, behavioural responses as well as internal ones.

Pituitary *growth hormone*, which affects many aspects of metabolism but more especially provides medium-term regulation of the blood glucose level, is controlled by GRH and GIH (somatostatin). These factors are probably mainly produced in the ventromedial hypothalamus, a region that has long been known to be associated with the control of *eating*. An animal with a lesion in the ventromedial area develops a voracious appetite, as if unable to sense when it has had enough, and as a consequence it becomes obese. Lesions in the lateral hypothalamus have exactly the opposite effect: appetite is reduced, the animal displays little interest in food and loses weight. For this reason, the lateral area is often described as a 'feeding centre', and the ventromedial area as a 'satiety centre'. Cells of the ventromedial area take up glucose at a particularly high rate; as a consequence, injections of the poisonous glucose derivative gold thioglucose cause specific localized lesions that result in hyperphagia. This and other observations have led to the attractive idea that together the ventromedial and lateral areas regulate feeding behaviour by monitoring the level of blood glucose, and that this information is also used in a negative feedback loop which regulates pituitary growth hormone release by means of GRH and GIH in response to fluctuations in blood glucose. In addition, the control of eating is of course also dependent on sensory information coming both internally from the digestive tract and externally from smell and taste. Thus we have here a clear example of a system in which internal information from both the blood and viscera is used in conjunction with external stimuli to produce an integrated response that is partly internal (the regulation of growth hormone, and also the production of saliva and other digestive secretions, and other autonomic effects) and partly external – the eating itself.

Another hypothalamic system associated particularly with the supraoptic region is that controlling the concentration and volume of the body fluids, once again through co-operation between hormonal regulation and behaviour. Certain cells in this region act as *osmoreceptors*, stimulating the release of ADH when the blood becomes too concentrated; autonomic afferents carrying information about blood volume from stretch receptors in the venous circulation also appear to contribute to the control of ADH by the hypothalamus. Other information that is relevant to the regulation of water balance comes from receptors in the subfornical region, just above the hypothalamus; they respond to the hormone angiotensin II that essentially signals a low average blood pressure, but are more concerned with the regulation of drinking than with the control of ADH. Again, autonomic afferents from the oesophagus and stomach are also believed to contribute to thirst and to the initiation and especially the termination of drinking: animals stop drinking long before their body fluids have yet become fully rehydrated. The effects of hypothalamic lesions suggest that like eating, drinking is controlled by two opposed systems located in different areas. Lesions in the supraoptic region produce excessive drinking (polydipsia), while those in the lateral hypothalamus reduce drinking as well as eating; electrical stimulation of the lateral nuclei, on the contrary, causes an animal to take in enormous amounts of water.

The *thyroid-stimulating hormone* (TSH) is controlled by TRH, associated with more ventral parts of the hypothalamus. The thyroid hormones have many interrelated effects on metabolism and growth, which are not well understood. One of its functions appears to be to cause a general increase in metabolic rate, helping to maintain body temperature under conditions of chronic cold. *Temperature regulation* is in fact another example of homeostasis achieved through a mixture of internal and external

Box 14.1 Hypothalamic control of the pituitary

Pituitary hormone	Control of release	Actions
Oxytocin	Neural	Milk ejection; Uterine contraction
Vasopressin (ADH)	Neural	Water retention; Vasoconstriction, reduced cardiac output
Growth hormone	GRH, GIH	Medium-term provision of metabolic energy. Promotion of growth
TSH	TRH	Stimulates thyroid; its hormones raise body temperature and have other miscellaneous effects
ACTH	CRH	Regulates levels of cortisol and androgens from the adrenal cortex; some effects on aldosterone as well
LH	LHRH	Stimulates ovulation or testosterone secretion
FSH	LHRH	Stimulates follicular growth or spermatogenesis
Prolactin	PRH, PIH	Stimulates milk secretion and maternal behaviour
MSH	MRH, MIH	Control of skin colour in some species; in humans, function unclear

responses: autonomically, hormonally, and also through overt behaviour such as curling up in the cold and seeking warmth (not to mention putting on or taking off one's clothes). Once again, the input to this system is partly neural and partly humoral: afferent signals from somatosensory warm and cold receptors, and from cells in the anterior hypothalamus that themselves respond to the temperature of the blood. Temperature regulation appears to be represented rather diffusely in the hypothalamus. Electrical stimulation at many points can produce fragments of temperature-regulating activity such as shivering, piloerection, vasoconstriction and sweating. Broadly speaking, the anterior half is concerned with mechanisms for losing heat in a hot environment and the posterior half with conserving heat when it is cold. More generally, there is a tendency for sympathetic responses to be found in the posterior half and parasympathetic in the anterior half. The fact that none of these effects is sharply localized simply reflects the high degree of interrelationship that exists between different homeostatic functions: a given response such as vasoconstriction may be caused by many diverse kinds of stimulus, and will in turn have a disturbing effect on several different homeostatic systems.

The endless multiplication of examples can soon become wearisome, and in any case leads far outside the scope of this book; the remaining pituitary outputs will be only mentioned very briefly. The *gonadotropic hormones* LH and FSH, jointly controlled by a single releasing factor (LHRFH), together with the pituitary hormone *prolactin*, are the means by which the brain influences the reproductive systems. What is particularly interesting about them is that gonadal steroids feed back on to receptors in the hypothalamus, not only influencing the production of the hormones themselves (and thus generating reproductive cycles) but also controlling sexual and maternal behaviour. They also illustrate very clearly how an essentially hormonal control system can be influenced by a host of different types of stimuli from the special senses. One need only think of the effects of light on the timing of ovulation and breeding seasons, of the effect of skin and other kinds of stimulation on sexual arousal, of the influence of the sound or smell of offspring on maternal behaviour, of pheromones on ovulation and mating, and so on. Similarly, the effects of the various kinds of internal and external stimuli that constitute 'stress' on the secretion of corticotropic hormone (ACTH), that regulates the secretion of corticosteroids from the adrenals and is controlled by CRH, are well known; ACTH is actually quite widely distributed in the

brain, including the superior colliculus, substantia nigra and amygdala. Finally, there are the *melanocyte-stimulating hormones* (MSH), regulating the pigmentation of the skin in certain species and released from the interstitial part of the pituitary, that are controlled in a similar way by MRH and MIH, under the influence predominantly of visual stimulation.

Limbic connections

The neural pathways to and from the hypothalamus are not well understood. In particular, although it is evident that the hypothalamus is, in Sherrington's words, 'the head ganglion of the autonomic system', it has not been possible to identify conclusively by what routes its autonomic functions are mediated. Its connections with the limbic system are clearer: it receives afferents from the hippocampal region through a massive fibre bundle (the *fornix),* and is interconnected through the medial forebrain bundle with many parts of the limbic system and reticular formation, including the areas controlling respiration and the cardiovascular system (Fig. 13.12). The *medial forebrain bundle* also carries afferent olfactory information. Some hypothalamic nuclei – notably the supraoptic and paraventricular – project to extraordinarily diverse areas, including the substantia nigra and the substantia gelatinosa of the dorsal horn.

The projection from the *amygdala* to the hypothalamus through the medial forebrain bundle is particularly interesting, as its organization seems to correspond rather nicely with the two fundamental types of emotion described earlier in this chapter, conservation and arousal (Fig. 14.11). The dorsomedial amygdala projects directly on to the lateral hypothalamus, and both regions seem, broadly speaking, to be concerned with arousal, the activation of a positive motivational drive. We have already seen that the lateral hypothalamus is associated with the initiation of eating and drinking behaviour, in the sense that lesions give rise to aphagia and adipsia, but they also produce a more general *depression*: dogs with lateral hypothalamic lesions are described as having a sad appearance, and are listless and somnolent. Lesions of the dorsomedial amygdala have similar effects, with perhaps more of the general, affective component; stimulation in this region may produce hissing and growling and other signs of positive arousal. The properties of the other half of this system, the lateral amygdala and its projection to the ventromedial hypothalamus, are completely different, and correspond more to conservation, the horizontal axis of Figure 14.8. Lesions in the

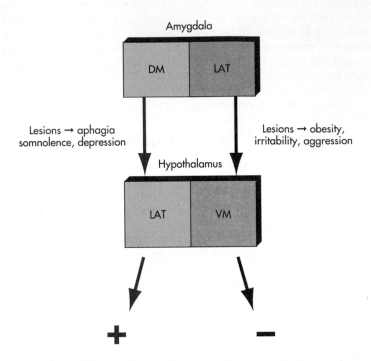

Amygdala

DM | LAT

Lesions → aphagia
somnolence, depression

Lesions → obesity,
irritability, aggression

Hypothalamus

LAT | VM

+   −

FIG. 14.11 Corresponding regions of amygdala and hypothalamus, broadly associated with arousal (+) and conservation (−). DM, dorsomedial; VM, ventromedial; LAT, lateral. (From data of Fonberg, 1972)

ventromedial hypothalamus, the 'satiety centre', produce overeating and obesity; again, similar effects are produced in the lateral amygdala but with a more general affective change as well, an increase in irritability and aggressiveness. Conversely, stimulation in this region of the amygdala produces passivity, and even sleep or stupor. Large bilateral lesions of the amygdala create an animal in which tropistic behaviour is greatly exaggerated (the *Klüver–Bucy syndrome*): everything in the environment seems indiscriminately attractive, and such a monkey will compulsively examine and try to eat such things as the bars of its cage and its own faeces, and even things like snakes that would terrify a normal animal. The same kind of hypertropism is seen in its sexual activity: the animal is markedly hypersexual and may try to copulate with members of its own sex, as well as inanimate objects.

More specifically sexual responses (as well as more general items of emotional expression such as pupil dilatation or changes in facial expression) may be elicited from the *cingulate gyrus,* a primitive cortical region of the limbic system which receives a projection from the hypothalamus by way of the mammillary bodies and anterior thalamus. Together with the nucleus accumbens, which appears to pro-

vide a link from the amygdala to the basal ganglia, it may provide the route to other cortical areas by which the hypothalamus generates overt behaviour. Other regions of the limbic system are described as *pleasure centres* in the sense that if an electrode is implanted in, for instance, the septal nuclei, and connected up so that when an animal presses a lever in its cage it receives a pulse of electrical stimulation through the electrode, then as soon as the animal discovers what the lever does, it will go on pressing it repeatedly, often in preference to 'really' pleasant stimuli such as food or sex. Of course, one cannot tell whether it is *feeling* pleasure as a result; but it is clear that the electrode must in a sense be by-passing the normal motivational mechanisms of the hypothalamus and in some way activating the tropistic input to the motor system directly. Other sites that have been found to produce direct motivation of this kind include parts of the amygdala and the hypothalamus itself. In some locations (dorsomedial thalamus, amygdala, hypothalamus) electrical stimulation has exactly the opposite effect: once the lever is pressed, it is never pressed again, presumably because the stimulus is evoking avoidance rather than positive tropism; but one has to be sure in such cases that the animal is not merely feeling pain.

SLEEP AND CORTICAL AROUSAL

There is a further aspect of the general emotional states of arousal and conservation that has yet to be considered. In addition to altering the visceral functions of the body, and to determining patterns of overt behaviour, they also regulate the activity of the thinking, cortical areas of the brain. Any system that works through association must have some way of regulating its sensitivity. Too sensitive, and it will tend to jump to conclusions, recognizing objects on insufficient evidence and wasting energy by making inappropriate responses; too cautious, and it may fail to respond to sensory signals that hint of predator or prey. In states of emotional arousal we generally find low cortical thresholds and over-excitability; in states of conservation (of which sleep is the most familiar example) thresholds are high and responses are hard to elicit.

It has been known for a long time that in parallel with the specific ascending pathways that project from the sensory receptors via the thalamus to the cerebral cortex, there is a second, more diffuse ascending system, consisting mostly of the ascending reticular formation and the diffuse nuclei of the thalamus (Fig. 14.12) that seems to be closely associated with the control of generalized states of activity, particularly of the cortex. This *reticular activating system* has extremely widespread inputs from all over the brain and from collaterals of ascending fibres, integrated over neurones with astonishingly large fields of projection (Fig. 14.13); through thalamic relays it seems to influence the neural circuits of the cerebral cortex, altering their level of activity by controlling different inflow. This activation may on some occasions be relatively local, acting rather like a spotlight to focus attention on a particular cortical region – as when a sudden sound at night alerts our auditory system – or more widespread, in the generalized states of arousal described earlier. It may well also

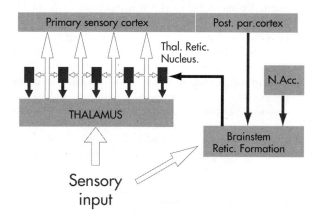

FIG. 14.12 Gating of afferent information to cortex by the thalmic reticular nucleus (red), driven in turn partly by the other thalamic nuclei and partly by the reticular activating system.

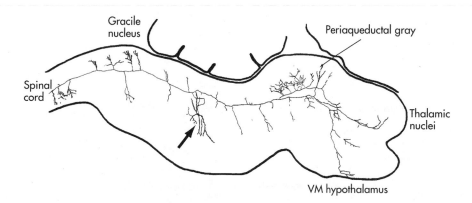

FIG. 14.13 Single cell (arrowed) from the nucleus magnocellularis of rat reticular formation, showing the distribution of branches of its axon to widespread areas of the brain. (Scheibel and Scheibel, 1957).

have a role in preventing cortical activity from getting out of hand. As we have seen, the presence of such a large degree of convergence and divergence amongst the neurones of the cerebral cortex (the average number of synapses on a neurone in the monkey's motor cortex is around 60 000) means that they are liable to fire each other off in a kind of explosive chain reaction: one can think of the reticular formation as acting rather like the damping rods in a nuclear reactor, altering the thresholds of the neurones in step with the level of incoming sensory activity, in such a way as to maintain a sufficient degree of sensitivity without triggering off the kind of neural explosion that is seen in epilepsy.

The general level of activity of the cortex may be measured by means of large electrodes attached to the scalp, which pick up the average electrical activity of very large numbers of cortical cells at once; a record of these potentials is called the *electroencephalogram* or EEG. Paradoxically, the largest potentials are not those recorded when the brain is active but when it is at rest. The reason seems to be that because cortical cells are so richly interconnected with one another, with multiple opportunities for feedback circuits that loop back on themselves, if left to their own devices they tend to lock into rhythmic oscillation, giving rise to waves of potential that run across the cortical surface like ripples on a pond. In a state of conscious quiet relaxation, these waves have a frequency of around 10 Hz, and are known as alpha waves (Fig. 14.14), most prominent near the occipital region. If the brain is aroused as a result of outside stimulation, this idling pattern is broken up into essentially random fluctuations of no particular frequency and small amplitude, just as the even flow of waves across a pond is disrupted by a shower of rain; the resultant EEG is then described as *desynchronized*. In sleep, which in many ways can be thought of as an emotional state akin to conservation, the EEG shows even more synchrony than that of the alpha rhythm in conscious rest: high-voltage waves of very low frequency, sometimes combined with bursts of high-frequency activity called spindles, are now seen (Fig. 14.14), a state called *slow-wave sleep* (SW sleep). The muscular tone of the body is much reduced, and the lack of cortical control is evident from the fact that primitive spinal responses like the Babinski sign may sometimes be evoked.

However, if one examines the EEG continuously throughout the course of a whole night's sleep, one finds that the slow-wave pattern of activity is not present all the time: there is in fact a slow cycle of changes in the type of EEG, in which the slow-wave activity is interrupted every two hours or so by long episodes in which the EEG resembles closely what is normally recorded in the waking state (Fig. 14.15). Yet the patient is actually more profoundly asleep – in the sense that he is harder to wake – during these episodes than he is in SW sleep, and for this reason these phases are called *paradoxical sleep*. About 20 percent of adult human sleep is of this kind, and this proportion is much increased in children and babies. Associated with the desynchronization of paradoxical sleep is a marked increase in bodily movement; the eyes in particular make large and rapid excursions, giving paradoxical sleep the alternative name

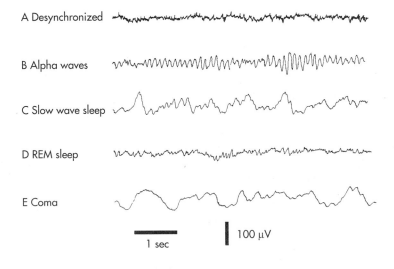

A Desynchronized

B Alpha waves

C Slow wave sleep

D REM sleep

E Coma

1 sec   100 μV

FIG. 14.14 Human electroencephalograms in different arousal states. (Penfield and Jasper, 1954; Roche, 1968)

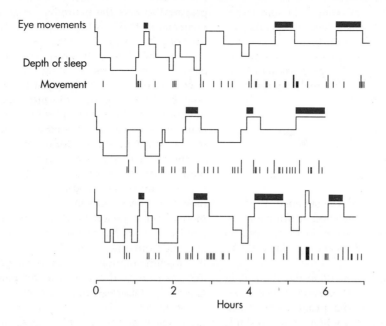

Eye movements

Depth of sleep

Movement

0   2   4   6

Hours

FIG. 14.15 Left, cyclic changes in a human subject during three different nights' sleep, showing correlation of periods of rapid eye movement with those of lightest sleep as determined by the EEG and increasing shallowness of the cycles as the night progresses. (After Dement and Kleitman, 1957)

of rapid eye movement, or REM sleep. A subject who is woken during REM sleep usually reports that he has been dreaming: the movements of the eyes and body may well reflect the contents of the dreams. It seems very likely that dreams are the result of the brain's associational mechanisms being allowed to free-wheel, without the check to fantasy that is imposed in the waking state by incoming messages about what the world is *really* doing. It is significant that waking subjects deprived of sensory input for sufficiently long periods often report dream-like hallucinations.

In sleeping animals, stimulation of the reticular activating system produces waking and, if continued, a marked state of general arousal. Lesions, on the other hand, put the animal in a permanent state of coma, with large-amplitude cortical waves; many general anaesthetics and sedatives act primarily on the reticular formation, as do such stimulants as amphetamine. The generation of the two types of sleep is thought to be under the control of two brainstem nuclei, the *locus ceruleus*, and the nuclei of the *raphe*. The cells of the locus ceruleus secrete noradrenaline, those of the raphe, serotonin; these control areas exert their influence over cortical arousal and over the brain as a whole partly through connections with the giant reticular neurones described earlier,

and partly through diffuse projections of their own, particularly to cerebral cortex. It is said that no cortical neurone is more than 30 μm away from a terminal of a cell in the locus ceruleus. Their activity increases with arousal, and is depressed in SW and REM sleep. There are mutual connections between these two areas and with the pontine reticular area that might be the cause of the periodic alternation of their activity that is characteristic of sleep.

The *functions* of sleep are far from clear; there are several well-attested instances of people who have succeeded in ridding themselves of the habit of regular periods of sleep, though it is generally believed that in such cases, instead of having all his sleep in one daily dose, the subject tends to drop off continually for periods of perhaps a few seconds without noticing it. When sleep deprivation is properly enforced, there is a steady decrease in the brain's efficiency, together with marked irritability, and eventually a state resembling psychosis results. Teleologically, it makes sense for an animal which cannot function efficiently at night to harbour its resources by entering a conservation state (just as hibernating mammals do during the winter). What is not clear is what the particular function of REM sleep, and its associated dreaming, might be: it is evident that less conservation of energy is taking place during it. It may be that dreaming is in some way *needed* by the brain, for if a subject is specifically deprived of REM sleep – by waking him up as soon as his EEG shows desynchronization – it is found that for several subsequent nights the proportion of time spent in REM sleep is increased to make up for it.

A LAST LOOK AT THE BRAIN

Our journey of exploration is almost ended. When it began, the goal of our ascent seemed unattainable, its heights unscalable and swathed in clouds of mystery. Yet here we are at the summit. Do things look different now?

If distance lends enchantment to the view, it is because it eliminates messy details; in this case the horribly numerous neurones that produce that rather queasy feeling we tend to get when we try to think about the brain. A glass of water contains far more molecules than the brain has neurones, but it seems quite simple to us because we ignore them. If we are

prepared to take the neurones for granted, to lump them all together and look at the brain in terms of the flow of patterns of information from one part of it to another, then trying to grasp what exactly it does becomes a much less daunting prospect. But we do, of course, have to *earn* the right to look at it in this way, by first mastering the intricacies of synaptic integration and the principles on which patterns of neuronal activity are recoded as they filter through from sensory input to motor output.

Figure 14.16 shows an attempt of this kind: the brain as seen from a very distant viewpoint. Fuzzy and oversimplified, to be sure, but it can at least help us get our bearings should we wish to examine it more closely. The left-hand side is sensory, the right-hand motor; its hairpin shape comes about because in going from sensory input to motor output we have first to climb to higher and higher hierarchical levels, and then descend again as motor patterns are progressively elaborated into their component parts.

At the top of the hierarchy comes the hypothalamus, which ultimately determines what we do; and it is here, as we have seen, that internal stimuli and responses are brought into contact with external ones. But side-by-side with this grand strategic

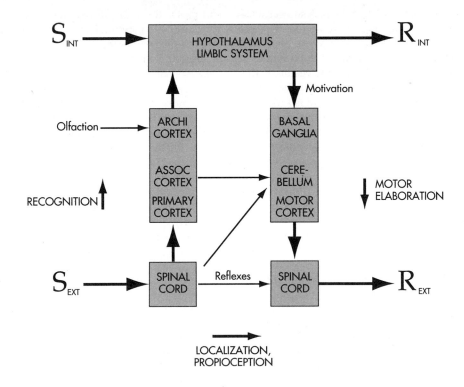

FIG. 14.16 A very distant view of the brain.

planning that requires the identification of possible goals through mechanisms of sensory recognition, we also require the humbler and simpler kinds of tactical co-ordination that are to do not with *what* objects are but *where* they are, where we are, and the effective execution of the generalized commands sent down from above. This requires pathways for localization and proprioception, often anatomically separate from the cortical mechanisms for recognition, that bypass the higher levels by cutting across from one side of the hairpin to the other. Some of these short-circuits – the stretch reflex, for example, which helps to ensure that limbs really are where we intend them to be – are at the lowest level of all, the spinal cord. Others, because they demand the integration of many different sources of information or because they imply a certain degree of learning, have to take place at higher levels such as the cerebellum. For simplicity, only input from the spinal cord is shown, but vision and hearing are organized in essentially the same general way. Olfaction is different: because it does not demand the analysis of patterns in the way that visual and auditory recognition do, and also because it provides purely motivational information with no localization component, it enters very near the top of the sensory hierarchy.

As a blueprint for a biological machine, Figure 14.16 seems plausible enough. But one may feel a little uneasy at the idea that such a scheme is a picture of *oneself*. Hasn't something been left out?

'Mind' and consciousness

'Nothing puzzles me more than time and space; and yet nothing troubles me less, as I never think about them' (Charles Lamb) – a reaction not very different from that of most neurophysiologists to problems of mind, brain, and consciousness. This is, of course, a field that has been thoroughly dug over since the days of Descartes and Hume and indeed long before, and philosophers have every right to question whether mere empirical physiologists can add much to such a hoary debate, in which the various arguments have been rehearsed so exhaustively. But recent developments both in neurophysiology and in computer science – for £20 I can purchase an electronic device hardly bigger than a packet of cigarettes that is the intellectual superior of half the animal kingdom – have so enlarged our notions of what classes of operation a physical system may in principle be capable of that a great deal of earlier thought on the subject is now merely irrelevant. In a nutshell, 'brain versus mind' is no longer a matter for much argument.

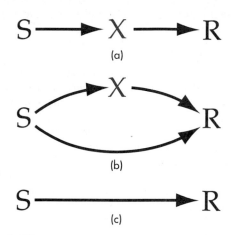

FIG. 14.17

Functions such as speech and memory, which not so long ago were generally held to be inexplicable in physical terms, have now been irrefutably demonstrated as being carried out by particular parts of the brain, and to a large extent imitable by suitably programmed computers. So far has brain encroached on mind that it is now simply superfluous to invoke anything other than neural circuits to explain every aspect of Man's overt behaviour.

Descartes' dualism, on the contrary, proposed some non-material entity – the 'ghost in the machine' – that was provided with sense data by the sensory nerves, analysed them within itself, and then responded with appropriate actions by acting on motor nerves (the mind thus having the same relation to the body as a driver to his car: Fig. 14.17a). Even a dualist must modify such a scheme to include the existence of certain automatic reflexes that obviously do not pass through the mind (Fig. 14.17b); but in fact modern neurophysiology goes further still. It admits no other path between stimulus S and response R than unbroken chains of neural connections (Fig. 14.17c): X, the ghost in the machine, has finally been laid to rest.

So is there still a problem, or have the philosophers been wasting their time? Indeed there is: that problem is *consciousness*. However sure I may be that (c) is a fair representation of *your* brain, there remains the obstinate and unshakable conviction that my brain is like (a). Though – after reading Freud – I might reluctantly agree that a great deal of what I do is not consciously willed, and that (b) is perhaps nearer the truth, nevertheless that there is *no X at all* is simply inconceivable. Now philosophers can have a great deal of fun with beliefs such as these, since the existence of my own consciousness is not something I can prove to other people in the way I can, for example, prove that I have hands. Clearly, its outward manifestations could easily be imitated by a machine (like Hebb's (1954) example of the calculator programmed to say 'I am multiplying' every time it multiplies). But this kind of scepticism is so self-consistent as to be utterly tautological: if, like Wittgenstein, we decide that the only criterion for consciousness must be overt, public behaviour, then of course we have nothing to say about it, because we have defined it out of existence. And for lazy neurophysiologists it provides a veneer of philosophical respectability for their unwillingness to think about the subject at all: Pavlov used to fine his students when he caught them using the words 'voluntary' or 'conscious'.

Yet to evade the problem by such specious materialism is perhaps no worse than to take the opposite extreme and accept consciousness as something much too mysterious and wonderful for a scientist even to begin to think about. Both attitudes contribute to the evident intellectual muddle that surrounds the whole subject. So how would a brash and simple-minded physiologist proceed? Once he had accepted the reality of the phenomenon, he might go on to relate it to the fabric of the brain in much the same way as he would in the case, say, of the sense of sight. It is clear, for example, that loss of a limb does not lead to blindness, whereas loss of the eyes does. By the use of inductive reasoning hardly more sophisticated than that, one may proceed into the brain itself and map out, almost neurone by neurone, the mechanism of the visual pathways. This kind of work has not of course been carried out systematically in the case of consciousness, if only because experiments of this sort on animals are useless to us. All the same, it is clear that we do in fact already know quite a lot about the functional anatomy of consciousness, even if we have little idea what consciousness actually *is*. We know, for instance, that while massive lesions of the cerebral cortex and its underlying fibres may blunt our perceptions, paralyse our limbs, impair our intelligence or even – as in the case of Phineas Gage – our morality, they have little effect on consciousness itself. Conversely, relatively slight injuries – perhaps a blow on the chin – that affect an area in the core of our brainstem (the same region of the reticular formation that is associated with arousal and sleep) can produce complete unconsciousness, even though the whole of the rest of the brain is unimpaired.

At a different level of description, it is clear that we are conscious of some kinds of brain activity but not others, and that the boundaries of this zone of awareness are not fixed. By and large it is what goes on at moderately high hierarchical levels that we are conscious of, although by introspection we can often learn to increase our awareness of lower levels. Curiously enough, we also tend to be relatively unconscious of the highest levels of all, those that control our motivations; and further, even the most complex mental processes can sometimes be carried out without being conscious of the fact at all. While reading through a difficult score at the piano, I have suddenly had the realization that for several bars I have been thinking about something entirely different, yet my brain had been getting on with the complex task of translating printed notes into finger movements perfectly well without me. Often, quite suddenly and unexpectedly when we were not thinking of it at all, we may find the solution to a problem that has baffled the most energetic conscious cerebration – perhaps, like Archimedes, in the bath or, like Coleridge with *Kubla Khan*, asleep! L. S. Kubie (1954) has gone as far as to say that there is nothing we can do consciously that we cannot also do unconsciously.

Thus consciousness is more associated with 'higher' functions than 'lower', yet not particularly affected by damage to precisely those regions of the brain that we know to carry out those higher functions; nor is it necessary to be conscious for those functions to be carried out perfectly adequately. The natural conclusion must surely be that the ghost in the machine is not an executive ghost, as it is in Figure 14.17 (a) and (b). It is rather a *spectator*, watching from its seat in the brainstem the play of activity on the cortex above it, perhaps able in some way to direct its attention from one area of interest to another but not to influence what is going on (Fig. 14.18).

But what about *free will*? An illusion. The ghost in such a scheme would observe the body's actions being planned, and see the commands being sent off to the muscles before the actions themselves began, and so one can well imagine how it might gain the impression that because it knew what was going to happen, that it was itself the cause. For X, the distinction between 'I lift my arms' and 'My arms go up', in which Wittgenstein epitomised the notion of voluntary action, would amount simply to the distinction

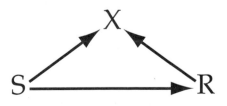

FIG. 14.18

between those actions which it observed being planned, and those – such as reflex withdrawal from a hot object – which it did not. There is no implied necessity here for us to be deterministic in our actions – to an outsider we may appear to have free will – since the physical processes linking S and R can be as random and essentially unpredictable as we please. Such a scheme seems more intellectually satisfying than Figure 14.17 (a) or (b) without conflicting with our own feelings about ourselves; unlike (c), it does not merely evade the issue. The most serious objection to it is perhaps that it is difficult to see what on earth X is *for*, since it can't actually do anything. Perhaps it does just occasionally intervene. But in any case, what is the audience at a concert for? Or the spectators at a football match? The idea that I am being carried round by my body as a kind of perpetual tourist, a spectator of the world's stage, is not – on reflection – so very unattractive. The moral is clear: *enjoy your trip!*

References

Dement, W. and Kleitman, N. (1957) Cyclic variations in EEG during sleep and their relation to eye movements, body motility and dreaming. *Electroencephalography and Clinical Neurophysiology* 9, 673–690.

Engel, G. L. and Schmale, A. H. (1972) Conservation–withdrawal: a primary regulatory process for organismic homeostasis. In *Physiology, Emotion and Psychosomatic Illness*, CIBA Symposium 8. Elsevier, Amsterdam.

Fonberg, E. (1972) Control of emotional behaviour through the hypothalamus and amygdaloid complex. In *Physiology, Emotion and Psychosomatic Illness*, CIBA Symposium 8. Elsevier, Amsterdam.

Gould, P. and White, R. (1974) *Mental Maps*. Penguin, Harmondsworth.

Hebb, D. O. (1954) The problem of consciousness and introspection. In *Brain Mechanisms and Consciousness*, ed. E. D. Adrian, F. Bretler, H. H. Jasper and J. F. Delafresnaye. Blackwell, Oxford.

Kubie, L. S. (1954) Psychiatric and psychoanalytic considerations of the problem of consciousness. In *Brain Mechanisms and Consciousness*, ed. E. D. Adrian, F. Bretler, H. H. Jasper and J. F. Delafresnaye. Blackwell, Oxford.

Penfield, W. and Jasper, H.H. (1954) *Epilepsy and the Functional Anatomy of the Human Brain*. Churchill Livingstone, London.

Roche (publ.) (1968) *Concepts of Sleep*. Roche Products Ltd, London.

Scheibel, M. E. and Scheibel, A. B. (1957) Structural substrates for integrative processes in the brainstem reticular core. In *The Reticular Formation of the Brain*, ed. H. H. Jasper, L. D. Proctor, R. S. Knighton, W. C. Wothay and R. T. Costello. Churchill, London.

Simon, H. (1981) *The Sciences of the Artificial*. MIT Press, Cambridge, Mass.

Wiener, S. I., Paul, C. A. and Eichenbaum, H. (1989) Spatial and behavioural correlates of hippocampal neuronal activity. *Journal of Neuroscience* 9, 2737–2763.

NOTES

Page 273 Neuropsychology Three excellent general books dealing with the topics covered in this chapter: Heilman, K. N. and Valenstein, E. (1979) *Clinical Neuropsychology* (Oxford University Press, Oxford); Walsh, K. W. (1994) *Neuropsychology, a Clinical Approach* (Churchill Livingstone, Edinburgh); Robbins, T. W. and Cooper, P. J. (1988) *Psychology for Medicine* (Edward Arnold, London).

Page 275 Hippocampal maps See for instance O'Keefe, J. and Nadel, L. (1978) *The Hippocampus as a Cognitive Map* (Clarendon, Oxford); Lopes da Silva, F. M. and Arnolds, D. E. A. T. (1978) Physiology of the hippocampus and related structures. *Annual Review of Physiology* 40, 185–216; O'Keefe, J. (1990) The hippocampal cognitive map and navigational strategies, in *Brain and Space*, ed. J. Paillard (Oxford University Press, Oxford).

Page 278 Hypothalamus Some useful accounts in this general area: Morgane, P. J. and Panksepp, J. (1979) *Handbook of the Hypothalamus* (Marcel Dekker, New York); Bloom, F. E., Lazerson, A. and Hofstadter, L. (1985) *Brain, Mind and Behaviour* (W. H, Freeman, New York); Donovan, B. T. (1985) *Hormones and Human Behaviour* (Cambridge University Press, Cambridge); Brown, R. E. (1994) *Introduction to Neuroendocrinology* (Cambridge University Press, Cambridge).

Page 281 Limbic connections See for instance Isaacson, R. K. (1982) *The Limbic System* (Plenum, New York); Bloom, F. E., Lazerson, A. and Hofstadter, L. (1985) *Brain, Mind and Behaviour* (W. H. Freeman, New York); Mogenson, G. J., Jones, D. L. and Yim, C. Y. (1980) From motivation to action: functional interface between the limbic system and the motor system. *Progress in Neurobiology* 14, 69.

Page 284 EEG First described more than 50 years ago: Adrian, E. D. (1944) Brain rhythms. *Nature* 153, 360–367.

Page 284 Sleep The classic account is Kleitman, N. (1939) *Sleep and Wakefulness* (University of Chicago Press, Chicago); a recent and comprehensive book is Cooper, R. (1994) *Sleep* (Chapman and Hall, London); Orem, J. and Bernes, C. D. (1980) *Physiology in Sleep* (Academic, New York) is a useful source of reference;

Hobson, J. A. (1990) *The Dreaming Brain* (Penguin, Harmondsworth) is a popular account, with an extended historical review of the study of dreaming.

Page 286 Consciousness By far the best of the more physiologically-oriented books in this area is Honderich, T. (1988) *A Theory of Determinism: the Mind, Neuroscience and Life-hopes* (Clarendon, Oxford); some of the issues have also been addressed in a stimulating recent article, Cotterill, R. J. (1994) Autism, Intelligence and the Brain. *Biologiske Skrifter det Kongelige Danske Videnskabernes Selskab* 45, 1–93. Walshe, F. M. R. (1972) The neurophysiological approach to the problem of consciousness, in *Scientific Foundations of Neurology*, ed. M. Critchley (Heinemann, London) is also well worth reading. A clear analysis of the basic problem can be found in Lewes, G. H. (1859) *The Physiology of Common Life* (Blackwood, London); Lewes was the writer George Eliot's husband. Finally, the musings of a scientific mystic (and poet): Sherrington, C. S. (1951) *Man on his Nature* (Cambridge University Press, Cambridge).

Page 288 Kubla Khan Coleridge recounts its composition, in a note prefixed to the first published edition (1816):

In the summer of 1797, the Author, then in ill health, had retired to a lonely farm-house between Porlock and Linton, on the Exmoor confines of Somerset and Devonshire. In consequence of a slight indisposition, an anodyne had been prescribed, from the effects of which he fell asleep in his chair at the moment that he was reading the following sentence, or words of the same substance, in 'Purchas's Pilgrimage': *Here the Khan Kubla commanded a palace to be built, and a stately garden thereunto. And thus ten miles of fertile ground were inclosed with a wall.*

The Author continued for about three hours in a profound sleep, at least of the external senses, during which time he had the most vivid confidence that he could not have composed less than from two to three hundred lines; if that indeed can be called composition in which all the images rose up before him as things, with a parallel production of the correspondent expressions, without any sensation or consciousness of effort. On awaking he appeared to himself to have a distinct recollection of the whole, and taking his pen, ink, and paper,

instantly and eagerly wrote down the lines that are here preserved. At this moment he was unfortunately called out by a person on business from Porlock, and detained by him above an hour, and on his return to his room, found, to his no small surprise and mortification, that though he still retained some vague and dim recollection of the general purport of the vision, yet, with the exception of some eight or ten scattered lines and images, all the rest had passed away like the images on the surface of a stream into which a stone has been cast, but, alas! without the restoration of the latter!

NEUROLAB

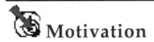

Motivation

Page 275

A not entirely serious implementation of a dynamic motivational map. The field of action is the black area at left, where an animal is represented by a mobile purple blob. You can create its motivational environment by selecting a type of goal (food, drink or sex) with the radio buttons at bottom right and then clicking where you like on the map; you can mix the types of goal to your taste. Then activate one of the check boxes at top right to determine which particular need or needs are motivating the animal. It will move down motivational gradients towards appropriate goals, which it then annihilates through its consummatory activity. You may also set up aversive stimuli that result in negative motivational gradients. Experiment with frustrating situations likely to evoke neurotic behaviour.

Hypothalamus

Page 278

This exhibit provides a simple self-test of the hypothalamic nuclei and their main functions. Click on the radio buttons round the window; the name of the corresponding area, and its salient functional features are shown on the right. Alternatively, click on the button to the right of the name window to display a list of names, and click on one of them; the location and functions will be displayed.

INDEX

References to NeuroLab are marked N; to supplementary notes, n.

Aberrations of eye 127–9, 144–6, N167
Absolute refractory period 34
Absolute threshold
    auditory 102, 111, n118
    olfactory 177
    Pacinian corpuscle 79
    visual 122, 134, 138, 140
Acalculia 253–4
Acceleration
    angular 99–100
    linear 95, 97–8
Accidental attributes of stimulus 266–7
Accommodation
    of lens 125, 128–9, 149, 162, N167
    of nerve 35, 39
Accretion 195
Accumbens, nucleus 239, 283
Acetylcholine 4, 44–6, 55–9, 239
ACTH 281
Action potential 18–39, N41
    biphasic 31–2
    composition of external medium, and 24
    compound 31–3, N42
    conduction velocity 19, 29–33, N42
    initiation 37–9
    mechanism of propagation 19–29
    monophasic 24, 32
    repetitive 37–9
Activation system, reticular 85, 283
Acuity N168
    auditory 110, n119
    pseudo- 143–4
    somatosensory 83
    vernier 143–4
    visual 124, 141–8, N168

Adaptation N70, N169
    bleaching 137, 139–141, N167–8
    chromatic 159, 169
    dark 53–4, 123–4, 133, 137–141, N167–8
    field 137–9
    functions of 52–54
    general mechanisms of 38–39, 48–52, N70
    in muscle spindle 91–3
    in Pacinian corpuscle 48–50, N70
    in vestibular system 98–100
    of joint receptors 94
    olfactory 177
    visual 123–4, 133, 137–141, N165, N167–9
ADH 278–280
Adiadochokinesis 234–5, 237
Adrenaline 276
Aerial perspective 163
After image 140, 159, N169
Ageing
    and accommodation 125–7, N167
    and touch 76–7
Agnosia 251–2
Agraphia 253–4
Akinesia 240
Albedo 122–3, 137, 159, 266–7
Alcohol
    effects on cerebellum 235
    effects on vestibular apparatus 222
Alexia 253–4
All-or-nothing law 33, 35–7
Alpha
    fibres 32–3, 205, 208, 211
    gamma co-activation 206, 211
    waves 284–5
Amacrine cells 131, 136–7, 172
Amnesia 258
    anterograde 261, 265
    retrograde 261, 264–5

Amoore's theory 178–9
Ampulla 95, 98
Amusia 253–4
Amygdala 8, 173, 258, 281–2
Anarthria 253–4
Anatomy of brain 5–8, 10–12, N17, N243, 286
Angiotensin n87
Angle expansion 269, n271
Angular acceleration, velocity 95, 98–100
Anomalies of colour vision 160
Anomia 253–4
Anopia, Anopsia 149
Anosmia 179
Anosognosia 252
Anoxia and nerve conduction 84
Anterior
    commissure 8, 172
    corticospinal tract 202–3
    spinothalamic tract 77–9, 85
    thalamus 249, 258, 260–1, 282
Anterograde
    amnesia 261, 265
    degeneration 11
Anterolateral
    chordotomy 78
    system 78–9, 85
Anxiety and frontal lobe 250
Apathy 240, 276–7, 281
Aphasia 251, 253–5
Appetite
    and hypothalamus 279, 281–2
    sodium 180
Apraxia 251–3
Aqueduct, cerebral 6, 8
Aqueous humour 125–6
Arch of Corti 107–8
Archicerebellum 232
Archicortex 258–261, 286
Argyll Robertson pupil 129
Army, as a hierarchy 196
Arousal 276–7, 281, 283–6
Ascending reticular activating system 85, 283
Aspartate 59, 137
Associated movements 240
Association
    and motivation 174, 273–4
    and recognition 267–270
    areas of cerebral cortex 247–8
    fibres of cortex 8, 227
    memory 263–5, 267–270
Astereognosis 84, 251
Astigmatism 127
Asymmetry of brain 255–8
Asynergia 234–5

Ataxia 234–5
Athetosis 240
Atropine 128
Attenuation 102
Audiometric curve 102
Audition 101–120, N119–120
Auditory
    localisation 114–8, N120
    meatus 130–1
    prostheses 113–4
    receptors 107–8, 110–3
Automatic gain control 54, 138–9
Autonomic
    effects of emotion 276–7, 281
    ganglia 5, 75
Axo-axonic synapses 63–4
Axon 7–9
    effect of diameter 20, 30–1, N42
    electrical properties of 19–20, 29–31
    hillock 59
    mechanism of conduction 18–28
    myelination 9–10, 30–1

Babinski sign 196–7, 284
Ballismus 240
Ballistic control 189–190, 237, N198
Barbiturates 64
Basal ganglia 228, 238–242
Basilar membrane 107–112, N120
Basket cells 234
Batting 192, n197
Bechterew nystagmus 222
Behaviour
    control of 173–5, 273–5, 277–282, 286–7
    olfaction and 173–5
    tropistic 273–5
Békésy, Georg von 109, n119, n183
Betelgeuse 144
Betz cells 228–9
Binocular
    cells in visual cortex 153, 163–4
    vision and depth perception 163–4
Bipolar cells of retina 9, 36, 131, 135–6, 154,
Bleaching of retinal pigment 137, 138–141, N168
Blind spot 130, N167, 252
Blobs 152–3
Body-image 252
Bowman's glands 170
Bradykinesia 240
Brain
    development and evolution of 3–7
    general topography of 6–7, 286–7
    left-right asymmetry 255–8

Brainstem
  and consciousness 288
  and decerebrate rigidity 203–4
  and saccades 194
  descending pathways 201–3
  visual responses 154, 164–5
Brightness 122–3
Broca's
  aphasia 253–4
  area 254, N271
Brodmann's areas N271
Bud, taste 181–2
Buttress reaction 215–6

Cable properties of axon 19–20, 29–31, N41
Calcium 39, 45–7, 667, 96, 111–2, 134, 139,
    N167, 263–4
Caloric vestibular stimulation 98, n100, 218
cAMP 45–6, 65, 175, 178, 181–2
Camphor 178
Canal of Schlemm 125
Candela 122
Capacitance
  of neural membrane 29–31
  of post-synaptic cell 44
Caudate nucleus 8, 238–9
Central aphasia 253–5
CCK 58, n87
Centre of gravity and posture 214–7
Centres 15
  of satiety 279, 282
  pleasure 173, 282
  speech 253–8
Cerebellum 6–8, 231–8
  afferent fibres 93–4, 233–4
  agenesis n242
  and co-ordination of visual and vestibular
    information 222, 237–8
  and motion sickness 222, 234
  and parametric feedback 212, 237–8
  and prism reversal 221, 237–8
  cell types 233–4
  disorders of 234–5, N243
  nuclei 232–3
  theories of action 235–8, N243
Cerebral
  aqueduct 6, 8
  blood-flow 14, 255
  cortex (see Cortex)
  dominance 255–8
  hemispheres 6
cGMP 45–6, 134–5, 139
Channels
  colour 155, 158–9

communication 52–4
ionic
  and resting potential 21–4
  in EPP 56–7
  in EPSP 57–8
  in IPSP 61–2
  in receptors 44–7, 51, 96, 110, 134, 175,
    181–2, N167
  ligand-gated 43–7, 54–8, 59–62
  NMDA 263–4
  role in action potential 21–8, N41
  voltage-dependant 25–8
Chemoreceptors 170–1, 175–6, 178–9, 181–2, 278–281
Chiasm, optic 149
Child prodigies n271
Chloralose 64
Chloride ions 23–4
  role in inhibition 61, 63
Cholinesterase 55, 58
Chorda tympani 180–1
Chorea 240
Choroid
  membrane 6
  of eye 126, 130–1
Chroma 155–7
Chromatic
  aberration 128, 144
  adaptation 159, 169
Chromophore 132
Ciliary
  ganglion 126
  muscle 125–6, 129
Cingulate gyrus 258, 282
Circuit
  equivalent 19
  local, nerve conduction 19–21, 29–31, N41
Circumvallate papillae 180–1
Civetone 175
Clarke's column 93–4
Clasp-knife reflex 93, 205–6
Classification
  dangers of 73–4
  neural mechanisms 265–270
  of colours 155–9
  of cutaneous stimuli 73–4
  of eye movements 194
  of nerve fibres 32–3
  of odours 176–8
  of receptors 47
  of visual neurones 154
Climbing fibres 233, 236–8
Cochlea 106–114
Cochlear
  hair cells 107–8, 110–3

microphonics 108, 110–1
nerve 107, 110–3, 116–7
nuclei 116–8
Coding
of auditory signals 105–6, 108–114
of nervous information 36–9, 52–4
of olfactory information 176, 269
of skin information 73–4
Cold
paradoxical 80
receptors 76, 79–80
Colliculi 6–8, 203
inferior 111, 117–8, 203
superior 148–150, 154, 160–2, 203, 241
Colour N169
anomalies 156, 159–160
blindness (see colour plates) 159–160, n166
complementary 158–9
constancy 159–160
contrast (see colour plates) 159
matching 156
mixing 155–8
opponent cells 150, 154, 158–9
space 156–7
triangle (see colour plates) 157–8
vision 122–4, 155–160
Columns
Clarke's 93–4
in motor cortex 227–8
in somatosensory cortex 84
in visual cortex 152–4
Coma 284
Comparator 190–3, 207–8
Complementary colours 158–9, N169
Complex cells 152–4
Compound action potential 31–3, N42
Computers 11–12, 16, 287–8
Conchae 170
Conditioning, Pavlovian 173, 262–3, N272
Conduction, nervous 18–39
anoxia and 84
passive 19–20, 29–31, N41
saltatory 30
speed of 19, 29–33, N42
Cones 108, 110, 123–4, 130–145, 155, 159–160
Confabulation 262
Conjunctiva 126
Conscious control of movement 228, 241–2
and cerebellum 235
Consciousness 257–8, 284, 287–9
Conservation 276–7, 281–2
Constancy, colour 159–60
Constant-field equation 22
Constructional apraxia 251–3

Context, sensory 236–7
Contrast 141–3, 146–8, 159
colour 159, N169
simultaneous 146, 159, N169
successive 159
Control systems 187–195, N198
Convergence
of eyes 129, 164, 191–2, 194, N199
of neural pathways 61, 80–1, 96, 110, 131,
134, 145–6, 171, 187–8, 200, 284
Convulsants 61, 64
Cornea 124–7
Cornsweet illusion N168
Corpus callosum 8, 256–8
Corpus striatum 7–8, 238–9
Corpuscle, Pacinian 47–50, 75–7, 94, N70
Corresponding points of retina 163
Cortex
cerebellar 232–4
cerebral 6–8, N271
auditory 117–8
cingulate 258, 282
entorhinal 173, 258, 260
frontal 248–250, 258
gustatory 180–1
hippocampal 173, 176–7, 258–63
motor 211, 226–231
olfactory 173, 176–7
parietal 247, 251–8
periamygdaloid 173, 181, 258, 260
prepyriform 173, 176–7, 258, 260
somatosensory 77–8, 84–5
temporal 160, 258–262,
visual 150–4, 160, 163–4, 267–9
Corti, arch of 107–8
Corticospinal tract 202–3, 211, 228–9
Cribriform plate 171–2
Crista 98
Cuneate nucleus 77–9, 81, 93–4
Cuneocerebellar tract 93
Cupula 98–9
Current
flow in action potential 19–21, 25–31
generator 38–9, 45, 51
inhibition 62–3
synaptic 38–9, 45, 59, 62–3
Cutaneous receptors 48–51, 74–7, 79–80, 94–5
adaptation in 48–51, 76–7, 79–80, 84
Cut-off frequency 143, 145–8
Cylindrical lens 127–8

Dale's hypothesis 60, 62, n69
Dark adaptation 53–4, 123–4, 133, 137–141, N167–8
Dark light 138–9

Dash-pot 49, 92, 99
Deafferentation 211, n212
Decerebrate
    preparation 203–5, 206–8
    rigidity 203, 206
Decibel 102
Decomposition of movement 234–5
Decorticate preparation 204
Degeneration, nerve 10–11
Degrees of freedom in colour vision 156–160
Deiter's nucleus 96, 202–3
Delayed reaction test 250
Dendrites 7–9, 54–5, 59, 264
Dendritic spines 55, 264
Dendro-dendritic synapses 54, 172
Denervation sensitivity 67
Densitometry, retinal 133, 139, 160
Dentate nucleus 232
Deodorants 177
Deoxyglucose 14
Depression
    emotional 240, 276–7, 281
    post-tetanic 65
Depth perception, visual 162–4
Dermatomes 74–5, n87
Descartes, René 287
Descending
    control of pain 85–6
    tracts 201–3, N212
Desynchronization of EEG 284
Detection
    disparity 163–4
    line 151–3, 267
    of visual targets 122–4, 141–8
Determinism 288
Deuteranopia 159
Development
    of brain 5–7
    of synaptic connections 66–8, 263–4
Diencephalon 6–7
Diffraction in eye 129, 145
Dioptres 124–5
Direction perception
    auditory 114–8, N120
    olfactory 172, n183
    visual 160–2
Disc, optic 130
Discos n118
Discrimination
    between auditory frequencies 110, n119
    between stimulus intensities 52–4
    colour 155–160
    somatosensory spatial 80–3
    visual spatial 141–8, N168

Disparity, retinal
    and vergence movements 191–2, 194, N199
    cortical detectors 153, 163–4
Distance perception
    auditory 114
    visual 162–4
Dominance
    in cerebral hemispheres 255–8
    ocular, in visual cortex 153
DOPA 240
Dopamine 59, 239–240
Dorsal column nuclei 77–9, 81, 279
Dorsal roots
    distribution to skin 74–5
    ganglia 5, 75, 77
Drawing
    and non-dominant hemisphere 257
    and parietal lobe damage 252
    and redundancy 83
    by children 255
    by split-brain patient 257
Dreaming 285–6
Drift 194, N225
Drinking 180, 279–280
Dualism 287–9
Dummy head recording n119
Dynamic
    gamma fibres 91–3
    range 53–4, 102, 123–6, 151–2
    vestibular reflexes 218–9
    vestibulo-ocular reflexes 218
Dysarthria 253–4
Dyslexia 253–4
Dysmetria 234–5, N243

Ear, structure 106–8
Eating 174, n183, 279–282
Ectoderm 4–5
Edinger-Westphal nucleus 126
Efference copy
    and knowledge of eye position 162, 220–1
    in internal feedback 193–4
    in postural control 224
Efferent fibres to sense organs 52, 91–3, 96, 110, 117
Effort, sense of 95, 231
Elastic element
    in muscle spindle 92
    in Pacinian corpuscle 49
    in semicircular canals 99
Electrical properties of axon 19–20, 29–31, N70
Electrical synapses 43–4, 96, 135–6
Electroconvulsive therapy (ECT) 264
Electroencephalogram (EEG) 284–5
Electromyogram (EMG) 208–210

Electro-olfactogram (EOG) 176
El Greco n166
Emboliform nucleus 232
Emmetropia 125–6
Emotional
    behaviour 275–8, 281–2
    content of speech 105
    effects on autonomic nervous
        system 129, 276–7, 281
    effects on pupil 129, n166, 276
    feelings 175, 276
Encapsulated sensory endings 47–51, 75–6, 94–5
Encephalization 4, 195
Endolymph 95, 97–9, 107–9
Endorphins 59, 86–7
Endplate, motor 55–7
Enkephalins 59, 86–7
Entorhinal cortex 173, 258–261
Epilepsy 61, 226, 256, 259
Equilibrium potential 22–3
Equivalent
    background 140
    circuit 19
Erotic stimulation of skin 85
Error
    in control systems 190–4, 209–210
    refractive 126–8, 144–5
Essential attributes of a stimulus 266–7
Eustachian tube 106
Evolution
    and olfaction 172–3
    of basal ganglia 238
    of brain 3–6
    of cerebellum 231–2
    of cerebral cortex 203, 230, 247–8
    of colour sense 159
    of labyrinth 95
    of limbic system 172–4, 258–9
Excitatory postsynaptic potential (EPSP)
    generation of 57–8
    summation of 58–9
Expressive aphasia 253–4
Extensor thrust 215
External ear 106
External meatus 106
Extrapyramidal pathways 228
Eye 124–137, N167–9
    movements 194, N198, N225
        and sleep 285–6
        miniature 194
        nystagmus 194, 218, 220–2
        saccades 161–2, 193–5, 241
        smooth pursuit 161, 194
        vergence 129, 164, 191–2, 194, N199

    vestibular 217–8
    position, knowledge of 162, 220–221
    structure 124–6, 129–137

Facilitation 65
Far point 125
Fastigial nucleus 232
Feedback
    and motor control 188, 190–5, 207–212
    in basal ganglia 239
    in cerebellum 234–7
    internal 162, 193–5
    negative
        in action potential 33–4
        in cochlear hair cells 111–3
        in control of muscle 188, 190–5, 206–212
        in olfactory bulb 171–2
        in pain 85–7
        in posture 214
        in voltage clamp 26
    inhibition 61–2, 81–3
    parametric 190–1, 211, 221, N243
    positive 33–4
Feedforward
    control 189–190, 224
    inhibition 83
Feet, role in upright posture 214–6, 223–4
Fibres of passage 11
Field adaptation 137–9
Fila olfactaria 171
Filiform papillae 180–1
Filter
    as model for recognition 266–270
    energy 46, 48–51, 91, 99
    high-pass 48–54, 91–92, 147
    second, in cochlea 111–3
Final common path 200
Firing frequency 36–9, 51, 59
Flaccid paralysis 228–9
Flexion reflex 200
Flicker fusion frequency 148
Flourens, Charles n198
Focusing by the eye 125, 128–9, 149, N167
Follow-up servo 207–8
Force
    control of 205–212, 230–1
    role in cutaneous sensation 76, 231
Forebrain 6–7
Formants 104–6
Fornix 8, 258, 260, 281
Fourier analysis in hearing 103–6, 108–114, N119
Fovea centralis 130
Free will 241–2, 288–9
Frequency

analysis by cochlea 103–6, 108–114
code of action potentials 36–9, 52–4, 59
cut-off 143, 145–8
fundamental 103
of sound 101–6, 108–114, 118
spatial 142–3, 146–8
temporal 148
Freud, Sigmund 287
Frontal leucotomy 85, 250
Frontal lobe 247–250
Fundamental frequency of a sound 103
Fungiform papillae 180–1
Fusimotor fibres 90, 92–3, 207–212

G-protein 45, 134, 182
GABA 59, 61, 64, 135, 137, 233, 239
Gage, Phineas 249–250, 288
Gain n166
control in retina 138–9
of stretch reflex 206, 209–210
Galvani, Luigi 18, n39
Gamma
amino butyric acid 59, 61, 64, 135, 137, 233, 239
fibres 32–3, 90, 92–3, 207–212
Ganglion
cell, retinal 131, 136–7, 145, 149, 154, 158–9
ciliary 126
dorsal root 5, 75, 77
nodose 74
spiral 107, 110
sympathetic 5, 75
Gap junctions 43–4
Gating
by presynaptic inhibition 65
in lateral geniculate 150
of pain 85–7
Gaze-holding and shifting 194
Generator current and potential 45–6, 48, 51
Geniculate
ganglion 180
lateral, nucleus 148, 150, 249
medial, nucleus 117–8, 249
Gennari, Francesco 150, n166
Glabrous skin 75
Glare 145–6
Glaucoma 125
Glial cells 9, 65
Global aphasia 253
Globose nucleus 232
Globus pallidus 238–9
Glomeruli
cerebellar 233
olfactory 171–2
Glutamate 59, 96, 135, 137, 239, 263–4

Glycine 59, 61
Goldmann constant field equation 22
Golgi
apparatus 47, 264
cells of cerebellum 234
silver stain 10, 131
tendon organ 90, 93–5, 205–6, 211
Gracile nucleus 77–9, 94
Granule cells
in cerebellum 9, 233
in olfactory bulb 171–2
Grasping
and motor cortex 229–231
sensory aspects 76, 79, n87
Gratings, as visual targets 142–3, 146–8
Gravity
centre of, and posture 214–5
direction of 97–8, 216–7
Grey matter 6
GRH 280–1
Grip
and motor cortex 229–231
sensory aspects 76, 79, n87
Guided systems 191–2
Gustation (see Taste)

Habituation 66, 260
Hair cells
cochlear 107–8, 110–3
olfactory 171–2, 175–6
vestibular 96–7
Hair follicle, innervation of 75–6
Handedness 256
Harmonics 102–5
Head
and auditory localisation 114–5
position, sense of 95, 97–8, 216–9
righting reflexes 216
tilt 97–8
Hearing 101–120, N119
Hebb, D. O. 263, n271, 288
Hebbian synapses 263–4
Heights, instability with n224
Helicotrema 107
Helmholtz, Hermann von 108, 130, 220–1, n166
Hemianopia 149
Henning's prism 178
Heraldry n166
Hermann grid 146
Heteronymous hemianopia 149
Hexachlorethane 178–9
Hibernation 276
Hierarchical organisation 195–7, 204, 223, 241–2, 253
High-pass filter 48–54, 91–2, 147

Hindbrain 6–7
Hippocampus 7, 258–262, 274–5
Histamine 85
Hodgkin, Sir Alan 27
Holism 12–14
Homonymous hemianopia 149
Homunculus 77–8, 226–7, 230
Hopping reaction 216
Horizontal cells 131, 135–6, 154, 172, N168
Horopter n167
Horseradish peroxidase 10
Hue 155–7
Humour, aqueous and vitreous 125–6
Huxley, Sir Andrew 27
Hydra 4
Hypercolumn 153
Hypercomplex cells 152, 154, N168
Hypermetropia 126, N167
Hypertropism 282
Hypophysis (see Pituitary)
Hypothalamus 7–8, 85, 126, 173, 181, 258,
　　　274–5, 278–282, 286, N290
Hypotonia 203, 228, 234–5

Idiots savants 254
Illuminance 122–3
Illusion
　　angle expansion 269, n271
　　Cornsweet N168
　　Müller–Lyer 163
　　phantom contour 268
　　Poggendorf 269
　　Ponzo 163
　　strip N168
　　waterfall 165, n167, N169
　　Zöllner 269
Image
　　after 140, 159, N169
　　body 252
　　retinal, quality of 126–9, 141–6
　　stabilised 137
Immobilisation response 85
Immunohistochemical stains 11, 57
Impedance matching, in ear 106
Impulse, nervous (see Action potential)
Inactivation, sodium 26–7, 34–5
Incense 175
Increment threshold 137–8, 140
Incus 106
Indole 177
Inferior
　　colliculus 6–8, 111, 117–8
　　ganglion 74
　　olive 237–8, 273

Inflow theory 220–1
Information 36–7, 52–4
Infra–red 121
　　theory of olfaction 179
Infundibulum 8
Inhibition
　　current 62–3
　　feedback 61–2, 81–3
　　feedforward 83
　　lateral (see Lateral inhibition)
　　presynaptic 63–5
　　reciprocal 60, 68
　　remote 63
　　synaptic 59–65
　　voltage 62–3
Inhibitory postsynaptic potential (IPSP) 60–1
Initiation
　　action potentials 37–9
　　movement 195–7, 240–2
Inner ear 107–8
Innervation
　　of cochlear hair cells 110
　　of muscle 200–1, 205
　　of muscle spindle 90–3
　　of skin 74–7, 79–81
　　of viscera 74–5, 85
　　reciprocal 60, 68
Insular cortex 180–1
Intelligence 247–8, 255
Intensity
　　coding of 36–7, 52–4
　　of sound 102, 104
Intention tremor 234–5
Interaural sound differences 104, 114–8, N120
Internal capsule 77, 79, 238–9
Internal feedback 193–5
　　in cerebellum 236–8
Interneurones 4
　　in cerebellum 233–4
　　in cerebral cortex 227
　　in dorsal horn 77
　　in olfactory bulb 171–2
　　in retina 131, 135–7
　　in spinal cord 60, 62
Interplexiform cells 131
Interpositus nucleus 232
Intrafusal fibres 91
Intraocular pressure 125
Iodoform 177
Ionic
　　distribution across membranes 21–5, N41
　　permeability channels (see Channels)
Iris (see Pupil)
Itch 74, 84–5

Jacksonian epilepsy 226
Jargon 254
Johnson, Dr Samuel n270
Joint receptors 94–5, 222–3, 230–1

Keller, Helen 177, n183
Kinaesthesia 94–5
Klüver–Bucy syndrome 282
Korsakov syndrome 261–2
KQ receptors 263–4
Krause end-bulb 76

Labyrinth 95–100, 106–14
Lanceolate endings 76, 106–8
Landolt C chart 143–4
Language, cerebral localisation of 253–5
Larynx 104–6, N119
Lashley, Karl 75–6, 248
Lateral
    corticospinal tract 202–3
    geniculate nucleus (LGN) 148, 150, 249
    inhibition 13, 80–3, 268–9, N168
        in cerebellum 234
        in cerebral cortex 228
        in cochlea 112–3
        in olfactory bulb 171–2, 176, 269
        in skin 80–3, 86–7
        in spinal cord 200
        in vision 135–6, 146–8, 268–9, N146, N168
    lemniscus 117
    line organ 95
    nucleus of hypothalamus 278–282
    olfactory tract 171–3
    posterior nucleus 249, 251
    reticulospinal tract 202
    spinothalamic tract 78–9
    ventricles 6
    vestibular nucleus 96, 202–3
Learning
    brain lesions and 258, 260–2
    cerebellar 234–8
    in motor system 190–1, 193–4, 211–2, 234–8
    in posture 221–2
    in visual system 262, 265–9
    possible mechanisms 66, 68, 262–5, N272
Left-handedness 256
Lemniscal system 77–9
Lemniscus
    lateral 117
    medial 77–9
Lens
    of eye 124–9, N167
    spectacles 126–8, 237–8, N167

Lesions, interpretations of effects 11, 14–16, 240–1, 248
Leucine, tritiated 11
Leucotomy, frontal 85, 250
Ligand-gated channels 43–7, 54–8, 59–62
Light
    adaptation 123–4, 133, 137–41, N165, N167–9
    measurement 122–3
    visible spectrum 121
Limbic system 258–9, 274–5, 277–8, 281–2, 286
    olfaction and 172–5
Linear
    acceleration 95, 97–8
    perspective 162–3
Line-detectors 152–4, 267, N272
Linespread function 141–3, N168
Load, compensation for 207, 209–12, 230–1
Lobotomy, frontal 85, 250
Lobster n40
Localisation
    cutaneous 80–3
    of function in brain 14–16, 247–8
    olfactory 172, n183
    sound 114–8, N120
    visual 160–4, 220–1
Locus ceruleus 285
Long-term
    depression (LTD) 65, 238
    memory (LTM) 264–5
    potentiation (LTP) 65, 238
Low-frequency cut
    spatial 143, 146–8
    temporal 148
Lower motor neurone 228–9
Luminance 123
Lux 122

Macrosmatic 170
Macula
    lutea, of eye 130
    of otolith organs 97–8
Macular sparing 150
Magnetic resonance imaging (MRI) 14
Malleus 106
Mammillary bodies 258, 260–1
Manipulation 76, 79, n87, 229–231
Maps
    collicular 118, 160–2
    motivational 273–5
    motor 14, 226–7, 229–230
    somatosensory 78, 84
Marr, David 236
Mass action 15–16, 248
Mechanoreceptors

in cochlea 107–8, 110–4
in joints 94–5, 222–3, 229
in muscle 90–2, 94–5, 205–212, 229
in skin 48–51, 75–7, 79–81, 85–6, 95
in tendons 92, 94–5, 205–6, 211
in vestibular system 96–100
Medial
    forebrain bundle 173, 258, 281
    geniculate nucleus 117–8, 249
    lemniscus 94, 77–9
    reticulospinal tract 202
Medulla 6–8, 201
    pyramids of 203
    raphe nucleus 87, 239, 285
Meissner's corpuscle 75–7, 79
Membrane
    axonal 19–20, 29–31
    basilar 107–110, 112, N120
    Reissner's 107
    tectorial 107–8
    tympanic 106–7
Memory
    and olfaction 173–4
    disorders of 260–2, 264–5
    long-term (LTM) 264–5
    mechanisms 262–270
    short-term (STM) 264–5
    types of 262, 264
Merkel's disc 75–6, 79
Mesencephalon 6–7
Mesopic vision 122–3
Metencephalon 6–7
Microelectrodes 14
Microphonic potential, cochlear 108, 110–1
Microsaccades 194, N225
Microsmatic 170
Microtubules 9, 66
Midbrain 6–7
Middle ear 106–7
Mind 287–9
Miniature
    endplate potentials 56
    eye movements 194
Mitral cells 171–2
Modalities, sensory
    of skin 73–4
    of taste 179, 181
Modulation, amplitude and frequency 37
Monochromat, rod 139, 160
Monosynaptic reflex (see Stretch reflex)
Mossy fibres 233, 236, 238
Moth lure 175, 179, n184
Motion perception, visual 137, 152, 164–5,
    219–221, N169

Motion sickness 222
Motivation 173–4, 273–5, 277, 281–2, N290
    olfaction and 172–5
    secondary 173–4, 273
Motivational maps 273–5
Motor
    aphasia 253–4
    cortex 211, 226–231
    homunculus 226–7, 230
    maps 14, 226–7, 229–230
    programs 189, 191, 195
    unit 200
Motor control
    and efference copy 192–5, 231, 237
    ballistic 189–90, 237
    guided 190, 193, 207–12
    hierachical 195–7, 204–5, 223, 241–2
    prediction in 190, 193
    programs for 189, 191, 195
    types of 187–199, N198
    servo–hypothesis 207–212, N213
Motor neurones 9, 200–3
    'lower' 228–9
    membrane adaptation in 38–9
    synaptic potentials in 57–9, 61–2
    'upper' 228–9
Movement
    control (see Motor control)
    parallax 163
    sense of 94–5, 98–100, 219–221
    sensitivity, somatosensory 77
    sensitivity, visual 137, 152, 164–5, 219–222
MRI 14
MSH 280–1
Müller-Lyer illusion 163
Muscle
    gradation of contraction 200
    innervation of 200–1, 205
    proprioceptors 90–6, 205–212, 229–230, 236
    spindles 90–3, 95–6, 205–212, 229–230
    stapedius 107
    tensor tympani 107
    tone 203, 206, 276–7
Musical instruments 104, 113
Musk 175, n183
Mydriasis 128
Myelin 9–10, 20, 30–1
Myopia 126, N167
Myotatic reflex 206–7

Nauta stain 11
Near
    point 125
    reflex 129

Neck reflexes 222–3
Need 274–6
Negative feedback (see Feedback)
Neglect 252
Nelson, Sir Horatio n183
Neocerebellurn 232
Neocortex 226–7, 258–9
Neostriatum 238
Nernst equation 22
Nerve
    calyx, chalice 96
    chorda tympani 180–1
    cochlear 107, 110–3, 166–7
    conduction 18–36
    growth factor 67
    net 4
    olfactory 171–2
    optic 149–50
    trigeminal 180
    vestibular 95–7
Nerve fibres (see also Axon)
    classification 32
Network, neural 11, 16, 187–8, N198, 248, N272
Neural
    codes 36–9
    network 11, 16, 187–8, N198, 248, N272
    plate, tube 5–6
Neurofilaments 9, 66
NeuroLab
    Instructions for use vii
    Action potentials N41
    Adaptation N169
    Anatomical pathways N243
    Basilar membrane N120
    Blind spot N167
    Cerebellar dysmetria N243
    Cerebellar learning N243
    Colour N169
    Compound action potential N42
    Conduction velocity N42
    Control systems N198
    Cortical regions N271
    Eye movements N198, N225
    Horizontal cells N168
    Interaural delay N120
    Ionic equilibria N41
    Lateral inhibition N168
    Line learning N267
    Linespread function and acuity N168
    Motivation N290
    Neural networks N198, N272
    Olfactory recognition N184, 272
    Pacinian corpuscle N70
    Parametric feedback N225

Passive conduction N41
Pavlovian condition N272
Phase locking N120
Photoreceptors N167
Postural stability N225
Receptive fields N168
Sound and Fourier analysis N119
Spinal tracts N212
Stretch reflex as a servo N213
Synaptic interactions N70
Time constants N70
Visual optics N167
Vowels N119
Neuromuscular junction
    denervation sensitivity 67
    mechanism 55–7
Neurones 3–4, 7–10, 18–39, 43–70
    summation in 58–9, 62–3
Neurotransmitters 3–4, 9, 11, 44–6, 54–62, 64, 239
Neurotubules 9, 66
Nitric oxide 59, 263–4
NMDA receptors 66, 238, 263–4
Nociceptors 74, 84–5
Node of Ranvier 9–10, 30
Nodose ganglion 74
Noise
    in axons 36–7, 52–4
    in motor system 189, 193
    retinal 138–140
    signal to noise ratio 53
    thermal, and olfaction 179
Nominal aphasia 253
Noradrenaline
    and sleep 285
    as neurotransmitter 45, 59, 128, 285
Nose, internal structure 170–1
Nucleus (see names of specific nuclei) 10
    accumbens 239, 283
    gigantocellularis 202, 283
    solitarius 180–1
Nystagmus N198, N225
    Bechterew 222
    caloric 98–9, n100, 218
    optokinetic 194, 220
    per-rotatory 218
    positional 222
    post-rotatory 218
    quick phase 218–9
    slow phase 218–9
    vestibular 194, 218–9

Occlusion 59
Ocular dominance columns 153

Olfactory
   bulb 171–3
   cilia 171
   cleft 170
   effects on behaviour 173–5
   epithelium 170–1
   pathways 172–4, 258
   receptors 171, 175–6, 178–9, N184
   sensitivity 177
   transduction 175–6, 178–9
   tract 171–3, 176
   tubercle 173
Olive
   inferior 233, 237–8
   superior 116–7
Olivocochlear bundle 110, 117
Ophthalmoscope 129–130
Opiates 86–7
Opsin 132, n166
Optic
   chiasm 149–150
   disc 130
   nerve 149–150
   radiation 150
   tract 149–150
Optics of eye 124–9, 141–2, 144–6, N167
Optokinetic nystagmus 194, 219–220
Orthograde degeneration 11
Osmoreceptors 280
Ossicles of middle ear 106
Otoconia 97
Otolith organs 95–6, 216–8
Outflow theory 221
Oval window 106–7
Overlap 80, 162–3
Oxytocin 59, 279
Oysters n40

Pacinian corpuscle 47–50, 75–6, 94, N70
Pain 74, 84–7
   and frontal lobe 85, 250
   and opiates 86–7
   as an emotion 85
   descending control 85–7
   gating theory 85–7
   receptors 84
   referred 85
Paleocerebellum 232
Paleostriatum 238
Panum's fusional area 164
Papillae 180–1
Paradoxical
   cold 80
   sleep 284–5

Parallax, movement 163
Parallel fibres 233, 236
Paralysis
   agitans 240
   flaccid 203, 228–9
   in stroke 203
   spastic 203, 228–9
Parametric feedback 190–1, 211–2, 221, N225
Paresis 228
Parietal cortex 248–9, 251–8
Parkinsonism 240–1
Passive conduction 19–20, 29–31, N41
Patch clamping 27–8, 175–6
Pattern-recognition 9, 13, 176, 237, 265–270
Patterns of activity
   at neurones 9, 13, 59, 187
   in cochlear units 110–4
   in skin 73–4
   olfactory 176
Pause cells 241
Pavlovian conditioning 173, 262–3, N272
PDE 134
Peep-show n167
Peptides as transmitters 11, 59, 136, n87, 279
Periamygdaloid cortex 173, 181, 258, 260
Periaqueductal grey 85–7
Periglomerular cells 171–2
Perilymph 107–9
Permeability, ionic
   and resting potential 21–4
   during action potential 24–8
   in receptors 44–7, 51, 96, 110, 134, 175,
      181–2, N167
   in synapses 56–8, 60–3
Per-rotatory nystagmus 218
Perseveration 240
Perspective 162–3
PET scans 14, 255–6
Phantom contours 268
Phase
   -locking 113, N120
   of sound waves 102–4, 114–6
Phenylephrine 128
Pheromones 174–5, 281
Photometry 122–3
Photons 121–2, 134
Photopic vision 122–3, 129
Photopigment of retina 132–4, 138–141, 160
Photoreceptors 108, 123, 130–5, 138–40, 145, 158–9,
   N167
Phrenology 15
Picrotoxin 61, 64
Pigment
   epithelium 130–1, 133

olfactory 171, 179
  retinal 132–4, 138–41, 160
Pinna 106, 114
Pitch 101, 104–5, 108–110, 113–4
Pituitary 8, 278–281
Placing reactions 216, 230
Planaria 4
Plasticity 14, 16, 262–5
  in cerebellum 235–8
  of cerebral cortex 16, 84, 231
  of vestibulo-ocular reflex 221–2, 235–8
Pleasure centres 173, 282
Poggendorf illusion 269
Pointspread function 141–3, N168
Pons 6–8, 148–9, 165, 201–2, 233, 285
Ponzo illusion 163
Position sense
  of eye 162, 193, 220–1
  of head 95–100, 216–9
  of limbs 94–5
Positional nystagmus 222
Positive supporting reaction 215
Positron emission tomography (PET) 14, 255–6
Posterior spinocerebellar tract 93–4
Post-rotatory nystagmus 218
Post-tetanic
  depression 65
  potentiation 66
Postural
  sway reaction 216
  vestibular reflexes 216–9
Posture 214–225, N225
  and basal ganglia 240
  and neck 222–3
  and cerebellum 234, 222
  criteria for upright 214–5
  in depression 276–7
  vestibular contributions 216–9, 221–2, 224
  visual contribution 219–222, 224
Potassium
  and action potential 21–6, 28, 33–5, 39
  and glial cells 65
  and membrane adaptation 39
  and resting potential 21–6
  and taste receptors 181–2
  role in inhibition 61–3
Potential
  action (see Action potential)
  cochlear microphonic 108, 110–1
  endplate (EPP) 55–7
  equilibrium 22, N41
  excitatory postsynaptic (EPSP) 57–8
  generator 38–9, 45, 51
  inhibitory postsynaptic 60, 62–3

miniature endplate 56
  resting 21–6
  reversal 48, 55, 57–8, 61
Potentiation 66
  long-term (LTP) 66, 263–5
Poverty of movement 240
Predictions
  in motivation 274
  in motor control 189–190, 193
  in posture 218, 224
Prepyriform cortex 173, 176–7, 258, 260
Presbyopia 125–7, N167
Pressure receptors 75–6, 79
  and posture 211, 214–6, 223–4
  and stretch reflex 229–231
Presynaptic inhibition 63–5
Pretectum 126, 148–9, 165
Primary
  afferent depolarization (PAD) 63–4
  colours 158–9
  odours, lack of 176–8
Prism
  Henning's 178
  reversal 221–2, 237–8
Procion yellow 10
Programs, motor 189, 191, 195
Prolactin 279–280
Proprioceptors
  Golgi tendon organs 90, 93–4, 205–6, 211, 230
  in neck 222
  joint receptors 94–5, 222–3, 230–1
  muscle spindles 90–3, 95–6, 205–212
  vestibular apparatus 95–100
  visual 148–9, 165, 219–220
Prosencephalon 6
Protanopia 159
Pulvinar nucleus of thalamus 148, 151, 249, 251
Pupil
  Argyll Robertson 129
  control of 128–9, 144–6
  effect on visual optics 128–9, 137, 144–6
  emotional influence 129, 276
Purkinje
  cell, cerebellum 9, 232–3, 236–8, 264
  shift 121, 124
Putamen 238–9
Pyramidal cells
  of hippocampus 260–1, 263
  of motor cortex 203, 226–9
Pyramidal tract 202–3, 211, 228–9
Pyramids of the medulla 203

Quick phase of nystagmus 219

Radiation
electromagnetic 121
optic 149–150
Range, dynamic 53–4
auditory 102
visual 123
of accommodation 125–6
Ranvier, node of 9–10, 30
Raphe nucleus 86–7, 239, 285
Rapid eye movement (REM)
sleep 285–6
Rate sensitivity
as function of adaptation 54
in muscle spindle 91
in joint receptor 94
Rebound 234–5
Receptive fields 80, N168
binocular 153, 163–4
in motor cortex 229
in temporal cortex 153–4, 259
in visual cortex 151–4
of bipolar cells 135–6, 154
of ganglion cells 136–7, 154
of hippocampal cells 260, 275
of lateral geniculate cells 150
of Purkinje cells 233
somatosensory 80–1, 86
Receptors 4, 44–54
adaptation in 48–54, 91–2, 99–100
auditory 107–8, 110–3
cold 76, 79–80
cutaneous 74–7, 79–81, 84–5
efferent control of 52, 91–3, 96, 110, 117
joint 94–5, 222
olfactory 171, 175–6, 178–9
pain 84–5
retinal 108, 123, 130–5, 138–140, 145, 158–9, N167
stretch 90–3, 95–6, 205–212, 229–230
taste 180–2
temperature 76, 79–80
transduction 44–8
vestibular 148–9, 165
Reciprocal innervation 60, 68
Recognition
disorders 251–2
of smells 176–8, 269
of sounds 103–6
of target neurones 66–8
of visual targets 149–154, 265–270
Recording methods 14
Recruitment 36–7, 104, 114, 200
Red nucleus 201–3, 228, 233
Red-green blindness 160
Reductionism 12

Redundancy
in neural coding 52, 82–3
in postural control 223
Referred pain 85
Reflex 200
clasp-knife 93, 205–6
conditioned 173, 262–3, N272
flexion 200
head righting 217
monosynaptic 57, 93, 206–212
myotatic 206–7
near 129
neck 222–3
pupillary 128–9, 144–6
righting 216
spinal 195–7, 200
stretch 57, 93, 206–212, 229
tendon jerk 206
vestibular 218–9
vestibulo-ocular 194, 217–9, 237–8, N243
wiping 195
withdrawal 85, 200, 289
Refractive
error 126–8, 144–5
index of parts of eye 124–5
power of eye 124–5
Refractory period 34
Regeneration
of action potential 21, 25–8
of tectal afferents in frog 67
of visual pigment 132–3
Reissner's membrane 107
Relative refractory period 34
Release 15, 195–7, 203, 229
Releasing hormones 279–280
REM sleep 285–6
Renshaw cells 62, 65, 200
Reproduction 174–5, 277, 280–1
Resolution, visual 141–6
Resonance
in cochlear hair cells 111–3
in olfaction 179
in speech production 104–6, N119
of outer ear 106
theory of basilar membrane 108–9
Resting potential 21–5
Reticular formation
activating system 85, 283
and decerebrate rigidity 203–5
medullary 201–4
nucleus gigantocellularis 202, 283
pontine 148–9, 201–2
raphe nucleus 86–7, 239, 285
Reticular lamina 108

Reticulospinal tract 201–2
Retina 129–137
Retinal (retinene) 132–3
Retinal receptors 108, 123, 130–5, 138–140, 145, 158–9, N167
Retrograde
    amnesia 261, 264–5
    degeneration of neurones 11
Reversal potential 48, 55, 57–8, 61
Rexed's laminae 77
Rhinencephalon 174, 176, 258
Rhodopsin 132–141
Rhombencephalon 6–7
Righting reflexes 216
Rigidity
    and basal ganglia disorders 240
    decerebrate 203–6
Rods 110, 122–4, 130–141, 145–6
Rotation
    reflex effects of 218–9, 222
    vestibular response to 95, 98–100
Round window 107
Rubrospinal tract 201–3
Ruffini end-bulb 94, 75–6, 79

Saccadic eye movements 161–2, 193–5, 241
Saccule 95, 97–8
Salt taste 179–181
Saltatory conduction 30
Satiety centre 279, 282
Saturation
    in colour-space 157
    of retinal receptors 134, 138
Scala
    media 107
    tympani 107
    vestibuli 107
Scanning speech 234–5
Schlemm, canal of 125
Schwann cell 9–10
Sclera 126
Scotopic vision 122–3, 129, 145
Second filter 111–3
Secondary motivation 123–4, 273
Semicircular canals 95, 98–100, 218–9
Sensory
    aphasia 253–4
    context 236–7
    homunculus 77–8
    modality 73–4
    receptors (see Receptor)
Septal nuclei 173, 258, 260–1, 282
Serotonin
    and sleep 285

    as neurotransmitter 59, 65, 239, 285
    in pain transmission 86–7
Servo N213
    assistance 211–2
    hypothesis, simple 207–210
Shadow
    and depth perception 162–3
    in auditory localisation 114–6
Shearing of skin 76
Sheep-detectors 154
Sherrington, Sir Charles 220, 281
Shock
    electroconvulsive 264
    emotional effects of 276–7
    spinal 195
Short-term memory (STM) 264–5
Sight (see Vision)
Signal flags n166
Signal to noise ratio 52–4
Silent areas 247
Sinus hairs 76
Sinusoidal
    gratings 141–3, 146–8
    sound waves 101–6
    flicker 148
Simple
    cells of visual cortex 151–2, 154
    servo hypothesis 207–210
Skin, receptors in 74–7, 79–81, 84–5
Sleep 276, 283–6
Slow phase of nystagmus 218–9
Slow-wave sleep 284–5
Smell 170–184
Smith predictor n197
Smooth pursuit 161, 194
Snellen chart 143–4
Sniffing 170, 177, n183
Sodium
    and salt taste 181–2
    appetite 180
    channels 22–8, 30, 33–5
    inactivation 26–7, 34–5
    refractoriness 34
    pump 23
Solitarius, nucleus 180–1
Somatosensory
    cortical areas 77–9, 85, 231
    modalities 73–4
    system 73–89
Somatostatin 59, n87, 279,
Sound 101–6, N119
    localisation 114–6, 118
    timbre 102–6, 114

Space
  colour (see colour plates) 156–7
  constant, of axon 19–20, 29–31, N41
  orientation of head in 95–8, 216–7, 219
Spasticity 203, 229
Spatial
  agnosia 251–2
  frequency 142–3, 146–8
  localisation of sound sources 114–6, 118
  localisation of visual targets 160–4
  pattern of activity in cochlea 108–14
  resolution 80–3
  summation 58–9, 63, N70
Spectacles 126–8, N167, 221
Spectrum
  of visual lights (see colour plates) 121
  of sound 102–6, N119
Speech N119
  disorders 251, 253–5
  localisation of cerebral areas 253–5
  mechanism 104–6, N119
  scanning 234–5
  spectrum 104–6, N119
Spherical aberration 128–9, 144–5
Spinal
  preparation 195, 200–1, 203
  reflexes 195–7, 200–1
  shock 195
Spinal cord 4–6, 200–1
  ascending tracts 77–9, 93, N88
  descending tracts 201–3, N88
  hemisection of 78
Spindle, muscle (see Muscle spindle)
Spines, dendritic 55, 264
Spinocerebellar tract, posterior 93–4
Spino-olivary tract 93–4
Spinothalamic tracts 77–9, 85
Spiral ganglion 107, 110
Split brain preparation 256–8
Squid axon 25–7, 30
Stability
  in standing 211–6
  of axon 33–4
Stabilised image 137
Stains for neural tissue 10–11, 57
Standing mechanisms 211–6
Stapedius 107
Stapes 106
Stars, visibility of 141, 144
Static
  gamma fibres 91–2
  vestibulo-ocular reflexes 217
Stellate cells 151, 263
Stepping reaction 216

Stereocilia 96–7, 110–3
Stereophony n119
Stimulation 14–15, 188
  of motor cortex 226, 229
  of temporal cortex 259
  of visual cortex 259
Stretch receptors (see Muscle spindles)
Stretch reflex 57, 93, 205–212, 229, N213
  and decerebrate rigidity 206
  gain 206, 209–210
Striate cortex (see Visual cortex)
Striatum, corpus 6–8, 238–9
Striosomes 239
Strip illusion N168
Stroke 203, n270
Strychnine 61
Stuttering 254, 270
Subiculum 260–1
Substance P 58–9, n87
Substantia
  gelatinosa 85, 281
  nigra 238–241, 281
Subthalamus 238–240
Summation
  olfactory 171
  spatial, in neurones 58–9, 63, N70
  temporal 59
  vestibulo-visual 221–3
Superior
  colliculus 6–7, 148–150, 154, 160–2, 203, 241, 281
  olive 116–7
Supraoptic nucleus 278, 280
Suspensory ligaments 125
Sympathetic ganglion 5, 75
Synapses 4, 7–8, 11, 43–68
  axo-axonic 63–4
  development 66–8
  dendro-dendritic 54, 172
  electrical 43–4, 96, 135–6
  Hebbian 262–4
  inhibitory 59–65
  interactions between 10, 58–9, 62–5, N70
  memory and 66, 68, 262–5
  NMDA 66, 263–4
  structure 54–6 58–9, 62–5
  summation 58–9, 62–5

Tactile agnosia 84, 251
Taste 179–182
  bitter 179, 181–2
  buds 180–1
  mechanism of 181–2
  modalities of 179, 181–2
  receptor responses 181

sour 179, 181–2
sweet 179, 181–2
TEA 26
Tectorial membrane 107–8
Tectospinal tract 201–3
Tectum (see Colliculi)
Telencephalon 6–7
Telephone exchange 16, n17, 231, 248
Teloreceptors 4
Temperature
   and conduction velocity 30, n40
   receptors 76, 179–180
   regulation 280–1
Temporal lobe 153–4, 248–9, 258–262
   stimulation of 259
   visual cells in 153–4
Temporal summation in neurones 59
Tendon
   jerk 206
   organ, Golgi 90, 93–5, 205–6, 211
Tension, muscle
   control of 205–212, 229–231
   receptors for 90, 93–5, 205–6, 211
Tensor tympani 107
Tetramethylammonium (TEA) 26
Tetrodotoxin (TTX) 26
Texture
   cutaneous 75, 79, 231
   gradient 162–3
Thalamus 6–8, 249
   and pain 85
   and taste 180–1
   nuclei of
      anterior 249, 258, 260–1, 282
      centromedian (CM) 228
      dorsomedial (DM) 249
      intralaminar 78, 201
      lateral geniculate 148, 150, 249
      lateral posterior 249, 251
      medial geniculate 116–8, 249
      pulvinar 148, 151, 249, 251,
      ventral posterolateral (VPL) 77–9, 93–4, 249
      ventral posteromedial (VPM) 180–1
      ventro–anterior (VA) 228, 239, 249
      ventrolateral (VL) 228, 233, 239, 249
Thermoreceptors 79–80, 281
Thiamine deficiency 261
Threshold
   absolute
      for Pacinian corpuscle 79
      for sound intensity 102, 111, n118
      for vision 122, 134, 138–140
      for olfaction 177
   for action potential 33–6

increment 137–8, 140
Tickle 74, 85
Tight junctions 43
Timbre 102–6, 114
Time constant of axonal membrane 29–31, n40
   N41, 56, N70
Time-differences, perception of
   auditory 115–6, 118, N120
   olfactory 172
Time intensity trade 116
Tinnitus 112
Tone, muscle
   and decerebration 203
   and depression 276–7
   and muscle spindles 206
   and vestibular system 203–4
Tongue
   and taste 180–1
   in speech 105, N119
Tonic
   muscle fibres 200
   neck reflex 222–3
   stretch reflex 206
   vestibular reflex 216–8
Touch 73–89
Tracts 10 (see under appropriate name)
Transduction 44–52
   gustatory 181–2
   in cochlea 110–4
   in Pacinian corpuscle 47–50
   olfactory 175–6, 178–9
   vestibular 96–100
   visual 108, 123, 130–5, 138–140, 145, 158–9, N167
Transmitters 4, 9, 11, 44–6, 54–62, 64, 239
   at neuromuscular junction 55–6
   evidence for 57–8
   in retina 135–7
Trapezoid body 117
Travelling wave 109, N120
Tremor
   at rest 240
   intention 234–5
   of eye muscles 194, N199
Triangle, colour (see colour plates) 157–8, N169
Trichromacy 155–9
Trigeminal nerve 180–1
Triple response 129
Tritanopia (see colour plates) 159–60, n166
Tropisms 273–5
TSH 280–1
TTX 26
Tuning curves 111–2
Two point discrimination test 83, 251
Tympanic membrane 106–7

Upper motor neurone 228–9
Utricle 95, 97–8

Velocity
    of nervous conduction 19, 29–33, N42
    sensitivity of semicircular canals 95, 98–100
Ventral horn cells (see Motor neurones)
Ventricles of brain 6–8
Ventromedial hypothalamus 278–282
Vergence movements 129, 164, 191–2, 194, N199
Vertical, sense of 97–8, 216–8
Vesicles, synaptic 45–7, 54–5
Vestibular
    apparatus 37, 95–100
    contribution to upright posture 216–9, 221–4
    influence on decerebrate rigidity 203–4
    nerve 95
    nuclei 96, 202–3, 223, 233
    nystagmus 194, 218–9
    projections to spinal cord 201–3
    reflexes 216–9
Vestibulo-cerebellum 237–8, 222
Vestibulo-ocular reflex (VOR)
    dynamic 194, 218–9
    plasticity 221–2, 235–8, N243
    static 194, 216–7
Vestibulospinal tract 201–3
Vibration
    and stretch reflex 91–2, 206
    sensitivity of Pacinian corpuscle 50
Viscera, sensory afferents from 74–5, 85
Viscous elements
    in muscle spindle 92
    in Pacinian corpuscle 49
    in semicircular canals 99–100
Vision 121–169
Visual
    acuity 124, 141–8, N168
    adaptation 123–4, 133, 137–141, N165, N167–9
    agnosia 251–2
    contrast 141–3, 146–8, 159
    contributions to posture 219, 222
    cortex 150–4, 160, 163–4, 267–9

optics 124–9, 141–2, 144–6, N167
    pathways 148–154
    pigment 132–4, 138–141, 160
    proprioception 148–9, 165
    receptors 108, 123, 130–5, 138–140, 145, 158–9, N167
    resolution 124, 141–8, N168
Vitamin A 133, 140, n166
Vitreous humour 124–5
Voice 104–6, N119
Voltage clamp 25–8
Voluntary movement 240–2, 288
von Békésy, Georg 109, n119, n183
Vowels 104–6, N119

Waking-sleeping cycle 284–5
Walking
    by new-born child 197, n198
    in cerebellar disorders 234–5
    mechanisms 195
Wallerian degeneration 11
Warmth receptors 79–80
Water, as a taste stimulus 179, 181
Waterfall illusion 165, n167, N169
Wavelength
    of sound waves 101, 115
    of visible lights 121
    and diffraction 144
    discrimination 155–160
WDR cells 86
Weber-Fechner relationship 138
Weight, sense of 95, 231
Wernicke's area 253–4
White matter 6
Wiping reflex 195
Withdrawal
    behaviour 276–7
    reflex 85, 200, 289
Word deafness 253–4

X-cells, Y-cells 137, 150, 154

Zöllner illusion 269